Extremity Replantation

A. Neil Salyapongse • Samuel O. Poore
Ahmed M. Afifi • Michael L. Bentz
Editors

Extremity Replantation

A Comprehensive Clinical Guide

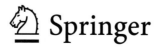 Springer

Editors
A. Neil Salyapongse, MD
Division of Plastic and
Reconstructive Surgery
Department of Surgery
University of Wisconsin
Madison, WI
USA

Samuel O. Poore, MD, PhD
Division of Plastic and
Reconstructive Surgery
Department of Surgery
University of Wisconsin
Madison, WI
USA

Ahmed M. Afifi, MD
Division of Plastic and
Reconstructive Surgery
Department of Surgery
University of Wisconsin
Madison, WI
USA

Division of Plastic Surgery
Cairo University Cairo
Egypt

Michael L. Bentz, MD
Division of Plastic and
Reconstructive Surgery
Department of Surgery
University of Wisconsin
Madison, WI
USA

ISBN 978-1-4899-7515-7   ISBN 978-1-4899-7516-4   (eBook)
DOI 10.1007/978-1-4899-7516-4
Springer New York Heidelberg Dordrecht London

Library of Congress Control Number: 2014955361

Printed on acid-free paper

Springer is part of Springer Science+Business Media (www.springer.com)

I dedicate this book to my father, Amorn Salyapongse,
whose lifelong passion for hand surgery and boundless
enthusiasm in the face of countless replant cases
fascinated me in my youth and continue to inspire me today.

A. Neil Salyapongse

To my family, Hannah, Anabelle, and Silas. Your wonderful
and wild ways keep me smiling. To my parents, Henry and
Nina. Your dedication, energy, and compassion inspire me.
And to Ted Goslow—colleague, teacher, and friend.

Samuel O. Poore

To my two favorite mentors, friends, and role models:
my mother, Karima, who showed me that you can be both
a good parent and a good physician, and my father, Medhat,
who completed his first replantation when I was 3 years old.

Ahmed M. Afifi

For Kim, Gretchen, Alex, and Eric.

Michael L. Bentz

Preface

Winter is coming. This certainty drives each of us to prepare for the inevitable occurrence that will threaten life and limb. It trains us to be seers, recognizing the patterns of disaster so that we might steer toward a better future. And, in contrast to the *lone wolf* surgeon stereotype, it leads us to value and encourage the abilities of a broadly experienced team. When the tragedy of extremity amputation comes, the best prepared and cooperative team offers the best chance of *survival and optimal function.*

When Kristopher Spring approached us about a book addressing replantation, we were struck by the fact that there had not been a comprehensive text covering the field for at least the past decade. Surely, an event that raises the health-care team's adrenaline levels almost as much as the patient's would spur some sort of survival guide; after all, countless individuals are now well prepared for the zombie apocalypse despite its relative infrequent occurrence compared to extremity amputation. We also recognized that the complexity of the subject matter ranging from the basics of nerve, bone, and tendon healing to the intricacies of maintaining vascular patency and providing appropriate postoperative rehabilitation therapy only provides bookends to a world of possible replantation scenarios.

In generating this guide, we have sought the wisdom and experience of a global team of authors, all of whom are well known in the fields of plastic and orthopedic surgery. Our goal has been to tease out specifics particularly relevant to different types and levels of amputation. As a result, while some elements of patient care and surgical technique may be present in each individual chapter, references to other chapters for commonalities are included, making the work function as a more coherent whole and, perhaps, leading an otherwise targeted reader to new knowledge they might not have anticipated needing to know.

Looking back on the process of assembling this book, I realize the importance of community not only in the care of the replant patient but also in the creation of the text. I am grateful for the excellent quality of the manuscripts received, for the insights that taught me new tricks, and for the encouragement and generous extension provided by our publisher. I would also like to thank the efforts of my coeditors and the guidance and direction of our developmental editor, Elizabeth Corra. Without the collective push forward, none of this would have come to fruition.

Ultimately, the proof of this guide's utility will be found in the battleground of the emergency departments, operating theaters, and rehabilitation units, where all our teams labor to provide the best outcomes for our patients. Winter is coming; it is best to be prepared.

Madison, WI, USA   A. Neil Salyapongse, MD

Contents

1 The History of Extremity Replantation 1
Wayne A. Morrison

**2 Principles of Musculoskeletal Repair
in Extremity Replantation** 9
Steve J. Kempton, Samuel R.H. Steiner,
and A. Neil Salyapongse

**3 Principles of Nerve Repair and Neural
Recovery in Extremity Replantation Surgery** 25
Sahil Kapur and Samuel O. Poore

4 Replantation of the Thumb 39
Matthew L. Iorio, Nicholas B. Vedder,
and Jeffrey B. Friedrich

5 Replantation of the Digits 49
Clifford Pereira and Kodi Azari

6 Replantation at the Level of the Radiocarpal Joint 67
Mauricio Kuri, Andrew Watt, and Gregory M. Buncke

7 Replantation of the Forearm or Arm 83
Michael Waters and Brian J. Harley

8 Optimizing Vascular Patency in Replantation 103
Andrew D. Navarrete and Michael L. Bentz

9 Toe-to-Hand Transplantation After Failed Replantation 117
Nidal F. ALDeek and Fu-Chan Wei

10 Heterotopic Digital Replantation 133
Cheng-Hung Lin and Fu-Chan Wei

11 Replantation in the Child and Adolescent 137
Joshua M. Abzug, Scott H. Kozin, and Dan A. Zlotolow

12 Lower Limb Replantation 145
Pedro C. Cavadas and Alessandro Thione

13 Management of Complications After Replantation 161
Guang Yang and Kevin C. Chung

14   Secondary Procedures in Replantation.................... 171
S. Raja Sabapathy, Jenny Tzujane Chen,
and Ahmed M. Afifi

**15   Rehabilitation Following Replantation
in the Upper Extremity**................................ 191
Sarah A. Ezerins, Carol J. Harm, Steve J. Kempton,
and A. Neil Salyapongse

Index 207

Contributors

Joshua M. Abzug, MD Department of Orthopaedics, University of Maryland Medical System, Timonium, MD, USA

Ahmed M. Afifi, MD Division of Plastic Surgery, University of Wisconsin Hospital and Clinics, Madison, WI, USA

Nidal F. ALDeek, MSc, MD Department of Plastic and Reconstructive Surgery, Chang Gung Memorial Hospital, Taipei, Taiwan

Kodi Azari, MD, FACS Section of Reconstructive Transplantation, Department of Orthopaedic Surgery and Plastic Surgery, David Geffen School of Medicine at UCLA, Los Angeles, CA, USA

Michael L. Bentz, MD Division of Plastic Surgery, University of Wisconsin Hospital and Clinics, Madison, WI, USA

Gregory M. Buncke, MD Division of Microsurgery, The Buncke Medical Clinic, San Francisco, CA, USA

Pedro C. Cavadas, MD, PhD Department of Reconstructive Surgery, Clinica Cavadas, Hospital de Manises, Valencia, Spain

Jenny Tzujane Chen, MD Division of Plastic Surgery, University of Wisconsin Hospital and Clinics, Madison, WI, USA

Kevin C. Chung, MD, MS Section of Plastic Surgery, University of Michigan Health System, Ann Arbor, MI, USA

Sarah A. Ezerins, OTR, MS Occupational Therapy Department, University of Wisconsin Hospital and Clinics, Hand and Upper Extremity Clinic, Madison, WI, USA

Jeffrey B. Friedrich, MD Division of Plastic Surgery, University of Washington, Seattle, WA, USA

Brian J. Harley, MD, FRCSC Department of Orthopedic Surgery, SUNY Upstate Medical University, Syracuse, NY, USA

Carol J. Harm, BS, OT, OTR, CHT Department of Occupational Therapy, University of Wisconsin Hospital and Clinics, Hand and Upper Extremity Clinic, Madison, WI, USA

Matthew L. Iorio, MD Division of Plastic Surgery,
University of Washington, Seattle, WA, USA

Sahil Kapur, MD Division of Plastic Surgery, University of Wisconsin
Hospital and Clinics, Madison, WI, USA

Steve J. Kempton, MD Division of Plastic Surgery, University of
Wisconsin Hospital and Clinics, Madison, WI, USA

Scott H. Kozin, MD Department of Orthopaedic Surgery,
Shriners Hospital for Children, Philadelphia, PA, USA

Mauricio Kuri, MD Division of Microsurgery, The Buncke Medical
Clinic, San Francisco, CA, USA

Cheng-Hung Lin, MD Department of Plastic and Reconstructive Surgery,
Chang Gung Memorial Hospital, Taipei, Taiwan

Wayne Morrison, MD, FRACS Department of Surgery,
St. Vincent's Hospital, Fitzroy, VIC, Australia

Australian Catholic University, Fitzroy, VIC, Australia

O'Brien Institute, Fitzroy, VIC, Australia

University of Melbourne, Parkville, VIC, Australia

Andrew D. Navarrete, MD Division of Plastic Surgery, University of
Wisconsin Hospital and Clinics, Madison, WI, USA

Clifford Pereira, MBBS, FRCS(Eng) Department of Plastic
and Reconstructive Surgery, David Geffen School
of Medicine at UCLA, Los Angeles, CA, USA

Samuel O. Poore, MD, PhD Division of Plastic Surgery, University of
Wisconsin Hospital and Clinics, Madison, WI, USA

S. Raja Sabapathy, MD, MCh, DNB, FRCS, MAMS Department
of Plastic Surgery, Hand and Reconstructive Microsurgery, and Burns,
Ganga Hospital, Coimbatore, India

A. Neil Salyapongse, MD Division of Plastic Surgery,
University of Wisconsin Hospital and Clinics, Madison, WI, USA

Samuel R.H. Steiner, MD Department of Orthopedics and Rehabilitation,
University of Wisconsin Hospitals and Clinics, Madison, WI, USA

Alessandro Thione, MD, PhD Department of Reconstructive Surgery,
Clinica Cavadas, Hospital de Manises, Valencia, Spain

Nicholas B. Vedder, MD Division of Plastic Surgery,
University of Washington, Seattle, WA, USA

Michael Waters, MD Department of Orthopedic Surgery,
SUNY Upstate Medical University, Syracuse, NY, USA

Andrew Watt, MD Division of Microsurgery, The Buncke Medical Clinic, San Francisco, CA, USA

Fu-Chan Wei, MD Department of Plastic Surgery, Chang Gung Memorial Hospital, Taipei, Taiwan

Guang Yang, MD Department of Hand Surgery, China-Japan Union Hospital of Jilin University, Changchun, Peoples Republic of China

Dan A. Zlotolow, MD Department of Orthopaedic Surgery, Shriners Hospital for Children, Philadelphia, PA, USA

The History of Extremity Replantation

Wayne A. Morrison

Introduction

The first successful digital replantation in 1965 by Tamai [1] (Fig. 1.1) heralded the clinical era of microsurgery. Soon microvascular surgical techniques would be applied to free tissue flap transfers, introducing a new sophistication in reconstructive surgery. But was it destiny or an even higher intervention that guided the healing hand of this Japanese surgeon to reattach an amputated part? For in certain Japanese cultural traditions, the dead should be buried with all body parts intact. This taboo continues to limit transplantation in Japan as evidenced by low donorship levels. In western culture, the procedure evoked the opposite reaction in some; to them the concept of bringing the dead back to life was in defiance of nature's ordinance. Even today, observing the death pallor suffusing progressively to pink upon revascularization of a major body part such as a limb or even more so a face evokes a certain horror and unease.

Despite this, the history of reattachment of parts has a strong religious association, and the first recorded case is fittingly in the Gospel of St. Luke (22, 50–51). As the Roman soldiers were arresting Christ accompanied by his apostles, a commotion ensued and "one of them smote the servant of the high priest and cut off his right ear....and he (Christ) touched his ear and healed him." In his fascinating and erudite article on early free grafting, Thomas Gibson [2] refers to the Biblical debate regarding this incident. While all the evangelists record the injury, only Luke mentions total severance and the miraculous healing. Gibson highlights that Paula Zacchias (1584–1659), poet, painter, and personal

W.A. Morrison, MD, FRACS
Department of Surgery, St. Vincent's Hospital, Fitzroy, VIC, Australia

Australian Catholic University, Fitzroy, VIC, Australia

O'Brien Institute, Fitzroy, VIC, Australia

University of Melbourne, Parkville, VIC, Australia
e-mail: Wayne.morrison@unimelb.edu.au

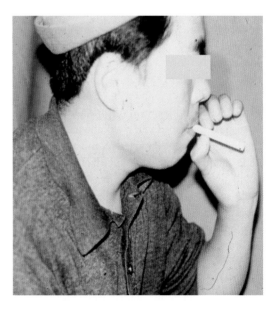

Fig. 1.1 World's first digital replant. Tamai 1965 (Used with permission from Kamatsu and Tamai [1])

A.N. Salyapongse et al. (eds.), *Extremity Replantation: A Comprehensive Clinical Guide*,
DOI 10.1007/978-1-4899-7516-4_1, © Springer Science+Business Media New York 2015

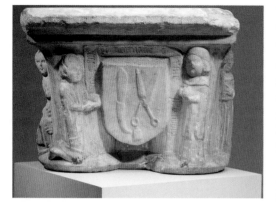

Fig. 1.2 Double capital depicting Saints Cosmas and Damian (guild of barber-surgeons) (Source: http://art.thewalters.org/detail/10296/double-capital-depicting-saints-cosmas-and-damian-guild-of-barber-surgeons/; In public domain)

physician to Pope Innocent X and founder of forensic medicine, in his treatise on miracles, concluded that if the ear was completely amputated before replantation it was a miracle of the First Order (one that could only occur supernaturally). However, if the ear was still attached by a tissue bridge, then it was a miracle of the Second Order (one that could possibly occur by a natural process). Harold Kleinert and team in Louisville had, 2 years prior to Tamai's replantation, revascularized digits, some with only minor skin bridges, using microsurgical technique [3]. Interestingly this same rigid canon distinction between complete and incomplete amputation was applied by modern-day inquisitors and denied Kleinert the award of First-Order Miracle status and the world's first acknowledgement. In the light of current knowledge, most would concede that proximal devascularizations attached solely by a small skin bridge or by tendons could only survive by a first-degree miracle. Many other legendary and miraculous reports of grafting, replantation, and transplantation have been recorded, the most famous of which involved the martyred physicians Cosmos and Damien (died 287 AD). They were indeed canonized for their good works including the transplantation of the leg of a Moor to replace that of a church worker after amputation for cancerous ulceration. They have since been adopted as the Patron Saints of barbers, physicians, and surgeons (Fig. 1.2 [4]). The miraculous replantation by St. Julius of the thumb of a church worker is the first recorded digital replantation and is celebrated in a painting in the church dedicated to the saint on the Isola San Giulio [5]. Saint Eligius of Noyon (590 AD), identified iconographically with a horse's leg at his side, is said to have successfully replanted all four limbs of a horse [6].

Renaissance Through Nineteenth Century

More credible evidence for surviving tissue reattachments by apparently natural means emerged in Renaissance times is detailed by Gibson and well summarized and elaborated on by Kocher [7] (*W J Surg* 1995) in his excellent review "History of Replantation." The famous case of the Italian physician Leonardo Fioravanti who successfully reattached the amputated nose of a Spanish gentleman lost after a quarrel with a soldier [8] offers an interesting protocol for preparing the amputated part "…I took it up and pissed thereon to wash away the sand and dressed it with balsama artificiato (dried blood powder) and bound it up and so left it to remain 8–10 days thinking that it would have come to matter, nevertheless when I did unbind it I found it fast conglutinated and then I dressed it only once more and it was perfectly whole." Balfour's report in 1814 of the reattachment of a carpenter's finger amputated at the PIP joint level is the most scientifically documented to that date [9]. Balfour was acutely aware of charlatan reports of the period and, sensitive to attracting similar skepticism, took the precaution of having affidavits sworn to verify the successful outcome. Some years preceding this incident Balfour had reattached three of his own son's fingertips which were caught in a door. He recorded that the finger was severed obliquely, spanning the proximal and middle phalanges, the longer side measuring 1.5 in., the shorter 1 in. from the tip. The part was cleansed and applied accurately to the opposing stump. No sutures were apparently used. The patient attended the following day but because of his doubts about its potential to survive sought advice from another physician with a view to having it removed. It was found to have adhered perfectly. Balfour next saw his patient 1 month later and noted that the nail had fallen off and the skin had desquamated but the finger was "the handsometh the man has and had recovered both heat and sensation."

Gibson [2] accredits Gottlieb Hoffacker [10, 11], doctor to the duelists of Heidelberg with the most critical and credible observations and hence the most valuable, in predicting success of free-grafting amputated parts. In analyzing the results of reported cases, including 16 amputated nose tips and lips sustained from dueling incidents that were his own, Hoffacker observed that contrary to common understanding, completely severed parts were not yet dead and the most predictable parameters for rescue were washing away blood, oblique amputation, and delay. The latter allowed bleeding to stop, the severed part to relax from its contracted state to its original dimension and for its blood vessels to reopen allowing lymph fluid exuding from the cut wound to reenter the now open ends. Replantation of the part facilitated accurate and maximum primary adhesion over the largest recipient area and favored first, rather than second, intention healing. These parameters appear obvious today as those which would most favor graft take, but it is of note that at this period, nearly 40 years before Revedin reported his skin grafting in 1870 [12], it was generally accepted that wounds could only heal by secondary intention.

Twentieth Century and into the Twenty-First Century

By the end of the nineteenth and beginning of the twentieth century, surgeons were experimenting with replantation and transplantation. In 1903 [13] Hopfner performed successful revascularization of canine limbs by vascular anastomosis, and Carrel and Guthrie [14] reported successful replantations though not without complications. Even before then, Briau, in 1896 [15], had anastomosed a canine carotid, and Halstead, in 1897

[16], had transfemorally amputated a dog's hind limb save for the femoral artery and transferred it to the opposite leg. He observed that subsequent division of the artery after 5 days did not result in death of the transplanted leg. Alexis Carrel who perfected the procedure in dogs and developed the foundations of vascular surgery and transplantation was awarded the Nobel Prize in Physiology and Medicine in 1912.

Although vascular repair had now been essentially mastered, its application for clinical replantation was a long way in the future. The safety of the procedure and the length of time that a part could be detached remained a mystery. Antibiotics and reliable bone fixation were unknown. In his excellent monograph, on "Major limb replantation and post ischaemia syndrome," Hans Steinau [17] outlines the relevant milestones in this field. World War I highlighted the phenomenon of crush syndromes and Volkmann's ischemia and their detrimental systemic effects including those following reversal of the ischemic insult. In 1930, Blalock [18], using canine hind limb tourniquet studies, disproved the theory that the toxins of ischemia produced "shock." Rather, he demonstrated the triggering factor to be extravasation of plasma from the circulation into the tissue and that this could be ameliorated by blood transfusion. In 1938, using the same model as Blalock, Allen [19] demonstrated that cooling to 2 °C dramatically decreased mortality. Further advancements were made During WW II by Bywaters [20] who demonstrated that postischemia syndrome was characterized by hyperkalemia, ECG changes, and renal damage from intravascular hemolysis.

Hall [21], in 1944, experiencing the mayhem of the war and the devastatingly high incidence of limb loss, published a detailed proposal and protocol for homologous transplantation of above-elbow amputations, 20 years before the first clinical replantation was performed.

Meanwhile canine limb replant studies were further developed in the 1960s with the work of Lapchinsky [22] in Moscow, and Snyder [23] and Eilsen [24] in the United States.

In 1962, Ronald Malt and McKhann [25] of Boston finally mustered the courage to try what had been technically feasible for many years and successfully reattached the above-elbow amputated arm of a 12-year-old boy. Chen Zong-Wei [26] independently pioneered replantation surgery in China and, in 1963, reattached completely amputated limbs. The following year, the first arm transplantation was performed in Ecuador in 1964 but quickly failed through lack of adequate immunosuppression.

In the meantime by 1960, microvascular surgery was being explored by Julius Jacobson and his student Ernest Suarez in Vermont [27], by Donaghy and Yasargil likewise for neurosurgery [28] and notably soon after by Harry Buncke for plastic surgery [29] in San Francisco. Jacobson had been appointed Professor and Director of the surgical research laboratory at the University of Vermont, and surgical research was, in many ways, the driver to perfect microvascular techniques. Small animal models were required to evaluate emerging clinical procedures such as portocaval shunting [30], transplantation, reperfusion injury, and drug development and opened up a new field of microvascular-based surgical research. Young, keen-eyed, hand-steady, and dexterous lab technicians were often the early masters of microsurgical technique. Many prior attempts at clinical replantation in the West and in China had failed because of the inadequacy of the tools necessary to achieve consistent results [31, 32]. In China polyethylene tubing was used as substitutes for suture anastomosis. The microscope already introduced for ENT and ophthalmology was greatly improved with Zeiss' introduction of the OPMI 1 in 1953. Jacobson noticed an OPMI 1 microscope abandoned in a corner of the surgical research lab that had been ordered by the ear surgeons for experimentation whose interests had since lapsed. Jacobson instantly realized the microscope's potential with its magnification of 25 times for the repair of small blood vessels. "The first experience in using the microscope for the performance of a vascular anastomosis can be likened to the first time the moon is looked at through a powerful telescope: a whole welter of unrecognized detail is seen" [33]. He reported 100 % patency of vessels 1.6–3.2 mm diameter

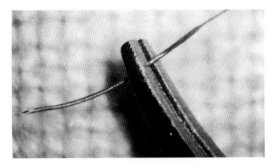

Fig. 1.3 The micro needle holder grasping the needle of a 19 μm metallized nylon microsuture (Used with permission from O'Brien [55])

[27], and soon the procedure was being adopted by others, and even smaller vessels were being repaired with high success rates [34]. The microscope was further enhanced by the insertion of a beam splitter so that two surgeons seated opposite each other could have the same view.

Sutures became finer and needles were perfected. Initially with Du Pont, Buncke designed metalized needles which were fashioned by dipping the tips of fine nylon thread into molten metal and polishing them to a point [35] (Fig. 1.3). Eventually the needles could be swaged onto threads in the same manner as larger sutures [36]. Micro-instrument development was also critical to the success of the microsurgical revolution. Needle holders [37] and scissors were modified from ophthalmology, jewelry forceps copied, and new vascular clamps invented [38]. Bob Ackland, working with Springler and Tritt, was instrumental in perfecting microsurgical instrumentation [36]. Many early attempts at automation were tried without gaining popularity. The stage was set for many to participate in this revolution, and soon thereafter, consistently high patency rates of vessels of the order of 1 mm diameter were published by Hayhurst and O'Brien [37]. Preeminent in this research arena was Harry Buncke who, after working with Tom Gibson in Glasgow in 1957, acknowledged that it was he who suggested the potential of small vessel anastomosis not only as a means of replantation but also for tissue transplantation [38]. Inspired by the work of Julius Jacobson, Buncke

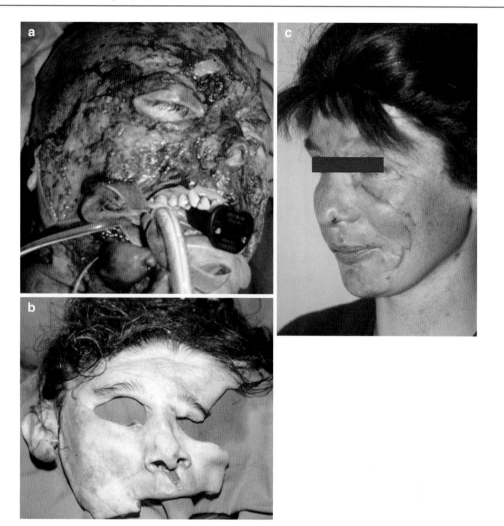

Fig. 1.4 (**a–c**) Total face and scalp avulsion. (**a, b**) Before replantation. (**c**) Three months after replantation

realized its application for the wider field of free tissue transfer and developed techniques of toe-to-hand transfers initially in monkeys [39] and then humans [40]. Tamai had spent time with Buncke and accredits his microvascular initiation to this period. In a historic clinical case, Buncke transferred omentum to repair a scalp defect by anastomosing the omental vessels to those in the scalp. To quote Buncke, "… It succeeded and the rest is history" [41].

For most surgeons, the opportunity to learn and apply microsurgery was in the emergency center. By now large experiences of clinical digital and limb replantations were being reported [42–51]. With increasing training, experience, and exuberance, replantation has now been applied to almost all tissues of the body, including lower limbs, scalp, tongue, and facial parts. In September 1997, we experienced an extraordinary case where a young woman's whole face and scalp were avulsed when her hair was caught in a milking machine. Only one other case of face replant has since been reported [52]. The part was avulsed in a very superficial plane leaving all major vessels *in situ* on the patient. Replantation was accomplished by anastomosing an upper labial branch of the facial artery and one supraorbital artery, and its success presaged the feasibility of facial transplantation which was to follow (Fig. 1.4a–c).

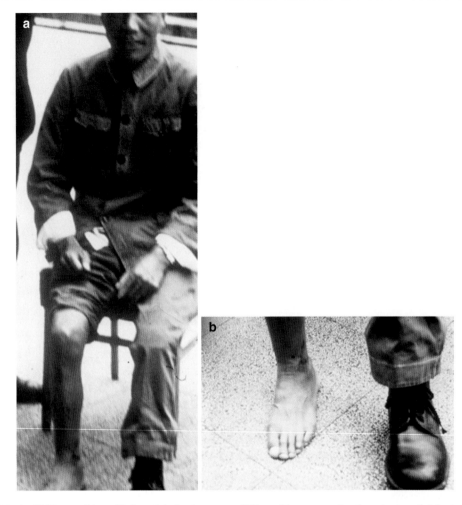

Fig. 1.5 (**a**, **b**) Transposition of left to right leg in a case of bilateral leg amputation (prosthesis to left leg). Case of Chen Zhong-Wei, MD (Courtesy of Family of Chen Zhong-Wei)

The technical advancements and refinements in replantation have been accompanied by significant opportunities for creativity. Where multiple digits and limbs have been amputated, the most suitable amputated part can be transposed to the most appropriate site (Fig. 1.5a, b). When the patient is unfit for formal replantation, the part can be temporarily banked by microvascular anastomosis in an ectopic site as reported by Godina [53]. Stroke victims have had their paralyzed hand transposed to the opposite side in situations where their surviving useful hand had suffered severe injury or amputation [54]. Reports of parts being salvaged from dog and crocodile stomachs (Fig. 1.6), the extraordinary survival times of digits preserved in the snow, and the frantic forensic identification for the ownership of multiple fingers avulsed following the breakage of a tug of war rope when 20 digits were placed collectively into a plastic bag (Guillermo Loda – personal conversation) all add color and excitement to the history of replantation.

To quote from Kocher's abstract in his article on History of Replantation: "Severed body parts from the fingers to extremities are now being routinely reattached at medical centres around the world. The dream of replantation traces its rich history from miracles and legends to early laboratory experiments and clinical attempts, culminating in today's common place procedure" [7].

Fig. 1.6 Arm being retrieved from crocodile belly (Photograph by Jerome Bien)

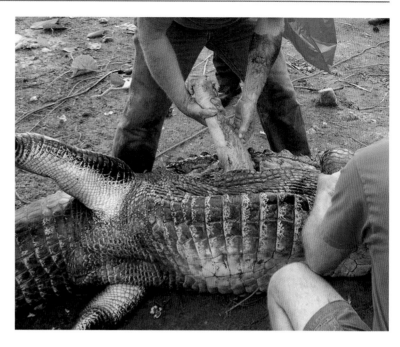

References

1. Kamatsu S, Tamai S. Successful replantation of a completely cut-off thumb: case report. Plast Reconstr Surg. 1968;42:374.
2. Gibson T. Early free grafting: the restitution of parts completely separated from the body. Br J Plast Surg. 1965;18:1.
3. Kleinert HE, Kasdan ML, Romero JL. Small blood vessel anastomosis for salvage of severely injured upper extremity. J Bone Joint Surg Am. 1963;45: 788.
4. Double Capital Depicting Saints Cosmas and Damian (Guild of Barber-Surgeons) [image on the internet]. 2013. Available from: http://art.thewalters.org/detail/10296/double-capital-depicting-saints-cosmas-and-damian-guild-of-barber-surgeons/.
5. Landi A. History of thumb reconstruction. In: Landi A, editor. Reconstruction of the thumb. Chapter 1. London: Chapman and Hall publishers; 1989.
6. Ei G. Die Legende vom abgeschmittenen Pferdebein. Tierarzti Umschau. 1956;11:152–4.
7. Kocher M. History of replantation: from miracle to mircrosurgery. World J Surg. 1995;19:462–7.
8. Fioravanti L. Tesaro Della Vita Humana. Venice: Appreso gli Heredi di M Sessa; 1570.
9. Balfour W. Two cases, with observations, demonstrative of the powers of nature to reunite parts which have been, by accident, totally separated from the animal system. Edinb Med Surg J. 1814;10:421.
10. Hoffacker W. Heidelb Clin Ann. 1828;4:232.
11. Hoffacker W. Medicinische Annalen. 1836;2:149.
12. Reverdin JL. Bull Soc Chir. 1870;10:511. 2 ser.
13. Hopfner E. Ueber gefassnacht, Gefasstrasplantationen und replantation von umputirten extremitaten. Arch Klin Chir. 1903;70:417.
14. Carrel A, Guthrie CC. Complete amputation of the thigh, with replantation. Am J Med Sci. 1906;131:297.
15. Hershey FB, Calnan CH. Atlas of vascular surgery. St Louis: C.V. Mosby Co.; 1967.
16. Halstead WS, Reichert FL, Reid MR. Replantation of entire limbs without suture of vessels. Trans Am Surg Assoc. 1922;40:160.
17. Steinau HU. Major limb replantation and postischemia syndrome: investigation of acute ischemia-induced myopathy and reperfusion injury. Berlin: Springer; 1987. p. 1–8. Chapter 1, Introduction.
18. Blalock A. Experimental shock: the cause of the low blood pressure produced by muscle injury. Arch Surg. 1930;20:959–96.
19. Allen FM. Resistance of peripheral tissues to asphyxia at various temperatures. Obstet Gynecol. 1938;67: 746–51.
20. Bywaters EGL. Ischemic muscle necrosis. JAMA. 1944;124:1103–9.
21. Hall RH. Whole upper extremity transplant for human beings: general plans of procedure and operative technic. Ann Surg. 1944;120:12.
22. Lapchinsky AG. Recent results of experimental transplantation of preserved limbs and kidneys and possible use of this technique in clinical practice. Ann N Y Acad Sci. 1960;87:539.
23. Snyder CC, Knowles RP, Mayer PW, Hobbs JC. Extremity replantation. Plast Reconstr Surg. 1960;26: 251.
24. Eiken O, Nabseth DC, Mayer RF, Deterling Jr RA. Limb replantation. Arch Surg. 1964;88:48.

25. Malt RA, McKhann CF. Replantation of severed arms. JAMA. 1964;189:716.

26. Chen ZW, Chen YC, Pao YS. Salvage of the forearm following complete amputation: report of a case. Chin Med J. 1963;82:632.

27. Jacobson JH, Suarez EL. Microsurgery and anastomosis of the small vessels. Surg Forum. 1960; 11:243.

28. Donalghy R, Ysargal M. Microvascular surgery. St. Louis: Mosby; 1967.

29. Buncke Jr HJ, Schulz WP. Experimental digital amputation and replantation. Plast Reconstr Surg. 1965;36:62.

30. Lee SH, Fisher B. Portacaval shunt in the rat. Surgery. 1961;50:668–72.

31. McDowell F. Replantation surgery in China. Report of the American replantation mission to China. Plast Reconstr Surg. 1973;52:476–89.

32. O'Brien BM. Replantation surgery in China. Med J Aust. 1974;2(7):255–9.

33. Donalghy RMP, Yasargil MG. Micro-vascular surgery. Stuttgart: Georg Thieme Verlag; 1967. p. 4.

34. Chase MD, Schwartz SI. Consistent patency of 1.5 mm arterial anastomoses. Surg Forum. 1962;13:220–2.

35. Buncke HJ, Schulz WP. Total ear reimplantation in the rabbit utilizing micro-miniature vascular anastomoses. Br J Plast Surg. 1966;19:15–22.

36. Acland R. A new needle for microvascular surgery. Surgery. 1972;71:130–1.

37. O'Brien B, Hayburst JW. Metallized microsutures and a new micro needle holder. Plast Reconstr Surg. 1973;52:673–6.

38. Buncke Jr HJ, Schulz WP. The suture repair of one-millimeter vessels. In: Donaghy RMP, Yasargil MG, editors. Micro-vascular surgery. St. Louis/Stuttgart: The C.V. Mosby Company/George Thieme Verlag; 1967. p. 24–35.

39. Buncke HJ, Buncke CM, Schulz WP. Immediate nicaladoni procedure in the rhesus monkey, or hallux-to-hand transplantation, utilizing microminiature vascular anastomoses. Br J Plast Surg. 1966;19:332–7.

40. Buncke HJ, McLean DH, Geroge PT, Creech BJ, Chater NL, Commons GW. Thumb replacement: Great toe transplantation by microvascular anastomosis. Br J Plast Surg. 1973;26:194–201.

41. Terzis J. History of microsurgery. Norfolk: Julia K. Terzis; 2009.

42. Sixth People's Hospital S. Reattachment of traumatic amputations, a summing up of experiences. Chin Med J (Engl). 1967;1:392–401.

43. Biemer E. Definitions and classifications in replantation surgery. Br J Plast Surg. 1980;33(2):164–8.

44. Chow JA, Bilos ZJ, Chunprapaph B. Thirty thumb replantations. Indications and results. Plast Reconstr Surg. 1979;64(5):626–30.

45. Lendvay PG. Replacement of the amputated digit. Br J Plast Surg. 1973;126(4):398–405.

46. Morrison WA, O'Brien BM, MacLeod AM. Evaluation of digital replantation-a review of 100 cases. Orthop Clin N Am. 1977;8(2):295–308.

47. Morrison WA, O'Brien BM, MacLeod AM. Digital replantation and revascularization. A long term review of one hundred cases. Hand. 1978;10(2):125–34.

48. O'Brien BM, MacLeod AM, Miller GD, et al. Clinical replantation of digits. Plast Reconstr Surg. 1973;52(5): 490–502.

49. Tsai TM. Experimental and clinical application of microvascular surgery. Ann Surg. 1975;2:169–77.

50. Tamai S. Twenty years' experience of limb replantation-review of 293 upper extremity replants. J Hand Surg Am. 1982;7(6):549–56.

51. Buncke Jr HJ. Microvascular hand surgery-transplants and replants-over the past 25 years. J Hand Surg Am. 2000;25(3):415–28.

52. Thomas A, Obed V, Muraka A, Malhotra G. Total face and scalp replantation. Plast Reconstr Surg. 1998; 102(6):2085–7.

53. Godina M, Bajee T, Baraga A. Salvage of mutilated upper extremity with temporary ectopic transplantation of the undamaged part. Plast Reconstr Surg. 1986;78(3):295–9.

54. May JW, Rothkopf D, Savage RC, Atkinson R. Elective coon-hand transfer: a case report with a 5 year follow-up. J Hand Surg Ann. 1989;14(1):28–45.

55. O'Brien BH. Microvascular reconstructive surgery. Edinburgh: Churchill Livingstone; 1977.

Principles of Musculoskeletal Repair in Extremity Replantation

2

Steve J. Kempton, Samuel R.H. Steiner, and A. Neil Salyapongse

"Firmitas, utilitas, venustas" (solid, useful, beautiful)

Marcus Vitruvius Pollio, De Architectura

Introduction

Although the Vitruvian Triad of "solid, useful, and beautiful" originated with the field of architecture, the principles have informed the disciplines of science and art, intersecting most notably in the anatomical studies of Renaissance masters including Michelangelo, Alberti, and Da Vinci (Fig. 2.1). Guidelines and techniques for extremity replantation laid out in the remainder of this book echo these principles, guiding restoration, or, when that is not possible, reconstruction (see Chap. 10) of the form necessary for useful function. Stable osteosynthesis following extremity amputation is the first step in returning patients to normal form.

S.J. Kempton, MD
Division of Plastic Surgery, University of Wisconsin
Hospital and Clinics, Madison, WI, USA
e-mail: skempton@uwhealth.org

S.R.H. Steiner, MD
Department of Orthopedics and Rehabilitation,
University of Wisconsin Hospitals and Clinics,
Madison, WI, USA
e-mail: ssteiner@uwhealth.org

A.N. Salyapongse, MD (✉)
Division of Plastic Surgery, University of Wisconsin
Hospital and Clinics, Madison, WI, USA
e-mail: a.salyapongse@uwmf.wisc.edu

This important first step provides a framework for soft tissue reconstruction and allows for the greatest chance of restoring normal function. While some joints, notably the radiocarpal and thumb metacarpophalangeal, tolerate immobility, the crux of *useful* reconstruction is restoration of motion. Muscles and tendons work in concert with the appendicular skeleton to provide stabilization and motion across joints. Disruption of the musculotendinous system always occurs in the setting of extremity amputation. Though the level of discontinuity can occur at any point along the muscle, most replants occur distal to the level of the wrist, placing the injury at the level of the tendon. Restoration of function hinges on solid healing of the tendon as well as useful excursion. In this chapter, we will provide general principles, as well as the basic biology on which they are founded, applicable to both osteosynthesis and tendon repair in the setting of extremity replantation.

Bone

Anatomy

Bone is a unique, well-organized, and dynamic tissue. Its composition and intricate structure make it resilient to stress while at the same time

A.N. Salyapongse et al. (eds.), *Extremity Replantation: A Comprehensive Clinical Guide*,
DOI 10.1007/978-1-4899-7516-4_2, © Springer Science+Business Media New York 2015

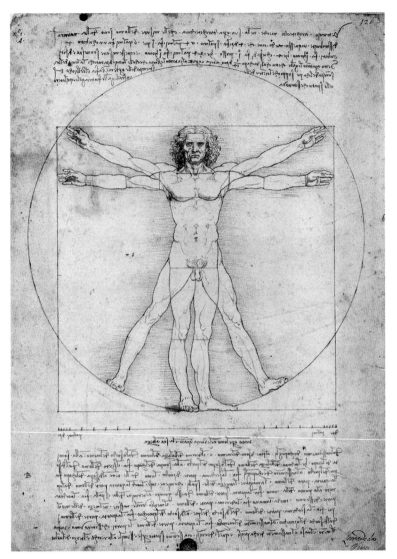

lightweight, making it ideal for mechanical support, motion, and grasp. It serves as attachment points for muscles, tendons, and ligaments and as a reservoir for calcium hemostasis. At the macroscopic level, there are two major forms of bone: cortical and cancellous. Cortical bone, also known as compact bone, comprises approximately 80 % of the skeleton and forms the cortex, or outer shell, of most bones. It is four times denser than cancellous bone [1]. The strength of cortical bone is due to its intricate architecture with the fundamental unit being the haversian system or osteon. The osteon is a cylindrical structure several millimeters long running parallel to the long axis of the bone. At the core of the osteon is a tubelike structure called the central or haversian canal, which houses capillaries and poorly myelinated nerve fibers. Surrounding the haversian canal are concentric rings called lamellae. In between lamellae are osteocytes, former osteoblasts now surrounded by a bone matrix and housed in a space termed lacunae. Branching from each lacunae and running approximately tangential to each lamellae are small channels called canaliculi. It is through these small channels that osteocytes send out extensive cell processes thereby establishing contact with nearby osteocytes.

Cancellous bone, also known as trabecular bone, has approximately one fourth the mass of cortical bone. It is softer, weaker, and more elastic. This is due in part to its structure consisting of branching bony struts or spicules that are organized into a loose network typically aligned along areas of stress. Relatively large spaces exist in between struts making cancellous bone quite porous. This gives it a larger surface area to volume ratio. Because bony turnover is proportional to the surface area available, cancellous bone has approximately eight times greater metabolic turnover than cortical bone.

At the microscopic level, there are two major forms of bone: woven and lamellar. Woven bone, also called primary bone, is the bone that is formed de novo, making it the initial tissue in bone formation. It can be either immature, as seen in the embryo and with fracture callus formation, or pathologic and formed by bony tumors. Woven bone is not stress oriented and is weaker and more flexible compared to lamellar bone.

Lamellar bone, considered normal bone, is formed after the remodeling of woven bone and can be either cortical or cancellous. It is highly organized and forms more slowly than woven bone.

Bone Healing

Unlike many other tissues of the body that form scar tissue during the healing process, fracture healing restores injured bone to its original state with the same biological and mechanical properties it once had. The main factors contributing to proper healing of bone include an adequate blood supply, progenitor cells, growth factors, and an extracellular matrix.

Bone blood flow is the major determinant to how well a fracture heals for it carries nutrients, oxygen, and other essentials to the injury site. Grossly, vessels damaged at or near the site of bone injury need to be repaired in order to provide adequate blood supply. At the microscopic level, angiogenesis takes place within the periosteal tissues and marrow space in order to provide

blood flow to the fracture site. The importance of the periosteal circulation for healing leads directly to the recommendation of minimal bone stripping when performing osteosynthesis during replantation.

Bone healing also requires the recruitment of progenitor cells. This occurs as mesenchymal stem cells are brought to the fracture site, both from surrounding soft tissue as well as from the systemic circulation [2]. These cells in turn differentiate into osteoblasts, osteoclasts, chondrocytes, and fibroblasts. The recruitment and differentiation of mesenchymal stem cells is dependent on growth factors present at the site of injury.

The extracellular matrix (ECM) provides the scaffolding for new bone formation. Collagen is the major component of the ECM. Types I and IV make up the majority of bone, where types II, IX, X, and XI make up the majority of cartilage. In addition to collagen, glycoproteins and proteoglycans also make up the ECM.

The repair process of bone can be classified into two major forms of healing: primary and secondary. The type of healing that occurs is determined by the means of fracture fixation and the strain (Δlength/original length) experienced across the fracture. Primary (direct) bone healing occurs predominantly via intramembranous ossification. This occurs when rigid fixation and absolute stability is achieved with the two ends of bone in contact with one another. With minimal motion or gapping at the fracture site, strain is typically less than 2 % and an intermediate cartilaginous callus does not form [3]. Instead, the haversian system of remodeling takes place; osteoclasts cross the fracture site via cutting cones, and osteoblasts occupy the canal left in their wake to later organize and become osteons. The two ends of the fracture are joined by lamellar bone.

Secondary (indirect) bone healing is the predominant form of fracture healing. It occurs primarily via enchondral ossification though in some cases intramembranous healing also plays a role [4]. Secondary or enchondral ossification refers to fracture healing that occurs via a cartilage callus intermediate. This callus develops because of greater motion and less stability at the fracture site resulting in greater strain, typically between 2 and 10 % [3]. This creates an environment optimal for undifferentiated mesenchymal cells to become chondrocytes and establish a soft callus. The amount of callus that develops is inversely proportional to the degree of fracture immobilization that is achieved. Angiogenesis occurs within the fracture callus, and over time as greater stability is achieved, chondrocytes undergo apoptosis and are replaced by osteocytes. Woven bone is initially formed within the soft callus transforming it into a hard callus. This later undergoes remodeling as woven bone becomes lamellar bone in response to mechanical stress. If the strain at the fracture site is too great, however, an environment is created unsuitable for osteocytes or chondrocytes [5]. Instead, fibroblasts, the initial cell type to populate the fracture site, persist and a fibrous nonunion develops.

Principles of Fracture Fixation

In the setting of replantation, fracture fixation is paramount in order to provide stability and protect the vascular repair. Different means of fixation create varying degrees of stability. As mentioned above, stability influences which type of bone healing, if any at all, will occur. In the upper extremity and the hand, the most common types of fixation include wire sutures, Kirschner wires, lag screws, plates, and external fixators. Fracture location and pattern, soft tissue status, wound contamination, and surgeon preference all influence the type of fixation used. Furthermore, osteosynthesis techniques useful in the acute setting differ from those employed for secondary or revisional surgery.

One of the most useful techniques for fixation in the setting of both replantation and secondary procedures, such as toe-to-hand transfer, is intraosseous wiring [6, 7]. While not as rigid as plate or lag screw fixation, intraosseous wiring has been successfully used for fracture fixation in the hand and for small joint arthrodesis for over 35 years. Union rates for fractures treated with

this technique are uniformly high, ranging from roughly 98.5–100 % [8–10]. The technique has the additional advantage of being applicable to very short (5 mm) bone segments such as may occur when amputations occur proximate to joints. In addition, the technique requires only minimal dissection in order to expose adequate bone surfaces, thus minimizing interference with blood supply to the bone via the periosteum.

Preparation for intraosseous wiring begins with shaping of the surfaces to be joined. In most cases, this will involve leveling of the proximal and distal segments so that the union line approximates a purely transverse fracture. The raw surfaces of the cortical bone should be as smooth and congruent as possible so as to maximize contact area and minimize motion following synthesis. Next, the soft tissues and periosteum are dissected minimally away from the free surfaces; the exposed bone should allow for 2 mm of distance between the intraosseous wires and the union site. Beginning with either the proximal bone stump or the distal, amputated segment, two holes are drilled utilizing either a 1 mm drill bit or a 0.045 in. diameter K-wire. Configuration of these bicortical tunnels may be either parallel or in a 90–90 (perpendicular) configuration (Fig. 2.2a–d); both have demonstrated equal union rates. The remaining segment is then aligned against the previously prepared bone fragment, and corrections for any malrotation are made. Tunnels are then made parallel to those in the original segment. 2-0 (28 gauge) stainless steel wires may then be passed through the tunnels. While one member of the team holds the bone segments in proper alignment, a second operator twists the free wire ends to tighten the loops. Final check of alignment should be confirmed prior to completely tightening the wires, as small adjustments in rotation may still be made. After trimming the wires, the free ends should be rotated down adjacent to the union site and away from any tendons.

Osteosynthesis via intraosseous wiring does provide adequate rigidity for early rehabilitation, and, since wires transgress neither tendon nor skin, the technique provides little resistance to

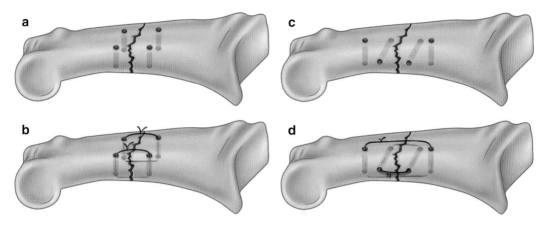

Fig. 2.2 (**a–d**) Diagrams of different intraosseous wire techniques. (**a**) In the parallel technique, holes are drilled equidistant from the fracture site and parallel to those in the opposite segment. (**b**) Wires are passed and twisted.

(**c**) In the 90–90 technique, holes on one side are drilled perpendicular to one another with mirror image holes drilled in the opposite segment. (**d**) Wires are passed between holes in the same plane

the gliding of surrounding soft tissues. Finally, the resources necessary for this technique (k-wires and stainless steel wire) are inexpensive and universally available. Limitations are primarily in the setting of amputation where the fracture line is long and oblique and where conversion to a transverse pattern would result in excessive shortening. In this setting, a single intraosseous wire may be combined with one or more K-wires.

Kirschner wires (K-wires) are a widely used fixation method, both temporarily prior to other means of fixation, and permanently until bony union occurs. Advantages of K-wire fixation include low cost, means of percutaneous application thus limiting soft tissue injury, speed of application limiting warm ischemia time, and ability to be easily removed once bony union occurs.

The degree of stability offered by K-wires is influenced by the pin diameter and configuration. For transverse phalanx fracture patterns, crossed wires offer the greatest stability to torsion, distraction, and bending [11]. For oblique fracture patterns, pins oriented perpendicular to the fracture line offer greater stability to torsion, distraction, and bending over crossed pins [11]. With regard to compression, however, pins oriented perpendicular to the shaft of the bone offer greater stability [12]. For oblique fracture

patterns, therefore, the application of multiple wires in different orientations provides the greatest stability. In the setting of significant bone loss not allowing for anatomic reduction, an intramedullary pin inserted prior to neurovascular repair allows for rotational adjustment and realignment of the vessels prior to additional wire placement [13].

There are disadvantages to K-wire fixation, however. Percutaneous wires have a significantly increased risk of pin tract infection [14–16], which may prompt early removal of hardware, potentially leading to instability at the fracture line. By nature of their placement, K-wires do not compress the fracture site; instead, they offer relative stability thus increasing the risk of nonunion and malunion compared to other means of more rigid fixation [17]. Finally, as noted above, K-wires may impede motion of soft tissue, including tendons, during rehabilitation.

An alternative to the intraosseous wire/ oblique K-wire technique for longer oblique fracture lines is to join the bone segments via lag screws. While providing some of the best rigidity and compression of any fixation method, the injury must meet specific criteria for lag screws to be applicable. The amputation line must be oblique enough to accommodate placement of at least two screws without encroaching on the free

Fig. 2.3 (**a**, **b**) Lag screw fixation. After drilling the gliding hole into the near cortex, a drill guide is inserted prior to drilling the thread hole into the far cortex (**a**). (**b**) Final screw placement with countersinking of the gliding hole demonstrates how screw head protrusion can be minimized

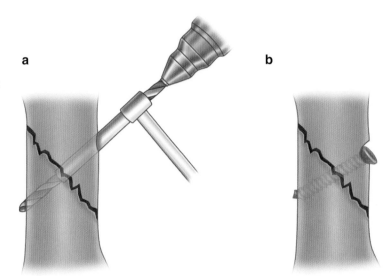

edge of the fracture line. Bone loss should be minimal so that good contact of cortical surfaces can be achieved nearly, if not completely, circumferentially. Finally, no comminution at the fracture site should be present. Lag screw application starts with the use of pointed reduction clamps to maintain reduction while aligning the drill perpendicular to the fracture line. The near cortex is drilled to match the outer thread diameter of the screw thereby creating a gliding hole. A drill sleeve or guide is placed into the hole, thus insuring both stages of drilling are in line. The far cortex is then drilled with the appropriately sized drill bit, typically to match the screw's core size, creating a thread hole. For example, placement of a 1.0 mm screw would require a 1.0 mm drill bit to create the gliding hole and a 0.8 mm drill bit to create the thread hole. Countersinking, or tapping of the outer surface of the near cortex to match the screw head size, is typically performed to decrease the amount of screw head protrusion and reduce surrounding soft tissue irritation.

The number of screws used is dependent on the length of the fracture line. A fracture line whose length is more than twice the diameter of the diaphysis typically requires two or more screws (Fig. 2.3a–b). When a screw is inserted close to the apex of a fragment, ensuring that the distance from the fracture line to the edge of the screw is no less than the diameter of the screw head will decrease the risk of fracturing off the fragment apex.

Open reduction and internal fixation with the use of miniplates and screws offers one of the most broadly applicable and stable forms of osteosynthesis for complex fractures in the small bones of the hand. At the level of the forearm or arm, rigid plate fixation, often with a dynamic compression technique, would be the standard for repair of the bony injury in the setting of amputation (see Chap. 7). Advantages also include adequate stability for early motion and rehabilitation [18–21]. Despite the versatility of the technique, it is rarely employed in the setting of primary replantation at the level distal to the wrist, largely because plate application requires extensive soft tissue dissection, potentially jeopardizing local blood supply to the union site, and longer operative time in what will already be a lengthy procedure. More commonly, plate and screw osteosynthesis will be used in the setting of secondary surgery for nonunion or malunion (see Chaps. 13 and 14).

While the majority of successful replantations will proceed to bony union, nonunions may still occur. Incidence of nonunion varies depending on the primary osteosynthesis technique employed, ranging from as low as 1.5 % with intraosseous wiring [10] to 9–19 % with K-wires alone [17]. Nonunions are defined by the lack of the potential to heal without further intervention and can be classified as either atrophic or hypertrophic. Atrophic nonunions lack any callus and are physiologically defined by a poor blood supply to the fracture site. Successful healing of an atrophic nonunion requires the use of cancellous bone grafts in addition to plate fixation. Cancellous bone graft is osteoconductive, acting as a structural framework or scaffold for new bone growth [22, 23]. If an autograft is used, harvested from the patient, and transferred at the time of surgery, the graft is also said to be osteoinductive, containing growth factors that stimulate osteoprogenitor cells to differentiate into osteoblasts during the process of new bone formation. Compared with cortical bone grafts, cancellous grafts heal more rapidly and are more resistant to infection [24].

Hypertrophic nonunions have an adequate blood supply to the fracture ends and an abundance of callus formation. They occur due to poor stability and excessive motion at the fracture site. In this setting, secondary surgery typically addresses take down of the fibrous nonunion and plate fixation with or without the use of a bone graft.

Successful bone healing, albeit in a malrotated or angulated position, occurs in anywhere between 2 and 14 % of replanted digits [17]. When faced with malunion and unacceptable bony alignment, secondary surgery requires a corrective osteotomy (see Chap. 14). In cases where significant bone loss occurred at the time of amputation, or if significant bone needs to be removed in order to correct alignment, corticocancellous grafts can be applied. Cancellous bone grafts alone are not enough to provide structural support and maintain alignment after correction is made [25]. Cortical bone, either autograft or allograft, is tailored and shaped to fill the bony void so that continuous cortical bone exists circumferentially around the site of correction. Typically, a plate is applied over the bone graft to help maintain its positioning and decrease the risk of shifting of the graft before it is fully incorporated.

Tendon

Tendon Anatomy

Knowledge of tendon anatomy is paramount to understanding tendon homeostasis and to performing successful tendon repair in the setting of replantation. Tendons play an essential role in the musculoskeletal system, transmitting tensile loads from muscle to bone, resulting in joint stabilization and movement. The primary cell type in tendon is the tenocyte. These fibroblast-like cells function to produce collagen and other extracellular matrix proteins. Type I collagen accounts for approximately 70 % of tendon composition. Other types of collagen (III, V, IX, X, XI, and XII) are present in lesser amounts and contribute to overall tendon homeostasis [26]. Tendons are sequentially composed of collagen molecules, fibrils, and fascicles arranged into parallel primary, secondary, and tertiary bundles. Each bundle is surrounded by an endotenon that contains both blood vessels and nerves [27]. An epitenon and paratenon layer surrounds the tendon unit with a thin layer of synovial fluid in between and function in tendon regeneration, repair, and gliding.

Tendons are well-vascularized structures with a distinctly different blood supply depending on the presence or absence of a synovial sheath. Extensor tendons and flexor tendons proximal to the A1 pulley of the hand receive their blood supply by way of segmental branches from nearby arteries coursing through adjacent connective tissue. Blood vessels enter the tendon unit through the para- and epitenon, forming a vascular network around each fibril to provide nutrition to individual bundles via the endotenon [28].

Digital flexor tendons distal to the A1 pulley are unique in that a synovial sheath is the source of nutrition. The flexor sheath is composed of a fibrous portion and a synovial portion with both visceral and parietal layers. Its primary mode of providing tendon nutrition is through a combination of local diffusion and direct vascular perfusion via specialized mesotenon called vincula. Segmental branches from adjacent digital arteries supply the vincula. Each flexor digitorum profundus (FDP) tendon has a short vincula attached to the middle phalanx and a long vincula attached to the proximal phalanx. The superficialis tendon (FDS) also has a short vincula and a long vincula which both arise at the level of the proximal phalanx. The blood supply from each vinculum enters the sheath on the dorsal surface [28].

Tendon Healing

The ability of tendons to hold tension for prolonged periods of time is the result of very low oxygen tension requirements. Consequently, tendons exhibit slow metabolic rates and slower healing [27]. Understanding the factors involved in tendon healing is necessary to optimize outcomes during and following repair.

Similar to wound healing, tendon healing has been divided into three distinct, but overlapping, phases: an inflammatory phase, a matrix production phase, and a remodeling and maturation phase. The inflammatory phase occurs within hours of injury, after initial hemostasis and clot formation. Neutrophils predominate early, followed closely by monocytes and macrophages at 24 h to phagocytose necrotic material. Cytokine release signals tenocyte activation for production of collagen III and early angiogenesis. Tendon strength during the inflammatory phase is defined by the strength of the suture itself [29]. The matrix production phase commences after a few days and lasts for approximately 4 weeks. Collagen III production is highest during this phase, however, also highly unorganized. Self-renewing tendon stem cells (TSCs) have recently been identified as prominent cells involved in initial collagen production [30]. The remodeling and maturation phase begins around week 4–6 with a decrease in tendon cellularity and transition of collagen type III to collagen type I. Tendon tensile strength is gained during this phase.

Collagen fibers become properly aligned in parallel to lines of tension and important collagen cross-linking occurs. The repaired tendon is considered to be at full tensile strength around 12 weeks [31]. Tendon healing continues up to approximately 1-year post injury [27].

Mechanical loading and early motion play important roles in tendon homeostasis and decreased adhesion formation and are, therefore, key considerations following tendon repair. Tenocytes are mechanoresponsive in that they can modify the extracellular environment during mechanical loading through formation and degradation of matrix proteins [26]. Immobilization following tendon repair has been shown to significantly decrease the strength of repair within the first 3 weeks [32]. It is likely that immobilization results in an upregulation of inflammatory gene expression [33, 34]. Notably, tendon use has been shown to increase the number of activated fibroblasts that aid in tendon repair and remodeling [35]. Numerous studies have shown that early mobilization increases tendon tensile strength and reduces adhesion formation [36–39]. The proposed mechanism of this is that physiological forces promote gene expression of type 1 collagen formation during healing and that tension causes the collagen to be deposited and aligned in a parallel fashion [40]. Excessive tendon loading, however, can result in tendon injury, highlighting the importance of proper loading to improve outcomes following tendon repair surgery [41].

Principles of Tendon Repair

Acute tendon injury in the setting of upper extremity replantation follows the same principles involved in repair of isolated tendon injury. In most cases of replantation distal to the wrist, tendon repair will immediately follow osteosynthesis. This facilitates repair from deep to superficial and avoids stress on vascular and neural repairs that could occur during tendon manipulation. When approaching the severed tendon, a strong and gap resistant repair is the most important factor as the primary function of the tendon is to transmit force. In the setting of aggressive rehabilitation efforts, repair techniques must adapt to withstand the high forces applied by early active mobilization. The goals of primary tendon repair include sutures easily placed in the tendon, secure knots, smooth juncture of tendon ends, minimal gapping, minimal interference with tendon vascularity, and sufficient strength throughout healing [42].

Overall repair strength is a composite of both core and peripheral sutures. While it is generally accepted that tendon repair strength is proportional to the number of suture stands that cross the repair site and caliber of suture used [43–47], one must balance this information with technical difficulty, vascular interference, and tissue trauma. Common two-strand techniques including modified Kessler, Pennington, Tsuge, or modified Pennington are sufficient for passive motion rehabilitation, however, not early active motion [48]. A variety of four and six strand repairs have been shown to be able to withstand early active motion. Many techniques have been described; however, head-to-head comparisons are difficult due to variation in study design. The most common repairs include the four or six strand modified Kessler, Tsuge, and Savage techniques. Double-stranded looped suture is often used and may reduce operative time, along with tendon handling and puncture (Fig. 2.4a–e).

Suture anchoring has a critical impact on the strength of repair. As discussed previously, tendon fibrils are aligned in parallel to provide maximum strength in the line of most tension. A suture passing perpendicular to these fibrils does not integrate fibril bundles into the repair and can easily fail by pulling out. This is commonly seen with a non-grasping Bunnell repair. Anchoring the suture with a loop around a bundle of fibrils has been shown to be more effective. A grasping loop configuration refers to the creation of an open loop as seen in the Kessler repair. A locking configuration forms a closed loop around fibril bundles as demonstrated by a locking Kessler or modified Pennington suture. Grasping loop suture techniques pull through tendon fibers with applied tension and tend to fail by way of suture pull through. Locking techniques tighten around fibers with tendons and tend to fail from suture breakage (Fig. 2.5). Studies have shown that locking configuration provides superior strength and gap resistance compared to grasping [49]. Core suture purchase length has demonstrated to be an important contributor to repair strength and gap resistance with 0.7–1 cm purchase length showing the best results [50, 51].

The ideal suture material should be strong, inextensible, and easy to knot and should cause minimal tissue response [52]. Suture strength is most important when using a locking loop configuration as failure is caused by breakage and not by suture pull through [53]. Caliber sutures of 4-0 or 3-0 are commonly used, with 3-0 caliber showing no advantage of strength of the intact repair [54]. Most sutures used in tendon repair are nonabsorbable synthetic sutures. Coated braided polyester, monofilament nylon, and monofilament polypropylene have the best biocompatibility and are the most commonly used. Coated braided polyester seems to provide increased tensile strength and better gap resistance than nylon or polypropylene [52, 55, 56]. Braided polyblend polyethylene suture (FiberWire®, Arthrex, Naples, FL) has been introduced with strength and stiffness similar to stainless steel, higher than coated braided polyester with no difference in gap resistance [53, 55].

Epitendinous or circumferential suturing placed at the time of primary tendon repair has been shown to enhance strength and gap resistance [57]. A monofilament polypropylene suture is commonly used and the addition of this suture may increase repair strength up to 50 % [58]. Despite a variety of techniques, studies have shown superiority in strength and lower glide resistance of running locking, cross-stitch, and an interlocking horizontal mattress epitendinous techniques [59, 60] (Fig. 2.6a–c). It is important to note that complex epitendinous repairs may increase glide resistance. Peripheral sutures are often the first to break, transmitting more force to the core suture, which may result in failure or increased gap formation.

Gap formation between repaired tendon ends occurs within a few weeks following repair when applied tension during early motion exceed the tolerance of the suture repair. This occurrence

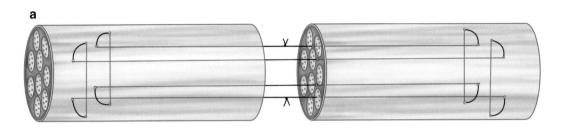

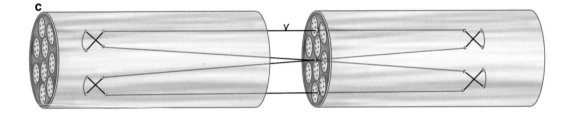

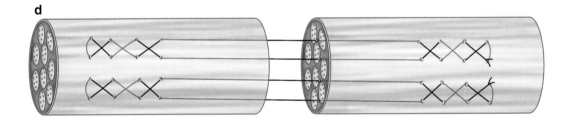

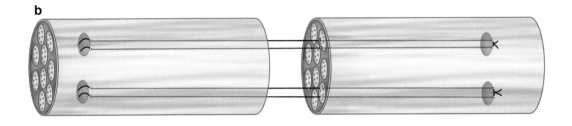

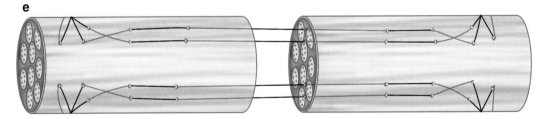

Fig. 2.4 (**a–e**) Common core suture techniques in tendon repair: (**a**) double modified Kessler; (**b**) double loop suture; (**c**) cruciate cross-stitch locked; (**d**) augmented Becker (MGH repair); (**e**) 4-strand Savage

Fig. 2.5 Diagram demonstrating tendon grasping (*top fibril*) and tendon locking (*bottom fibril*) techniques

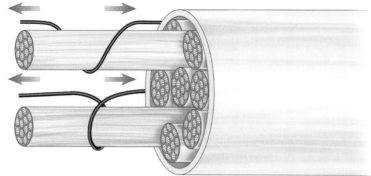

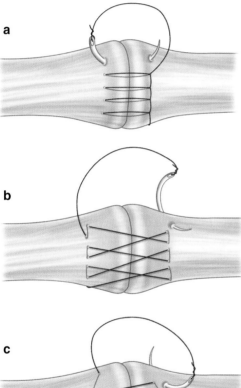

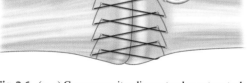

Fig. 2.6 (**a–c**) Common epitendinous tendon suture techniques: (**a**) simple running locking; (**b**) cross-stitch; (**c**) interlocking horizontal mattress

can result in poor outcomes due to decrease healing time and the potential for increased tendon adhesion formation. A repair gap greater than 3 mm is considered by most to be the upper limit before encountering negative results. This is proposed to be due to delayed healing, adhesion formation, and increased resistance to gliding [61, 62], all of which result in increased risk of postoperative rupture and range of motion impairment. However, reports of tendon gapping of 5–7 mm and up to 10 mm [63] have been reported with good results and no need for tenolysis. While somewhat unclear, a gap between tendon ends should be as small as possible to provide the best chance at good outcomes.

Manipulation of the mechanical environment of healing tendon may exert a biologic effect through the mechanotransduction mechanism and hold promise for promoting a repair process that restores normal tendon structure and function. These principles form the basis for rehabilitation principles (see Chap. 15). Disuse following immobilization has been associated with decreased levels of extracellular matrix protein expression, alterations in tenocyte morphology, and loss of normal extracellular matrix architecture, resulting in impaired function and healing capacity. The ideal postoperative exercise/rehabilitation program avoids injury to repair but provides a biologic stimulus for homeostasis and function [64, 65].

While the principles remain the same, slight differences exist in extensor tendon repair due to inherent differences from flexor tendons. Extensor tendons are smaller and flatter than flexor tendons. This reduced cross-sectional area and collagen cross-linking is most evident in distal extensor zones. As a result, extensor tendon repairs are only about 50 % as strong as flexor tendon repairs with the same suture technique

[66]. It has been suggested that the strength and quality of extensor tendon repair comparing traditional two-stranded techniques is not significantly different in the small, thinner, tendons compared to more proximally [67]. More recent studies have shown that a modified Bunnell and augmented Becker repairs are stronger with less incidence of suture pullout [67, 68]. These suture types have shown benefit to use as a core suture in zone III through zone VIII repairs. Additionally, Lee and colleagues showed that the use of a running, interlocking, horizontal mattress suture is comparable in strength to a modified Bunnell and Becker, however, has significantly less tendon shortening [69]. Zone IX injuries are often best managed with multiple figure of eight sutures [70].

Despite bony shortening during replantation, fraying and avulsion injuries may result in the need for additional tendon debridement. Flexor tendons can tolerate limited (easily 10 mm) shortening without loss of finger motion or even greater shortening at the cost of full extension. Extensor tendon shortening may be less well tolerated, as a decrease in MCP flexion can occur, resulting in decreased grip strength. Every effort should be made during tendon repair to balance the flexion and extension forces and avoid over-tensioning of the extensor repair. This balance may be best assessed by a combination of inspecting the finger cascade during tenodesis and by gently, passively flexing the fingers to the palm following osteosynthesis and tendon repair. Repairs that are too tight or gap during gentle passive motion at the time of repair are unlikely to tolerate the forces required for rehabilitation.

Secondary Tendon Reconstruction

Tendon reconstruction using tendon grafting may be required following replantation in the setting of attritional rupture of primarily repaired tendons or in the presence of segmental tendon loss as a result of extensive initial injury. Common donor tendons associated with minimal donor site complications include palmaris longus, plantaris, and extensor digitorum longus to the second toe. While palmaris longus is the most commonly used due to its convenient location in the upper extremity, plantaris and toe extensors can provide up to 35 cm of usable graft length.

During placement of the graft, a Pulvertaft end-to-side weave is the suture method of choice and a bone anchor may be used at the distal juncture if reconstruction of the tendon and bone interface is required. Tendon graft incorporation is commonly associated with considerable peritendinous necrosis and subsequent adhesion formation. However, peritendinous adhesions are found much less with placement of intrasynovial donor tendons. Following a brief period of immobilization, early digital range of motion is critical to obtain the best range of motion, as outcomes are often inferior to primary repair [71].

Tendon transfers may be performed as an alternative to tendon grafting or if tendon grafting is not an option. Specific tendon transfers are beyond the scope of this chapter; however, general principles of tendon transfer should be applied. In the acute setting of replantation, "spare parts" transfers where useful proximal tendons from a nonreplanted digit are available to power a replanted digit can be useful. Examples include the use of flexor tendons in a heterotopic replantation (see Chap. 10). When expendable motors are not easily available acutely, plans may be made for delayed transfer. Prerequisites for delayed tendon transfer include stable wounds, good passive range of motion of the involved joints, and available donors. Such delays are often best performed after the first few months when scars have softened and the soft tissues have stabilized.

Conclusion

Survival of a replanted digit may represent the culmination of technical and technological advances in microsurgery, but *successful* replantation relies on trauma principles developed by generations of hand surgeons. Understanding the processes by which bone and tendons heal led to current recommendations for osteosynthesis and tendon repair. As technological advances in the biology of musculoskeletal healing evolve, it is likely that the principles presented here will be refined, but, as evidenced by the consistency of recommendations for musculoskeletal repair over the past few decades, it is almost certain that these techniques will still be applicable.

References

1. Simon SR, ed. Orthopaedic basic science. Amer Academy of Orthopaedic, 1994.
2. Granero-Molto F, Weis JA, Miga MI, et al. Regenerative effects of transplanted mesenchymal stem cells in fracture healing. Stem Cells. 2009;27(8):1887–98.
3. Perren SM. Evolution of the internal fixation of long bone fractures. The scientific basis of biological internal fixation: choosing a new balance between stability and biology. J Bone Joint Surg Br. 2002;84(8):1093–110.
4. Gerstendfeld LC, Alkhiary YM, et al. Three-dimensional reconstruction of fracture callus morphogenesis. J Histochem Cytochem. 2006;54(11):1215–28.
5. Green E, Lubahn JD, Evans J. Risk factors, treatment, and outcomes associated with nonunion of the midshaft humerus fracture. J Surg Orthop Adv. 2005;14(2):64–72.
6. Gordon L, Monsanto EH. Skeletal stabilization for digital replantation surgery. Use of intraosseous wiring. Clin Orthop Relat Res. 1987;214:72–7.
7. Gingrass RP, Fehring B, Matloub H. Intraosseous wiring of complex hand fractures. Plast Reconstr Surg. 1980;66(3):383–94.
8. Lister G. Intraosseous wiring of the digital skeleton. J Hand Surg Am. 1978;3(5):427–35.
9. Zimmerman NB, Weiland AJ. Ninety-ninety intraosseous wiring for internal fixation of the digital skeleton. Orthopedics. 1989;12(1):99–103.
10. Yim KK, Wei FC. Intraosseous wiring in toe-to-hand transplantation. Ann Plast Surg. 1995;35(1):66–9.
11. Viegas SF, Ferren EL, Self J, et al. Comparative mechanical properties of various Kirschner wire configurations in transverse and oblique phalangeal fractures. J Hand Surg Am. 1988;13(2):246–53.
12. Tencer AF, Johnson KD, Kyle RF, et al. Biomechanics of fractures and fracture fixation. Instr Course Lect. 1993;42:19–55.
13. Touliatos AS, Soucacos PN, Beris AE, et al. Alternative techniques for restoration of bony segments in digital replantation. Acta Orthop Scand Suppl. 1995;264:19–22.
14. Rafique A, Ghani S, Sadiq M, et al. Kirschner wire pin tract infection rates between percutaneous and buried wires in treating metacarpal and phalangeal fractures. J Coll Phys Surg Pak. 2006;16(8):518–20.
15. Hargreaves DG, Drew SJ, Eckersley R. Kirschner wire pin tract infection rates: a randomized controlled trial between percutaneous and buried wires. J Hand Surg Br. 2004;29(4):374–6.
16. Lakshmanan P, Dixit V, Reed MR, et al. Infection rate of percutaneous Kirschner wire fixation for distal radius fractures. J Orthop Surg (Hong Kong). 2010;18(1):85–6.
17. Whitney TM, Lineaweaver WC, Buncke HJ, et al. Clinical results of bony fixation methods in digital replantation. J Hand Surg Am. 1990;15(2):328–34.
18. Chen SH, Wei FC, Chen HC, et al. Miniature plates and screws in acute complex hand injury. J Trauma. 1994;37(2):237–42.
19. Dabezies EJ, Schutte JP. Fixation of metacarpal and phalangeal fractures with miniature plates and screws. J Hand Surg Am. 1986;11(2):283–8.
20. Jones WW. Biomechanics of small bone fixation. Clin Orthop Relat Res. 1987;214:11–8.
21. Takigami H, Sakano H, Saito T. Internal fixation with the low profile plate system compared with Kirschner wire fixation: clinical results of treatment of metacarpal and phalangeal fractures. Hand Surg. 2010;15(1):1–6.
22. Buckwalter JA, Glimcher MJ, Cooper RR, et al. Bone biology. I: structure, blood supply, cells, matrix, and mineralization. Instr Course Lect. 1996;45:371–86.
23. Buckwalter JA, Glimcher MJ, Cooper RR, et al. Bone biology. II: formation, form, modeling, remodeling, and regulation of cell function. Instr Course Lect. 1996;45:387–99.
24. Freeland AE, Rehm JP. Autogenous bone grafting for fractures of the hand. Tech Hand Upper Extrem Surg. 2004;8(2):78–86.
25. Stevenson S. Enhancement of fracture healing with autogenous and allogeneic bone grafts. Clin Orthop Relat Res. 1998;355:S239–46.
26. Wang JH-C, Guo Q, Li B. Tendon biomechanics and mechanobiology-a minireview of basic concepts in recent advancements. J Hand Ther. 2012;25(2):133–40.
27. Sharma P, Maffulli N. Biology of tendon injury: healing, modeling, and remodeling. J Musculoskelet Nueronal Interact. 2006;6(2):181–90.
28. Manske PR, Lesker PA. Flexor tendon nutrition. Hand Clin. 1985;1(1):13–24.
29. Strickland JW. The scientific basis for advances in flexor tendon surgery. J Hand Ther. 2005;18(2):94–110.
30. Tan Q, Lui PP, Lee YW. In vivo identity of tendon stem cells and the roles of stem cells in tendon healing. Stem Cells Dev. 2013;22(23):3128–40.
31. Cooper C. Fundamentals of hand therapy: clinical reasoning and treatment guidelines for common diagnoses of the upper extremity. 2nd ed. St. Louis: Mosby Elsevier; Copyright 2013.
32. Hitchcock TF, Light TR, Bunch WB, et al. The effect of immediate constrained digital motion on the strength of flexor tendon repairs in chickens. J Hand Surg Am. 1987;12(4):590–5.
33. Eliasson P, Andersson T, Aspenberg P. Rat Achilles tendon healing: mechanical loading and gene expression. J Appl Physiol. 2009;107(2):399–407.

34. Uchida H, Tohyama H, Nagashima K, et al. Stress deprivation simultaneously induces over-expression of interleukin-1beta, tumor necrosis factor-alpha, and transformation growth factor-beta in fibroblasts and mechanical deterioration of the tissue in the patellar tendon. J Biomech. 2005;38(4):791–8.

35. Szczodry M, Zhang J, Lim C, et al. Treadmill running exercise results in the presence of numerous myofibroblasts in mouse patellar tendons. J Orthop Res. 2009;27(10):1373–8.

36. Groth GN. Pyramid of progressive force exercises to the injured flexor tendon. J Hand Ther. 2004;17(1):31–42.

37. Manske PR, Gelberman RH, Vande Berg JS, Lesker PA. Intrinsic flexor-tendon repair. A morphological study in vitro. J Bone Joint Surg Am. 1984;66(3):385–96.

38. Zhao C, Amadio PC, Zobitz ME, An KN. Gliding characteristics of tendon repair in canine flexor digitorum profundus tendons. J Orthop Res. 2001;19(4):580–6.

39. Silva MJ, Boyer MI, Gelberman RH. Recent progress in flexor tendon healing. J Orthop Sci. 2002;7(4):508–14.

40. Davidson CJ, Ganion LR, Gehlsen GM, et al. Rat tendon morphologic and functional changes resulting from soft tissue mobilization. Med Sci Sports Exerc. 1997;29(3):313–9.

41. Schultz GS, Davidson JM, Kirsner RS, et al. Dynamic reciprocity in the wound microenvironment. Wound Repair Regen. 2011;19(2):134–48.

42. Strickland JW. Flexor tendon injuries: II. Operative technique. J Am Acad Orthop Surg. 1995;3(1):55–62.

43. Savage R. The search for the ideal tendon repair in zone 2: strand number, anchor points and suture thickness. J Hand Surg Eur Vol. 2014;39(1):20–9.

44. Taras JS, Raphael JS, Marczyk SC, et al. Evaluation of suture caliber in flexor tendon repair. J Hand Surg Am. 2001;26(6):1100–4.

45. Shaieb MD, Singer DI. Tensile strengths of various suture techniques. J Hand Surg Br. 1997;22(6):764–7.

46. Komanduri M, Phillips CS, Mass DP. Tensile strength of flexor tendon repairs in a dynamic cadaver model. J Hand Surg. 1996;21A:605–11.

47. Silfverskiold IL, Anderson CH. Two new methods of tendon repair: an in vitro evaluation of tensile strength and gap formation. J Hand Surg. 1993;18A:58–65.

48. Bainbridge LC, Robertson C, Gilles D, et al. A comparison of post-operative mobilization of flexor tendon repairs with "passive flexion-active extension" and "controlled active motion" techniques. J Hand Surg Br. 1994;19(4):517–21.

49. Hotokezaka S, Manske P. Differences between locking loops and grasping loops: effects on 2-strand core suture. J Hand Surg. 1997;22(6):995–1003.

50. Cao Y, Zhu B, Xie RG, et al. Influence of core suture purchase length on strength of four-strand tendon repairs. J Hand Surg. 2006;31(1):107–12.

51. Tang JB, Zhang Y, Guo R. Core suture purchase affects strength of tendon repairs. J of Hand Surg. 2005;30(6):1262–6.

52. Trail IA, Powell ES, Noble J. An evaluation of suture materials used in tendon surgery. J Hand Surg. 1989;14B:422–7.

53. Miller B, Dodds SD, DeMars A, et al. Flexor tendon repairs: the impact of fiberwire on grasping and locking core sutures. J Hand Surg. 2007;32A:591–6.

54. Viinikainen A, Goransson H, Huovinen K, et al. A comparative analysis of the biomechanical behavior of five flexor tendon core sutures. J Hand Surg. 2004;29B:536–43.

55. Lawrence TM, Davis TRC. A biomechanical analysis of suture material and their influence on a four-strand flexor tendon repair. J Hand Surg. 2005;30A:836–41.

56. Vizesi F, Jones C, Lotz N, et al. Stress relaxation and creep: viscoelastic properties of common suture materials used for flexor tendon repair. J Hand Surg. 2008;33A:241–6.

57. Dona E, Gianoutsos MP, Walsh WR. Optimizing biomechanical performance of the 4-strand cruciate flexor tendon repair. J Hand Surg Am. 2004;29(4):571–80.

58. Viinikainen A, Goransson H, Ryhanen J. Primary flexor tendon repair techniques. Scand J Surg. 2008;97:333–40.

59. Moriya T, Zhao C, An KN, et al. The effect of epitendinous suture technique on gliding resistance during cyclin motion after flexor tendon repair: a cadaveric study. J Hand Surg Am. 2010;35(4):552–8.

60. Kubota H, Aoki M, Pruitt DL. Mechanical properties of various circumferential tendon suture techniques. J Hand Surg Br. 1996;21(4):474–80.

61. Gelberman RH, Boyer MI, Brodt MD, et al. The effect of gap formation at the repair site on the strength and excursion of intrasynovial flexor tendons. An experimental study on the early stages of tendon-healing in dogs. JBJS. 1999;81(7):975–82.

62. Zhao C, Amadio PC, Tanaka T, et al. Effect of gap size on gliding resistance after flexor tendon repair. JBJS. 2004;86(11):2482–8.

63. Silfverskiold KL, May EJ, Tornvall AH. Gap formation during controlled motion after flexor tendon repair in zone II: a prospective clinical study. J Hand Surg Am. 1992;17:539–46.

64. Reeves ND, Maganaris CN, Ferretti G, et al. Influence of 90-day simulated microgravity on human tendon mechanical properties and the effect of resistive countermeasures. J Appl Physiol. 2005;98(6):2278–86.

65. Yasuda T, Kinoshita M, Abe M, et al. Unfavorable effect of knee immobilization on Achilles tendon healing in rabbits. Acta Orthop Scand. 2000;71(1):69–73.

66. Standard of care: flexor/extensor tendon lacerations of the forearm, wrist, digits. The Brigham and Women's Hospital, Inc. Department of Rehabilitation Services. Copyright 2007.

67. Newport ML, Tucker RL. New perspectives on extensor tendon repair and implications for rehabilitation. J Hand Ther. 2005;18(2):175–81.

68. Woo SH, Tsai TM, Kleinert HE, et al. A biomechanical comparison of four extensor tendon repair techniques in zone IV. Plast Reconstr Surg. 2005;115(6): 1674–81.

69. Lee SK, Dubey A, Kim BH, et al. A biomechanical study of extensor tendon repair methods: introduction to the running-interlocking horizontal mattress

70. extensor tendon repair technique. J Hand Surg Am. 2010;35(1):19–23.

70. Matzon JL, Bozentka DJ. Extensor tendon injuries. J Hand Surg. 2010;35A:854–61.

71. Moore T, Anderson B, Seiler JG. Flexor tendon reconstruction. J Hand Surg. 2010;35(A):1025–30.

Principles of Nerve Repair and Neural Recovery in Extremity Replantation Surgery

Sahil Kapur and Samuel O. Poore

Introduction

Peripheral nerve injury is an extremely common event affecting both civilian and military populations, resulting from blunt trauma and sharp lacerations. Nerve laceration and injury is an obvious and concomitant event in cases of amputation, and successful replantation is not only highly contingent upon revascularization, fixation of bone, and (possible) repair of tendons and muscle but also upon accurate and precise nerve repair and neural rehabilitation. Failure of nerve repair results in an extremity or digit that is insensate, intolerant to changes in temperature, and subject to substantial neuropathic pain. All of these significantly debilitating clinical findings directly impact the aim of replantation: functional recovery. Therefore, when replanting an amputated digit or extremity, a basic understanding of the technical aspects of nerve repair is essential including the type of repair required (e.g., epineural vs. fascicular), the appropriate selection of a conduit when necessary, and a thorough knowledge of methodologies for assessing functional recovery.

While the focus of this chapter is on the repair of nerves that specifically accompanies amputation, the lessons learned from disparate cases and causes of nerve injury comprise much of the backbone of our knowledge of peripheral nerve regeneration and rehabilitation and thus are highly valuable for the larger field. In the civilian population, peripheral nerve injury occurs in about 2.8 % of all trauma cases [1]. In blunt trauma scenarios, such as falls and motor vehicle accidents, nerve pathology is related to crush or stretch-type injury. Sharp laceration of nerves occurs in about 30 % of extremity trauma cases. A 16-year retrospective study of 456 peripheral nerve injury cases by Kouyoumdjian et al. found that about 70 % of peripheral nerve injuries occur in upper extremity trauma and most commonly involve the ulnar nerve [2].

The incidence of peripheral nerve trauma in the military population is about five to ten times greater than the civilian population. Pathology in this population is caused mainly by shrapnel from blast events [3]. With the advent of improved core body armor, seen in the recent military action in the Middle East, the ratio of injuries leading to wound vs. death has doubled. This translates into a much higher rate of peripheral trauma and peripheral nerve injury [4]. Long-term comorbidity to the individual and cost to the health care system are significant because even

S. Kapur, MD • S.O. Poore, MD, PhD (✉)
Division of Plastic Surgery, University of Wisconsin Hospital and Clinics, Madison, WI, USA
e-mail: kapur.sahil@gmail.com;
poore@surgery.wisc.edu

A.N. Salyapongse et al. (eds.), *Extremity Replantation: A Comprehensive Clinical Guide*,
DOI 10.1007/978-1-4899-7516-4_3, © Springer Science+Business Media New York 2015

after repair of nerve gaps using autografts, significant functional benefit is seen in less than 60 % of patients. Furthermore, aberrant regeneration leads to long-term comorbidities such as neuropathic pain [5–7].

This chapter will provide a concise guide to nerve repair in replantation and in doing so will discuss the following: the basic biochemistry of nerve injury and regeneration, the microsurgical techniques of nerve repair, methods for managing conditions involving nerve gaps, and an analysis of functional outcomes.

Types of Nerve Injury: Biology and Electrophysiology

Nerve fibers can contain purely sensory axons, motor axons, or a combination of the two types. Myelinated or groups of nonmyelinated axons are surrounded by an endoneurial connective tissue layer. These groups are collectively called fascicles, each of which is surrounded by perineurium. Internal epineurium forms the connective tissue in between fascicles and external epineurium forms the outermost layer of the nerve fiber. Endoneurium is longitudinally oriented whereas the perineurium and epineurium are transversely oriented [8]. The blood supply exists in the form of plexuses of microvasculature running longitudinally along the epineurium.

Transverse branches from these plexuses pass through the internal epineurium and perineurium to connect with the capillary network of the endoneurium (Fig. 3.1) [4].

In developing an understanding regarding the classification of nerve injury, one must pay homage to both H. J. Seddon and Sir Sydney Sutherland. In a landmark paper (1943) based on the patterns of injury sustained by soldiers during World War II, Seddon classified nerve injury into three types: neurapraxia, axonotmesis, and neurotmesis. Later, in 1951, Sunderland subcategorized neurotmesis into three separate types [8]. While the two classification schemes are often confused, they are complementary in that both base their taxonomies on damage to the nerve's anatomic layers (Table 3.1, Fig. 3.2).

Neuropraxia (Sunderland Type I)

This category of nerve injury involves a brief, focal period of stress, ischemia, radiation, or electrical injury to the nerve, which results in conduction properties with or without changes in myelin structure. The resulting conduction block also leads to changes in motor recruitment properties of the target muscle. While conduction of signals originating proximal to the lesion is attenuated, signals originating distal to the lesion do not show any attenuation. These attenuation

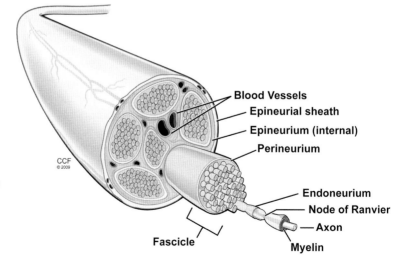

Fig. 3.1 Cross section of a nerve fiber demonstrating axons, fascicles along with the surrounding connective tissue layers: endoneurium, perineurium, and epineurium (Reprinted with permission from the Cleveland Clinic Center for Medical Art & Photograph © 2009–2014. All Rights Reserved)

Blood Vessels
Epineurial sheath
Epineurium (internal)
Perineurium
Endoneurium
Node of Ranvier
Axon
Fascicle
Myelin

CCF
© 2009

Table 3.1 Classifications and descriptions of nerve injury

Seddon classification	Sunderland classification	Description of injury
Neurapraxia	Grade I	Segmental demyelination without axonal injury
Axonotmesis	Grade II	Loss of continuity of axon without damage to outer layers (endoneurium, perineurium, epineurium)
Neurotmesis	Grade III	Loss of continuity of axon and endoneurium with intact perineurium and epineurium
	Grade IV	Loss of continuity of axon, endoneurium, and perineurium with intact epineurium
	Grade V	Loss of continuity of the entire nerve trunk

properties of the signal can help localize the lesion using electrodiagnostic testing. Nerve recovery is generally complete by 12 weeks (Fig. 3.2) [4].

Axonotmesis (Sunderland Type 2)

This category of nerve injury results in damage to the axon but leave the basal lamina, endoneurium, and all the outer layers of the nerve intact. The axonal damage is followed by Wallerian degeneration of the distal axonal stump and regeneration of the proximal axonal stump [9, 10]. Motor end plates degenerate by 12–18 months following injury after which the muscle cannot be reinnervated and muscle atrophy is irreversible. Since axons regenerate at rate of 1–3 mm/day, the proximity of a lesion to the motor end plate is predictive of recovery (Fig. 3.2) [11].

Neurotmesis (Sunderland Types 3, 4, and 5)

In type 3 nerve injury, the endoneurium is damaged along with the axon, but the perineurium

and epineurium are intact. Type 4 lesions involve damage to the endoneurium and perineurium, but the epineurium and the continuity of the nerve itself is not interrupted. Type 5 lesions involve the epineurium and can disrupt the continuity of the nerve. Type 4 and 5 lesions can lead to the development of significant scar tissue that will impede regeneration. Successful regeneration may require debridement of scar tissue and microsurgical repair of the nerve segments [12]. The distal nerve stumps in type 2–5 lesions continue to conduct for at least 1 week. Compound muscle action potentials can be elicited for 7 days, whereas nerve action potentials can be elicited for up to 10 days. Electrodiagnostic testing during this time period can be useful finding the location of the lesion [4]. Mackinnon introduced a type 6 injury classification, which is defined as nerve injury that comprises two additions to the previously discussed subtypes. *Specific to amputation and replantation, all nerve injuries are categorized as neurotmesis (Sunderland Type 5)* (Fig. 3.2).

Wallerian Degeneration and Axonal Regeneration

A full review of Wallerian degeneration and the biochemical events accompanying axonal regeneration is not within the intended scope of this chapter and is readily available elsewhere [13, 14]. Nevertheless, several key events should be highlighted. The first is that following axonal disruption, Wallerian degeneration (retrograde axonal degeneration) within the distal and proximal stumps and axonal regeneration of the proximal stump begins within a few hours. Retrograde axonal degeneration of the proximal stump stops at the first proximal internode in mild injuries but may continue for a few centimeters proximally in more major injuries [15]. This becomes important in the assessment of nerve regeneration because the "regeneration front" actually occurs proximal to the site of repair. The second important concept is that the transection of a peripheral nerve heralds a panoply of events which contribute to both axonal degradation

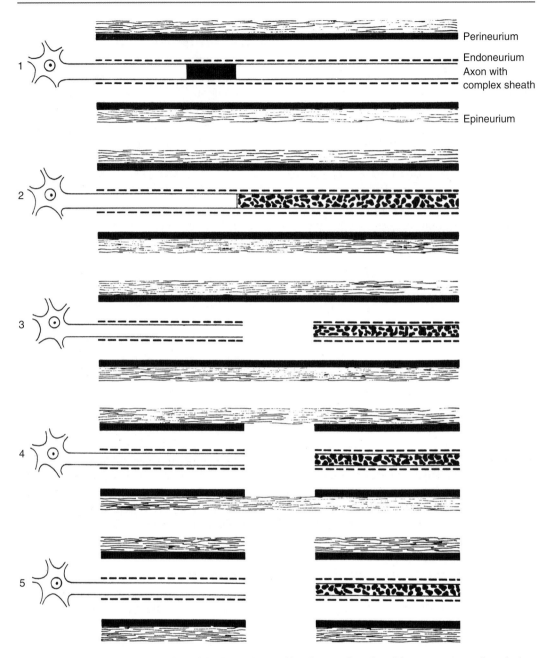

Perineurium

Endoneurium
Axon with
complex sheath

Epineurium

Fig. 3.2 Diagrammatic representation of the Sunderland classification of nerve injury. Each of the five categories of nerve injury demonstrates an increasing level of nerve fiber damage. Severity of damage corresponds to the layers of connective tissue that have been injured (Used with permission from Sunderland [8])

(Wallerian degeneration) and axonal regeneration. Wallerian degeneration begins with the prompt buildup of intracellular calcium and the activation of calpains and phospholipases necessary for cytoskeletal degradation within the proximal and distal stumps [4, 14, 16–18].

Wallerian degeneration and the acute inflammatory events that accompany it set the stage for axonal regeneration, which is heralded by the remarkable transformation of Schwann cells from supportive cells to proliferative cells. This transformation includes the decreased production of normal Schwann cell proteins (PMP22, P0, and connexin-32) and the production of axonal growth factors (GAP-43, neuregulin) [19, 20].

Transection of the peripheral nerve leads to chromatolytic changes within the cell that ultimately indicate a switch in the cellular process program from a transmitting mode to a growth mode. Within the next 12 h, there is an increased production of neutrophils, growth-associated proteins (GAP-43), insulin-like growth factors (IGFs), and glial-cell-derived neurotrophic factors (GDNFs), as well as a plethora of other proteins that promote axonal sprouting, growth cone development, and neurite formation [21, 22].

Extracellular matrix proteins (laminin and fibronectin) produced by Schwann cells form the connective tissue pathways between the nerve stumps. Schwann cells migrate along these pathways and form bands of Bungner. As proximal stump axons begin to regenerate, Schwann cells within the distal nerve stump secrete growth factors (BDNF, GDNF), which serve as a chemoattractant gradient guide for the growth cones. Topographical cues provided by the specific cell adhesion molecules present on the connective tissue pathways aid in growth cone attachment and migration [13]. When Schwann cells are contacted by these regenerating axons, they alter their phenotype and begin producing myelin to encase the newly growing axon.

The greatest obstacles for the regenerating axons include bridging a gap between the proximal and distal segments and overcoming the presence of scar tissue. Even if axons reach the endoneurial tubes of the distal stump, functional recovery is dependent on whether the axons can reach the motor end plates to reestablish functional neuromuscular junctions before the end plates degenerate. Hence, in replantation the reduction (or avoidance) of intraneural scar tissue is of critical importance. Motor end plates begin

to degenerate at 18–24 months. Whole muscle fibrosis can begin as early as a few weeks after injury. Schwann cells maintain their ability to promote regeneration for about 18 months. After this time period, they lose their ability to promote regeneration but are still able to myelinate growing axons. Sprouting axons attempt regeneration for up to 12 months following injury [4].

Types of Nerve Repair

Throughout the long and storied history of replantation and nerve repair, one principle which has stood the test of time above all others is the concept of *tension free repair* as championed by Millesi [23]. The inflammatory response induced by Wallerian degeneration, the cocktails of cytokines and growth factors produced by Schwann cells, and the advanced methods of rehabilitation are of minimal importance if peripheral nerves are repaired under tension. Specific techniques of peripheral nerve repair are based on the nature of injury and the condition of the nerve as well as on the size of the nerve (e.g., sciatic vs. digital). Amputations can result in avulsion injuries, crushing injuries, or clean guillotine-like lacerations. Regarding operative sequence, it is our preference in digital replantation to repair the nerve after the digit has been revascularized and before the venous anastomosis.

Epineural Repair

If the injury is a clean-cut injury without contusion, the standard of care is to perform an end-to-end epineural repair (Fig. 3.3). *The first goal of the epineural repair is coaptation of the nerves without tension* [24, 25]. Because the bone has often been shortened to facilitate replantation, primary repair without tension is usually not difficult. *The second goal is to reduce the formation of regeneration inducing scar tissue* (*see above*). This is achieved by the epineural placement of sutures, performing minimal intraneural

Fig. 3.3 Epineural repair
of nerve with sutures passing
only through external and
internal epineurium and
without violation of the
perineurium (Reprinted with
permission from the
Cleveland Clinic Center
for Medical Art &
Photograph © 2009–2014.
All Rights Reserved)

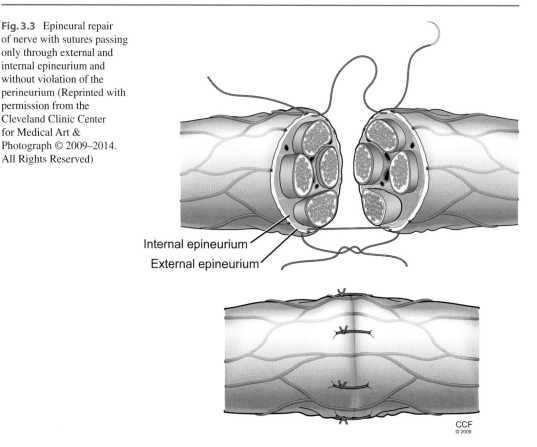

Internal epineurium
External epineurium

dissection, and using as few stitches as necessary to perform the repair. While the number of sutures needed to coapt a nerve is far smaller than what is needed, for example, in the arterial repair, it depends partly on the nerve being repaired. Four to eight simple interrupted sutures are used to approximate the two ends [12]. For digital nerves, usually three stitches are adequate and for larger nerves more stitches might be necessary. Nerve repair should be performed using an operative microscope for two reasons. First, the operative microscope aids in carefully placing stitches in the epineurium only, thus reducing the internal scar tissue which impedes regeneration, and secondly, magnification significantly aids in identifying the superficial vessels that are visible along the longitudinal aspects of the nerve segments (vasa nervorum). Aligning these vessels is an excellent method for the alignment of the fascicles, which significantly reduces misdirected axonal regeneration [26]. While it is not our preferred method, some groups have successfully performed sutureless epineural repair using fibrin glue [27].

Epineural Sleeve Repair

Epineural sleeve repair is a variation of epineural repair that is used when there is some contusion associated with the tips of the transected nerve stump (Fig. 3.4). The repair calls for peeling back the epineural sheath on the distal nerve stump and trimming back the contused fascicles by 2 mm. The fascicles are aligned using cues from the vasa nervorum, and the distal epineural sleeve is then sutured to the proximal sleeve. This repair is potentially advantageous compared to standard epineural repair, because it moves the suture lines away from the regenerating fascicular ends. There are no clinical comparisons that have proven significant statistical advantage of this variation to standard epineural repair methods [26].

Fig. 3.4 Epineural sleeve repair requires peeling back the epineurium and trimming back of the contused fascicles followed by placement of epineural sutures away from the location of the regenerating fascicles (Reprinted with permission from the Cleveland Clinic Center for Medical Art & Photograph © 2009–2014. All Rights Reserved)

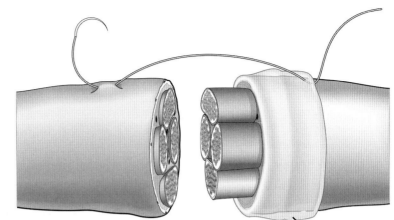

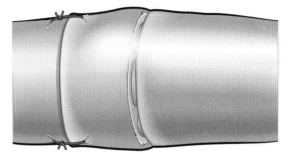

Epineural sheath sleeve

CCF
© 2009

Fig. 3.5 Fascicular repair or grouped fascicular repair involves aligning the fascicles by placing sutures in the perineurium (Reprinted with permission from the Cleveland Clinic Center for Medical Art & Photograph © 2009–2014. All Rights Reserved)

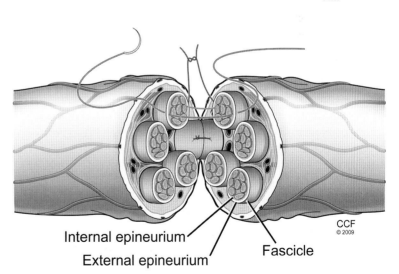

Internal epineurium

External epineurium

Fascicle

CCF
© 2009

Fascicular Repair

Nerve ends can also be coapted using fascicular or grouped fascicular repair (Fig. 3.5). In this case, the individual fascicles are aligned using perineural sutures, or groups of fascicles are aligned using sutures within the internal epineurium. Even though the technique provides superior fascicular alignment, it requires the use of at least two sutures per fascicle, which causes intraneural scar development and the reduction of blood flow that can worsen the final result. The method has fallen out of favor because clinical studies show no advantages of this technique over epineural suturing [26]. For nerves that are partially injured, however, there might still be a role for limited fascicular repair.

End-to-Side Repair

If one of the severed nerve segments is not available for coaptation, an end-to-side repair can be performed. The evidence on the overall clinical outcome is highly variable. Some of the variability in the outcome is related to the lack of a clear understanding of how axons from the donor nerve pass into distal segment, thus begging the need for further inquiry both in the laboratory and in the clinical setting [28]. Recent evidence comparing end-to-side repair with conventional (end-to-end) repair techniques indicates that end-to-side repair have functionally inferior outcome and should be used only as salvage procedures [29].

Nerve Conduits

Despite the bony shortening that often accompanies extremity or digital replantation, there are several scenarios where Millesi's critical tenet of tensionless repair is not possible. These include injuries involving segmental loss of the nerve, crushing injuries, and nerve avulsions. Also, when the nerve cannot be repaired primarily, there is significant contraction, making direct end-to-end tensionless repair unfeasible. While not typically a problem in the acute repair setting of a replant, the proximal and distal nerve stumps in clean-cut lacerations can contract by 4 % in the first week, 8 % in 3 weeks, and up to 28 % if left unrepaired over an extended time period [30]. Direct repair of contracted nerve segments place a high level of tension on the nerve. The increased tension leads to nerve ischemia and ultimately fibrosis of the nerve segment [26].

Nerve Autografts

When direct repair of a transected nerve is not possible, a nerve graft, nerve conduit, or nerve transfer needs to be considered in order to achieve functional restoration. The gold standard of reconstructing a nerve gap is with a nerve autograft. Autografts provide resident Schwann cells as well as the microarchitecture necessary to guide sprouting axons. Some of the candidates for autograft harvest include sural nerve (30–50 cm), dorsal cutaneous branch of the ulnar nerve (4–6 cm), superficial branch of the radial nerve (20–30 cm), lateral antebrachial cutaneous nerve (10–12 cm), and the medial antebrachial cutaneous nerve (10–12 cm). Autograft harvest, while imperative in some cases, should be used cautiously as it can lead to significant donor site morbidity, which includes hypesthesia at the donor site, increased neuroma formation in the donor nerve, and (usually) a separate incision [12].

It is our preference to use the sural nerve for autograft as it is a relatively easy harvest site, can be harvested by a separate team while the recipient site is being prepared, and results in relatively minimal donor site morbidity. On the other end of the spectrum, using the sensory branch of the radial nerve should be avoided at all costs as numbness and paresthesias associated with its harvest can be devastating to the patient. In selecting a nerve for autografting, several principles should be followed. First, size is important. Larger grafts can lead to central neural necrosis, and increased scar tissue formation, which can impede regeneration. Secondly, sensory nerve autografts containing small diameter fibers can lead to mediocre functional outcome due to the mismatch of size. Thirdly, a risk-benefit analysis should be performed for each donor site and the one with the least morbidity should be selected. Since there are limited options for autografts, research has been carried out to better understand the potential of biological and artificial conduits to fill nerve defects [31].

Biological Conduit Repair

Given the limited options of nerve autografts as well as the well-known morbidity in using them, multiple candidate materials for biological nerve conduits have been explored including arteries, veins, skeletal muscle, and epineurium. Veins have also been successfully used as inside-out or turn-over grafts. The collagen, laminin, and Schwann cells, which are found on the adventitia of veins, contribute to the increased speed of axonal regeneration found in turn-over vein grafts when compared to standard vein grafts [32]. Combination biological grafts containing vein, filled with skeletal muscle, have been found to be useful in filling nerve gaps ranging from 0.5 to 6 cm. Skeletal muscle tissue contains longitudinally oriented basal lamina which facilitates contact adhesion of migrating Schwann cells and ingrowing axonal fibers. Additionally filling the vein with muscle prevents the graft from collapsing [31]. Tendon grafts, which have similar longitudinal microarchitecture, have also been shown to be effective nerve conduits [33]. Epineural grafts are derived from neural tissue and produce large amounts of laminin B2 and VEGF, which augments Schwann cell attachment and axonal growth. Furthermore, epineural grafts are less immunogenic than the other biological conduit materials and could therefore even serve as an effective allograft. [26] It is our preference, when there is a limitation of nerve autograft or when the risks of harvest outweighs the benefits, to use turn-over vein grafts as they are relatively easy to harvest, are in abundant supply, and can usually easily be found in the same surgical field as the nerve that is being repaired (e.g., in forearm for cases of digital nerve reconstruction).

Artificial Conduits

Artificial nerve conduits were initially made of flexible, non-immunogenic but nonbiodegradable materials such as silicone and PTFE. Silicone conduits tend to develop a capsule of circumferentially oriented smooth muscle myofibroblasts, which constricts the conduit and the growing nerve segment [34]. Morbidities caused by the scarring and constriction of ten requires reoperation for removal of these conduits. Furthermore, silicone is nonpermeable and does not allow the exchange of larger biomolecules that may be beneficial to the growing axon [15]. Given the limitation of these early artificial conduits, newer conduit materials have been utilized including synthetic biodegradable materials such as aliphatic polyesters and polyphosphoesters as well as naturally occurring biodegradable materials such as collagen, hyaluronic acid, and fibrin. Aliphatic polyesters include various biodegradable non-immunogenic polymers such as polyglycolic acid (PGA), poly-(lactic acid) (PLA), polycaprolactone (PCL), poly-lactidecoglycolide (PLGA) copolymer, poly-(L-lactic acid) (PLLA), and poly-(3-hydroxybutyric acid) (PHB) [15]. PGA is a commonly used material in sutures and mesh. It is broken down by hydrolysis within 90 days. PGA tubes are commercially marketed to bridge sensory nerve gaps less than 30 mm (Neurotube, Synovis Life Technologies Inc., USA). The copolymerization process used to synthesize aliphatic polyesters such as PLGA and PLLA can be altered to vary degradation times, thermal properties, mechanical performance, and wettability of these materials. The permeability of these materials which is important to maintain the nutrient exchange and as well as growth factor leakage from the conduits can also be adjusted by adjusting the crystallinity of these synthetic materials [31].

Naturally occurring biodegradable conduits are made up of ECM components and therefore provide substrates with improved binding capabilities and structural support to the regenerating axons. Candidate substrates that fall in this category include decellularized allografts, collagen conduits, hyaluronic acid conduits, fibrin-based conduits, and agarose-based conduits. Decellularized conduits contain most of the native microarchitecture of a nerve but have been processed to remove immunogenic cells. Processing modalities include chemical decellularization, thermal decellularization, freeze-thawing, and cold preservation [35–38]. These substrates have significant advantages from a topographical perspective and have led to the development of new commercially available conduits.

Collagen is an abundant naturally occurring ECM component that is widely used in conduit production. Since it is highly conserved among mammalian species, it is relatively non-immunogenic. A large variety of conduit designs have proven to be beneficial, regeneration-promoting constructs. These include smooth empty conduits [39], conduits containing aligned collagen fibers [40], conduits containing electrospun collagen fibers [41], and those that contain freeze-dried aligned collagen gels [42]. Collagen has multiple integrin-mediated interactions with its environment, and therefore, it can mainly be used in the PNS where collagen is abundant but not in the CNS [43]. This led to the development of hyaluronic acid-based constructs which could be used to promote regeneration in the PNS as well as the CNS.

Given that autografts contain a niche environment of cytokines and growth factors with temporally and spatially varying picomolar concentration gradients that provide regeneration cues to the ingrowing axons similar to the proximal and distal stumps of the transected nerve, many groups have attempted to create conduits by varying the concentration and release kinetics mimicking the regenerative milieu [44–48]. While the experimental data on these conduits – filled with various growth factors, cytokines, Schwann cells, and stem cells – has demonstrated great promise, there has been very little translation from the bench to bedside and no such product is currently available for clinical use [49–52]. Nevertheless, the world of synthetic and natural-based conduits continues to grow, and there are currently 11 such conduits available (Table 3.2). Two particular conduits are worth special mention as they have been studied extensively and have produced particularly encouraging clinical data. This includes NeuraGen® (Integra, Plainsboro, NJ; collagen type 1 NGC) which has demonstrated similar efficacy to autograft for defects up to 2 cm and Neurotube (Synovis, St. Paul, MN) (PGA), the most clinically studied

Table 3.2 FDA-approved devices for peripheral nerve repair

Name	Material
Axogen Avance® Nerve Graft (Alachua, FL)	Decellularized ECM (human peripheral nerve)
Axogen AxoGuard® Protector (Alachua, FL)	Decellularized ECM (human peripheral nerve)
Axogen AxoGuard® Nerve Connector (Alachua, FL)	Decellularized ECM (human peripheral nerve)
Integra NeuraGen® (Plainsboro, NJ)	Collagen
Integra NeuraWrap™ (Plainsboro, NJ)	Collagen
Polyganics Neurolac® (Groningen, The Netherlands)	Poly(Dl-lactide-e-caprolactone)
Stryker NeuroMend (Kalamazoo, MI)	Collagen
Synovis Neurotube (St. Paul, MN)	Polyglycolic acid

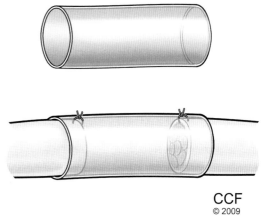

CCF
© 2009

Fig. 3.6 Bridging of two nerve segments with a nerve conduit (Reprinted with permission from the Cleveland Clinic Center for Medical Art & Photograph © 2009–2014. All Rights Reserved)

synthetic conduit. A new conduit made from decellularized nerve grafts, Avance® (Axogen, Alachua, FL) has demonstrated improved rates of nerve regeneration when compared to the currently available collagen-based nerve conduit, NeuraGen® (Integra, Plainsboro, NJ) [53]. The bottom line is that choosing the correct indication for one of these products and using it properly (Fig. 3.6) are probably more important than the product itself.

Nerve Allografts

In cases of nerve defects that exceed 3 cm, most current conduits fail despite major advances in conduit material, biochemical gradient, and in-conduit microstructure fabrication. Nerve allografts therefore continue to be a promising candidate for reconstruction. Allografts represent a much more abundant source than autografts and provide more options with respect to the nature of the native nerve fibers being regenerated (sensory or motor). Nerve tissue is less immunogenic than skin, muscle, or bone, yet the absence of any immunosuppression can lead to immunologic destruction and graft failure. Factors that improve graft take include MHC matching, graft pretreatment, optimal tolerance induction, and immunosuppressive medications. Multiple methods used for pretreating allografts prior to implantation include irradiation, cryo-preservation, lyophilization, freeze-thawing, predegeneration, and cold storage. Of these methods, cold storage of a graft proved to be the most efficacious. Cold storage of a graft for about 7 days at 5 °C in UW solution not only decreased graft antigenicity but also preserved Schwann cell viability [54]. Following graft placement, the patient is started on an immuno-suppressive regimen, which is continued until regenerating axons reach their targets. Immunosuppressive regimens using FK-506 have been shown to be more effective than earlier cyclosporine-based protocols. When appropriate immunosuppression was combined with cold storage graft pretreatment, the effects were synergistic and regeneration through the allograft was superior to the gold standard [55]. Tolerance induction agents such as nonselective T-cell depleting agents (polyantilymphocyte globulin (ALG) and antithymocyte globulin (ATG), anti-CD3 monoclonal antibody (muromonab), and anti-CD52 Campath-1H monoclonal antibody) have also been used to deplete recipient T cells in order to further promote graft take [26]. Nevertheless, the feasibility of long-term immunosuppression required for nerve allografting is questionable, and thus, there is a move towards decellularized nerve allografts and one such product is currently available for clinical use (Avance® Axogen, Alachua, FL).

Assessing Outcomes

The ultimate functional outcome following peripheral nerve repair and rehabilitation depends on multiple intrinsic and extrinsic factors. Intrinsic factors (over which a surgeon has no control) include the nature of nerve injury (clean cut vs. crush or avulsion-type injury), context of injury (isolated injury vs. major trauma requiring reconstruction and replantation), age of the patient, medical comorbidities, and social behavior. These also include certain postoperative factors such as the nature of occupational/hand therapy, densensitization therapy, and the general psychological context of the patients injury and recovery. Extrinsic factors that the surgeon can alter to improve outcome include the type and technique of nerve repair and the timing of repair. Multiple published tools and tests for assessing motor and sensory recovery include grip and pinch strength measurement with the Jamar dynamometer, Rotterdam intrinsic hand meter, Semmes-Weinstein monofilaments, Moberg's pickup test, Jebsen-Taylor hand function test, static two-point discrimination and moving two-point discrimination, Sollerman hand function test, shape identification test (STI), visual analog scale, Medical Research Council scale, Cold Sensitivity Severity questionnaire, McGill Pain Questionnaire, the disability of arm shoulder and hand (DASH) questionnaire, and cold intolerance severity score [56].

The wide range of available tests makes the assessment and reporting process difficult especially when trying to compare results across different groups. Despite this variability, a few conclusions can be made with regard to recovery rates of various nerves. Studies involving direct coaptation of severed ulnar and median nerves at the wrist level have shown improved motor recovery of the median nerve compared to the ulnar nerve [57]. For the same level of transection, motor axons in the ulnar nerve have to travel to more distal muscles (interossei), whereas motor axons in the median nerve are required to travel a much shorter distance to reach the thenar musculature [58]. Furthermore, muscles in the hand innervated by the ulnar nerve are thought to be more resistant to reinnervation. From a sensory standpoint, functional outcomes between median and ulnar nerves are similar.

When peripheral repairs are performed using isografts, their functional improvement is shown to vary based not only on the level of injury and conditions of injury but also on the biological properties of the nerve and its effector muscles. Nerve repair using isografts at proximal mid-arm and mid-thigh levels demonstrate improved recovery in radial and tibial nerves compared to ulnar and peroneal nerves. Injuries at intermediate levels (between mid arm and proximal forearm/between mid thigh and proximal leg) demonstrate better recovery for musculocutaneous, radial, and femoral nerves than for median, ulnar, and tibial nerves. Distal nerve injuries (distal forearm and hand/distal leg and foot) result in similar functional recovery for all the peripheral nerves [59]. Nerve-muscle pairs that require fewer axons (distributed over a smaller cross-sectional area of the nerve) to be regenerated to achieve adequate effector function (radial and tibial nerve vs. ulnar nerve) have better outcomes [60]. Pure motor nerves have better recovery than mixed nerves because of the lower cross-innervation potential.

Nerves with fewer fascicles, fewer interfascicular connections, and less intervening interfascicular connective tissue (radial, musculocutaneous, and axillary nerves) demonstrate better recovery potential. The topography of the nerve cell bodies in the spinal cord has also been implicated in having an effect of nerve recovery potential. Nerves in which cell bodies localized within the anterior horn of the spinal cord (radial nerve) show better recovery potential compared to nerves with cell bodies scattered over a greater volume within the anterior horn of the spinal cord (peroneal nerve) [59]. Sensory recovery has been shown to be similar for all nerves at distal as well as proximal injuries. With respect to digital replants, studies show that clean-cut injuries tend to have better outcomes than crush and avulsion injuries and that thumbs tend to exhibit more useful two-point discrimination compared to fingers [61].

Despite the array of available tests, one must be able to quickly assess regeneration in the clinical setting as patients often ask, "Is my nerve regrowing?" or "When will my finger not be numb?" One of the most effective methodologies is to follow an advancing Tinel sign, which should be measured in millimeters from the site of injury. The Tinel sign should advance approximately 1.0 mm per day, which translates to 1.0 in. per month.

Despite the remarkable ability for peripheral nerves to regenerate, success in recovery is multifaceted and requires a team approach with the patient at the center of that team. Positive outcomes begin with sound clinical decisions based on data (tensionless repair and avoidance of scar tissue), steadfast rehabilitation, the performance of secondary nerve grafting or alloplastic reconstruction when necessary, and the maintenance of a calm and reassuring demeanor to patients as they eagerly await the goal of (potentially) full functional recovery after replantation with neural reconstruction.

Conclusion

Beginning with the early work of the neuroscience pioneer Roman y Cajal (1928) and his observations that regenerating axons preferentially grow towards the distant stump of a transected nerve, and continuing with the work of Seddon and Sunderland in the middle of the twentieth century, today there continues to be significant advances in nerve repair techniques and technology. Progress in the field of material science and microfabrication has fueled the development of conduits that are much more conducive to growth. Advances in transplantation research has led to the development of shorter and improved immune suppression protocols necessary for the widespread adoption of nerve allografts. And the utilization of growth factors, cytokines, Schwann cells, and stem cells, though widely studied, is still in their infancy. Despite these significant advances in the laboratory, no significant progress has been made to accelerate nerve regeneration beyond 1.5 mm/day or to extend the lifespan of denervated motor end plates beyond 18 months in humans. In an era of increasing extremity trauma, continued research in nerve repair and rehabilitation is necessary to fully realize the functional benefit of the replanted extremity.

References

1. Noble J, Munro CA, Prasad VS, Midha R. Analysis of upper and lower extremity peripheral nerve injuries in a population of patients with multiple injuries. J Trauma. 1998;45:116–22.
2. Kouyoumdjian JA. Peripheral nerve injuries: a retrospective survey of 456 cases. Muscle Nerve. 2006;34: 785–8.
3. Maricevic A, Erceg M. War injuries to the extremities. Mil Med. 1997;162:808–11.
4. Campbell WW. Evaluation and management of peripheral nerve injury. Clin Neurophysiol. 2008;119: 1951–65.
5. Nicholson B, Verma S. Comorbidities in chronic neuropathic pain. Pain Med. 2004;5 Suppl 1:S9–27.
6. Taylor RS. Epidemiology of refractory neuropathic pain. Pain Pract. 2006;6:22–6.
7. Lee SK, Wolfe SW. Peripheral nerve injury and repair. J Am Acad Orthop Surg. 2000;8:243–52.
8. Sunderland S. The anatomy and physiology of nerve injury. Muscle Nerve. 1990;13:771–84.
9. Koeppen AH. Wallerian degeneration: history and clinical significance. J Neurol Sci. 2004;220:115–7.
10. Stoll G, Muller HW. Nerve injury, axonal degeneration and neural regeneration: basic insights. Brain Pathol. 1999;9:313–25.
11. Burnett MG, Zager EL. Pathophysiology of peripheral nerve injury: a brief review. Neurosurg Focus. 2004;16:E1.
12. Matsuyama T, Mackay M, Midha R. Peripheral nerve repair and grafting techniques: a review. Neurol Med Chir. 2000;40:187–99.
13. de Ruiter GC, Spinner RJ, Verhaagen J, Malessy MJ. Misdirection and guidance of regenerating axons after experimental nerve injury and repair. J Neurosurg. 2014;120(2):493–501.
14. Gaudet AD, Popovich PG, Ramer MS. Wallerian degeneration: gaining perspective on inflammatory events after peripheral nerve injury. J Neuroinflammation. 2011;8:110.
15. Deumens R, et al. Repairing injured peripheral nerves: bridging the gap. Prog Neurobiol. 2010;92:245–76.
16. Lunn ER, Brown MC, Perry VH. The pattern of axonal degeneration in the peripheral nervous system varies with different types of lesion. Neuroscience. 1990;35:157–65.
17. Wang MS, et al. Calpain inhibition protects against Taxol-induced sensory neuropathy. Brain J Neurol. 2004;127:671–9.
18. Touma E, Kato S, Fukui K, Koike T. Calpain-mediated cleavage of collapsin response mediator protein(CRMP)-2 during neurite degeneration in mice. Eur J Neurosci. 2007;26:3368–81.
19. Webber C, Zochodne D. The nerve regenerative microenvironment: early behavior and partnership of axons and Schwann cells. Exp Neurol. 2010;223:51–9.
20. Zanazzi G, et al. Glial growth factor/neuregulin inhibits Schwann cell myelination and induces demyelination. J Cell Biol. 2001;152:1289–99.
21. Fu SY, Gordon T. The cellular and molecular basis of peripheral nerve regeneration. Mol Neurobiol. 1997; 14:67–116.
22. Tanabe K, Bonilla I, Winkles JA, Strittmatter SM. Fibroblast growth factor-inducible-14 is induced in axotomized neurons and promotes neurite outgrowth. J Neurosci. 2003;23:9675–86.
23. Millesi H, Meissl G, Berger A. The interfascicular nerve-grafting of the median and ulnar nerves. J Bone Joint Surg Am. 1972;54:727–50.
24. Ornelas L, et al. Fibrin glue: an alternative technique for nerve coaptation–part I. Wave amplitude, conduction velocity, and plantar-length factors. J Reconstr Microsurg. 2006;22:119–22.
25. Dvali L, Mackinnon S. Nerve repair, grafting, and nerve transfers. Clin Plast Surg. 2003;30:203–21.
26. Siemionow M, Brzezicki G. Chapter 8: current techniques and concepts in peripheral nerve repair. Int Rev Neurobiol. 2009;87:141–72.
27. Ornelas L, et al. Fibrin glue: an alternative technique for nerve coaptation–part II. Nerve regeneration and histomorphometric assessment. J Reconstr Microsurg. 2006;22:123–8.
28. Bontioti E, Dahlin LB. Chapter 12: mechanisms underlying the end-to-side nerve regeneration. Int Rev Neurobiol. 2009;87:251–68.
29. Kettle SJ, Starritt NE, Glasby MA, Hems TE. End-to-side nerve repair in a large animal model: how does it compare with conventional methods of nerve repair? J Hand Surg Eur Vol. 2013;38:192–202.
30. Trumble TE, Shon FG. The physiology of nerve transplantation. Hand Clin. 2000;16:105–22.
31. Siemionow M, Bozkurt M, Zor F. Regeneration and repair of peripheral nerves with different biomaterials: review. Microsurgery. 2010;30:574–88.
32. Tang J, Wang XM, Hu J, Luo E, Qi MC. Autogenous standard versus inside-out vein graft to repair facial nerve in rabbits. Chin J Traumatol. 2008;11:104–9.
33. Brandt J, Dahlin LB, Kanje M, Lundborg G. Spatiotemporal progress of nerve regeneration in a tendon autograft used for bridging a peripheral nerve defect. Exp Neurol. 1999;160:386–93.
34. Dahlin LB, Anagnostaki L, Lundborg G. Tissue response to silicone tubes used to repair human median and ulnar nerves. Scand J Plast Reconstr Surg Hand Surg/Nordisk plastikkirurgisk forening [and] Nordisk klubb for handkirurgi. 2001;35:29–34.

35. Khaing ZZ, Schmidt CE. Advances in natural biomaterials for nerve tissue repair. Neurosci Lett. 2012;519:103–14.

36. Sondell M, Lundborg G, Kanje M. Regeneration of the rat sciatic nerve into allografts made acellular through chemical extraction. Brain Res. 1998;795: 44–54.

37. Dubovy P, et al. Laminin molecules in freeze-treated nerve segments are associated with migrating Schwann cells that display the corresponding alpha-6beta1 integrin receptor. Glia. 2001;33:36–44.

38. Evans PJ, et al. Cold preserved nerve allografts: changes in basement membrane, viability, immunogenicity, and regeneration. Muscle Nerve. 1998;21: 1507–22.

39. Kehoe S, Zhang XF, Boyd D. FDA approved guidance conduits and wraps for peripheral nerve injury: a review of materials and efficacy. Injury. 2012;43: 553–72.

40. Yoshii S, Oka M, Shima M, Taniguchi A, Akagi M. Bridging a 30-mm nerve defect using collagen filaments. J Biomed Mater Res A. 2003;67:467–74.

41. Wang Y, et al. The promotion of neural progenitor cells proliferation by aligned and randomly oriented collagen nanofibers through beta1 integrin/MAPK signaling pathway. Biomaterials. 2011;32:6737–44.

42. Bozkurt A, et al. In vitro assessment of axonal growth using dorsal root ganglia explants in a novel three-dimensional collagen matrix. Tissue Eng. 2007;13: 2971–9.

43. Novak U, Kaye AH. Extracellular matrix and the brain: components and function. J Clin Neurosci. 2000;7:280–90.

44. Pfister LA, Papaloizos M, Merkle HP, Gander B. Nerve conduits and growth factor delivery in peripheral nerve repair. J Peripher Nerv Syst. 2007;12: 65–82.

45. Chen YS, et al. Peripheral nerve regeneration using silicone rubber chambers filled with collagen, laminin and fibronectin. Biomaterials. 2000;21:1541–7.

46. Xu X, et al. Peripheral nerve regeneration with sustained release of poly(phosphoester) microencapsulated nerve growth factor within nerve guide conduits. Biomaterials. 2003;24:2405–12.

47. Wang S, et al. Acceleration effect of basic fibroblast growth factor on the regeneration of peripheral nerve through a 15-mm gap. J Biomed Mater Res A. 2003;66:522–31.

48. Hoke A, et al. Schwann cells express motor and sensory phenotypes that regulate axon regeneration. J Neurosci. 2006;26:9646–55.

49. Mosahebi A, Woodward B, Wiberg M, Martin R, Terenghi G. Retroviral labeling of Schwann cells: in vitro characterization and in vivo transplantation to improve peripheral nerve regeneration. Glia. 2001;34: 8–17.

50. Bryan DJ, et al. Influence of glial growth factor and Schwann cells in a bioresorbable guidance channel on peripheral nerve regeneration. Tissue Eng. 2000;6: 129–38.

51. Hermann A, et al. Efficient generation of neural stem cell-like cells from adult human bone marrow stromal cells. J Cell Sci. 2004;117:4411–22.

52. Amoh Y, et al. Implanted hair follicle stem cells form Schwann cells that support repair of severed peripheral nerves. Proc Natl Acad Sci U S A. 2005;102: 17734–8.

53. Brooks DN, et al. Processed nerve allografts for peripheral nerve reconstruction: a multicenter study of utilization and outcomes in sensory, mixed, and motor nerve reconstructions. Microsurgery. 2012;32: 1–14.

54. Evans PJ, et al. Regeneration across cold preserved peripheral nerve allografts. Microsurgery. 1999;19: 115–27.

55. Jensen JN, Brenner MJ, Tung TH, Hunter DA, Mackinnon SE. Effect of FK506 on peripheral nerve regeneration through long grafts in inbred swine. Ann Plast Surg. 2005;54:420–7.

56. Galanakos SP, Zoubos AB, Johnson EO, Kanellopoulos AD, Soucacos PN. Outcome models in peripheral nerve repair: time for a reappraisal or for a novel? Microsurgery. 2012;32:326–33.

57. Ruijs AC, Jaquet JB, Kalmijn S, Giele H, Hovius SE. Median and ulnar nerve injuries: a meta-analysis of predictors of motor and sensory recovery after modern microsurgical nerve repair. Plast Reconstr Surg. 2005;116:484–94; discussion 495–86.

58. Kim DH, Han K, Tiel RL, Murovic JA, Kline DG. Surgical outcomes of 654 ulnar nerve lesions. J Neurosurg. 2003;98:993–1004.

59. Roganovic Z, Pavlicevic G. Difference in recovery potential of peripheral nerves after graft repairs. Neurosurgery. 2006;59:621–33; discussion 621–33.

60. Kim DH, Ryu S, Tiel RL, Kline DG. Surgical management and results of 135 tibial nerve lesions at the Louisiana State University Health Sciences Center. Neurosurgery. 2003;53:1114–24; discussion 1124–15.

61. Maricevich M, Carlsen B, Mardini S, Moran S. Upper extremity and digital replantation. Hand (N Y). 2011;6:356–63.

Replantation of the Thumb

4

Matthew L. Iorio, Nicholas B. Vedder, and Jeffrey B. Friedrich

Initial Assessment

The thumb has a significant impact on the overall function of the hand, essentially half the function of the hand, and conversely, its absence can result in major impairment and disability. It is for this reason that amputations of the thumb should be strongly considered for replantation when the part is salvageable and the patient is medically stable [1, 2]. Functional impairment following the loss of the thumb will reliably degrade the overall function of the hand with a loss of 50 % of grasp, 30 % of pinch, and 20 % of hook strengths [3]. Given these factors, the thumb has been assigned a relative value of impairment of 40 %, further emphasizing the dictum that the thumb should be replanted in all situations possible [4, 5].

The functional outcome of replantation is not simply the product of the viability of the replanted thumb but also the level and nature of the injury [6]. A retrospective review of 46 patients at an average of 10.3 years following thumb replantation was able to identify level of injury as the major determinant of ultimate result. Using the modified Burton scale (which is based on objective range of motion and strength, socioeconomic

and subjective assessments), amputations distal to or at the interphalangeal joint (IP) level had the best outcomes. More proximal amputations through the proximal phalanx, metacarpal, and the carpometacarpal joint (CMC) had the poorest outcomes. This is partly attributable to the distal joint stiffness that occurs following a digital replantation but also to the progressive loss of function and sensory discrimination following a more proximal injury.

The mechanism of injury is a significant predictor of ultimate function, both in regard to strength and range of motion. Avulsion and crush injuries affect both the functional outcome and the feasibility of performing the replantation. In a retrospective review of 65 replanted thumbs, the failure rate for avulsion injury was 38 %, compared to 14 % for all other mechanisms [5, 7]. Pinch and grip strength are significantly worse following crush and avulsion injuries when compared to sharp injuries. Given the different fibroelastic properties and collagen composition of tendon, nerve, and vessel, each will have an element of elastic denaturing and injury following a thumb avulsion. To the surgeon, this implies several different levels of injury, debridement, and repair. Frequently, especially with avulsion injuries, the flexor pollicis longus will be ripped from the musculotendinous junction, essentially mandating some element of interphalangeal joint stabilization or arthrodesis at the time of replantation (Fig. 4.1). The digital vessels will stretch and rupture at their weakest point, which is the area

M.L. Iorio, MD (✉) • N.B. Vedder, MD
J.B. Friedrich, MD
Division of Plastic Surgery,
University of Washington, Seattle, WA, USA
e-mail: mattiorio@gmail.com; vedder@uw.edu;
jfriedri@uw.edu

A.N. Salyapongse et al. (eds.), *Extremity Replantation: A Comprehensive Clinical Guide*,
DOI 10.1007/978-1-4899-7516-4_4, © Springer Science+Business Media New York 2015

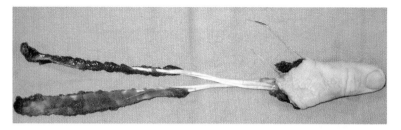

Fig. 4.1 A thumb avulsion injury that resulted in disruption of the flexor and extensor systems from their proximal muscle bellies. Additionally, the digital nerves are noted to disrupt proximally from the hand, whereas the digital vessels are most likely damaged much more distally within the part

of the smallest cross-sectional resistance, or essentially the more distal vessel. Therefore, the digital vessel stump may actually be further distal than the bony amputation level and involve vessels beyond the interphalangeal joint [8]. Digital nerves, however, tend to avulse proximally, often in the forearm, making anatomic reconstruction of the nerves difficult, if not impossible.

The above listed factors can render avulsion trauma a relative contraindication to replantation. Additional factors or contraindications may include a severely contaminated part, multilevel neurovascular and soft tissue injury, and severe intercalary crush defects. Even in these settings, however, a successfully replanted part may still offer a stable post for opposition and grasp. Therefore, if significant soft tissue damage or contamination is present and ongoing tissue necrosis and debridement is expected, the thumb should be considered for ectopic banking on the ipsilateral or contralateral radial artery. This can be performed in an end-to-side manner quickly, with some soft tissue stabilization to prevent early avulsion. Once the soft tissues of the hand have stabilized, the still viable thumb can then be successfully replanted and reconstructed [9].

Preoperative Management

The initial patient evaluation should be guided by the nature of the injury and should first ensure a hemodynamically stable patient following an appropriate trauma evaluation. If paramedics in the field consult the provider, the recommendation should be for a clean dressing to the hand to minimize ongoing contamination and blood loss.

Direct pressure can be held over point of bleeding and, except in extreme cases or major arterial injury, the use of tourniquets in the field should be discouraged. In addition to significant tourniquet pain, prolonged upper extremity tourniquet use can expose the patient to the risk of compressive neuropathy, hemodynamic instability following lactic acid production in the ischemic limb, and the potential for additional tissue or limb loss. The part itself should be placed in moistened gauze in a plastic bag, preferably on ice. If this is not possible, simply wrapping the amputated digit in saline-soaked gauze will help to cool it. The part should not be directly placed within the ice, and dry ice should never be utilized, both of which can cause severe thermal injury to the part. Additionally, tetanus booster should be updated and antibiotics administered. Intravenous pain medications should be used as necessary.

Upon presentation, the amputated part and injured hand should have radiographs obtained to determine the presence of any residual foreign bodies and define the quality of the bone fragments (Fig. 4.2). In some crush or high-energy injuries, severe fracture comminution will guide the operative plan and patient discussion towards aggressive shortening or immediate arthrodesis. If replantation is agreed upon, the amputated part should precede the patient to the operating room. This will give the surgeon a valuable chance to carefully examine the part and begin preparation for replantation prior to the start of anesthesia. This will have the added benefit of decreasing the overall ischemia time. The amputated digit should be cooled, with whatever is available, throughout this process.

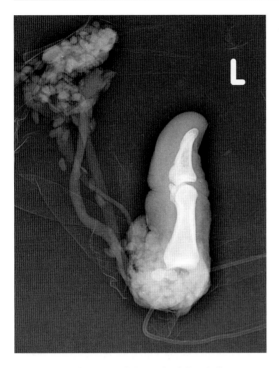

Fig. 4.2 A radiograph of the avulsed thumb demonstrating an intact articular surface and no other occult fractures

Time to return to work or the ability to return to the same occupation postoperatively should be strongly weighed and discussed with the patient when considering revision amputation verses replantation. A linear relationship between an increasingly proximal level of injury and a decrease in the likelihood of the patient's return to their pre-injury job should be expected and discussed. This finding was based on a review of 111 thumb amputations where more proximal amputations up to the level of the thumb metacarpophalangeal joint had the lowest rates of return to work with nearly 50 % of patients reporting that they were unable to return to work. Revision amputation through the proximal phalanx or metacarpal will give the patient a diminished ability to grasp large objects and to perform fine motor tasks such as buttoning a shirt [10].

Technique

The first step in any amputation is a thorough debridement and irrigation of the injury site and amputated part. Following an amputation,

particulate matter or organic debris can be deposited throughout and beneath various structures. Failure to recognize foreign contamination and thoroughly remove this debris may result in early infection with subsequent vascular thrombosis and loss of the replanted part [11]. If a small, viable dorsal skin bridge remains intact following a near-complete amputation, this bridge should be preserved as small veins may be present within this segment that will provide some element of venous outflow. Midlateral incisions on the amputated part can allow for exploration of the volar structures, including the flexor sheath and neurovascular bundles. Again, this can be performed on the back table prior to arrival of the patient in the operating room. The ulnar and radial neurovascular bundles should be identified, and the quality of the digital arterial and nerves should be inspected. Additionally, any dorsal veins should be identified and dissected. As the veins are in the superficial subcutaneous tissue, the dorsal skin should be sharply dissected off of the extensor tendon as one unit, including the dorsal veins. The veins can then be carefully identified by bleeding at the edge of the skin and dissected from the underlying subcutaneous tissue. One should be mindful to avoid aggressive trimming of vessel and nerve ends in the initial "tagging" stage. Prolonged operative time and the frequent handling of vessels can create a desiccated, crushed vessel end that needs secondary debridement and trimming. In this way, the vessel has been shortened twice and may increase the level of difficulty for primary anastomosis or vein grafting. The final trimming of the end of the vessel or the nerve, then, should be saved until immediately prior to anastomosis or coaptation.

Osteosynthesis

Replantation of the thumb, especially in conjunction with a multi-digit amputation, should proceed in a stepwise manner to maximize efficiency and prevent frustration. In that regard, osteosynthesis should be performed prior to any of the soft tissue or anastomotic work, as the tension on these repairs cannot be properly assessed until the part is rigidly fixed. The proximal and distal

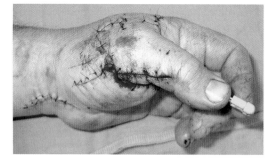

Fig. 4.3 Replantation of the thumb in the patient with the avulsed thumb, demonstrating a loose closure, k-wire stabilization, and functional positioning of the replanted thumb

bone segments should be shortened and squared to maximize bony contact and minimize postoperative instability or the need for prolonged immobilization. This step should be emphasized, as it may be tempting to "key-in" a fracture segment, but in a long oblique or multifragment injury, comminution and bone loss may prevent anatomic reduction and further complicate fixation [12]. If the bone ends are cleanly squared off with the use of a rongeur or sagittal saw, viable bone contact is maximized, fixation is straightforward, and operative time for this step is minimized. It should also be remembered that the skeletal shortening needed for successful replantation is not trivial: 7–10 mm of bone shortening is reasonable and will often allow for replantation without the use of vein and/or nerve grafts. Bone shortening is *far* preferable to vessel/nerve grafting, and the limited skeletal shortening will be of negligible functional consequence.

Osteosynthesis can be achieved in a variety of methods. Following adequate surface preparation, the most frequently utilized techniques include crossed Kirschner wires or 90-90 interosseous wiring (Fig. 4.3). Crossed Kirschner wires may be the most adaptable technique in that it is rapid and can be slightly adjusted at later stages in the replantation without significant jeopardy to the neurovascular or tendon repairs. Additionally, longitudinal Kirschner wires may be utilized, though difficulties with rotational stability and bone compression may occur. Bone shortening and Kirschner wire fixation can also be performed reliably to the thumb on the back table.

Interosseous wiring aims to create two perpendicular, transverse bone tunnels for stable fixation. A 0.045 or 0.054 Kirschner wire is drilled perpendicularly through the base of the amputated part. Following this the wire is slowly backed out, and a 20-gauge needle is passed as a guide for the 22-, 24-, or 26-gauge cerclage wire. A perpendicular tunnel is created in the same method on the amputated part, and another cerclage wire passed through. Following this, the technique should be repeated on the proximal stump and the corresponding cerclage wires passed through these bone tunnels. At this point, an assistant should slowly tighten down the wires while the segment is held in the desired position. An advantage of crossed interosseous wiring is the ability to only partially tighten the construct to allow some increased exposure of the ulnar border of the thumb by hinging the part open. This allows the surgeon to perform the microsurgery with increased exposure but with the ability to minimize tension or redundancy on the vessels by reliably checking the position of ultimate fixation.

If the amputation is through the joint, the articular cartilage should be removed from the residual joint surface and the joint fused. Fusion can be quickly performed with additional crossed Kirschner wires. However, unlike the other digits, the ultimate position of osteosynthesis can be more difficult to accurately position. In terms of function, the carpometacarpal joint permits motion about axes of flexion/extension and abduction/adduction and has the capability of 10–20° of rotation. It is the most important joint with regard to overall range of motion of the thumb. In the event of destruction of this joint or an amputation through the plane of the carpometacarpal joint, fusion should be performed with the thumb fixed in 40° palmar abduction, 15-degree extension, and 120° metacarpal pronation [13]. The goal is to have the resulting replanted thumb in a position that facilitates opposition to the ulnar digits.

The more distal joints allow less of this multiaxis or circumduction type of motion, but they do contribute to overall postoperative function. The metacarpophalangeal joint provides mostly flexion and extension, as well as a small amount of thumb abduction and adduction. This joint is capable of approximately 5° of extension, 100° of flexion, and 0–20° of abduction/adduction. The interphalangeal joint of the thumb is a hinge joint that is capable of approximately 15–20° of extension and 80° of flexion [3, 13]. Ideally, the thumb should be placed in a position such that it overlaps the second phalanx on the index finger in the composite fist position.

Tendon Repair

Following the bone repair, attention should then be turned to the extensor and flexor tendon repairs. The extensor system of the thumb is complex, with three separate tendons inserting at sequential points along the axis of the thumb. The abductor pollicis longus (APL) and extensor pollicis brevis (EPB) travel in the first extensor compartment and insert into the base of the first metacarpal and proximal phalanx, respectively. The extensor pollicis longus (EPL) is located in the third extensor compartment and inserts in a broad expansion at the base of the distal phalanx. All three tendons provide some element of thumb extension at their individual joints, though the EPL may be able to provide extension throughout the arc of motion at the interphalangeal, metacarpophalangeal, and carpometacarpal joints, in addition to radial abduction and retropulsion of the thumb. For these reasons, the EPL should be repaired whenever possible, whereas the EPB and APL may be sacrificed in more severe injuries [3]. Extensor tendon repairs can be performed in the same manner as the flexor tendons, but given the decreased work of extension and likelihood of rupture, a single Kessler or horizontal mattress stitch may be all that is necessary. It is often best to perform extensor tendon repair early so that it is not later forgotten, as extensor repair *cannot* be performed after vein repair.

Flexor tendon repairs should follow using a technique that will allow early passive motion, given the inherent stiffness and scarring that will follow the trauma. In this regard, a looped stitch and a double Tsuge configuration, or any type of locking suture, can achieve this goal. Specifics of tendon repair and healing are addressed in

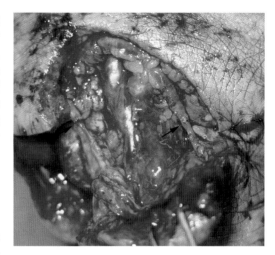

Fig. 4.4 Thumb replantation using two subcutaneous dorsal veins (*arrows*) for outflow

Chap. 2. Regardless of the technique chosen, a total of four core strands should be employed. If possible, the distal half of these core sutures can be placed through the flexor tendon in the amputated part during the initial back table evaluation. This will help to further decrease operative time.

Microvascular Repair

Following the initial debridement and inspection, the digital nerves and vessels should be identified and tagged with 8-0 nylon to prevent time spent "reidentifying" the same structure later in the case. Generally, dorsal subcutaneous veins are of a slightly larger caliber and may be more straightforward to utilize (Fig. 4.4). Additionally, the ulnar digital artery is larger in caliber than the radial digital artery and may be easier to repair [2]. However, when only one digital artery can be repaired, the largest available digital artery should be repaired to establish the most robust blood flow possible. At a minimum, two veins should be repaired whenever possible when replanting the thumb; however, in our practice, we prefer to connect as many veins as we can find. When the hand has been severely crushed or when there are multilevel lacerations, the digital vessels may not be suitable for replantation. In this setting, vein grafting should be utilized to bridge the larger of the two digital arteries in the

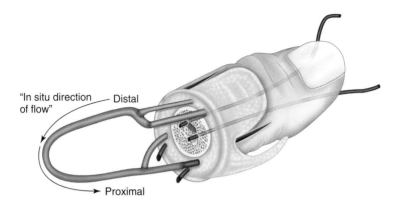

"In situ direction of flow" — Distal

Proximal

Fig. 4.5 Back-table preparation of the amputated thumb, with midlateral incisions for exposure, and early placement of k-wires and tendon stitches. Additionally, a vein loop is constructed by anastomosing the distal end of a vein graft to the dorsal veins within the part and the proximal end to the digital artery. Once osteosynthesis and the tendon repairs are performed, the vein loop can be transposed to the dorsal branch of the radial artery and halved for microvascular repair to the corresponding inflow and outflow vessels

amputated part (usually the ulnar digital artery) to the dorsal branch of the radial artery in the anatomic snuffbox. This branch of the radial artery can be sacrificed for an end-to-end anastomosis or an end-to-side fashion, depending on the individual circumstances and vessel size discrepancy. The artery may be repaired prior to the vein for several reasons. First, this technique will allow the rapid resumption of arterial supply and oxygenation to the digit, and if the veins are left to bleed, it allows the surgeon to both identify bleeding veins as good outflow vessels, and ischemia-related metabolic products are washed out of the digit [2].

If considerable soft tissue damage had occurred or multiple digits are injured, this step of microvascular reconstruction can begin on the back table. Following the initial steps of debridement, bone shortening and structure tagging, a long segment of vein graft can be utilized to reconstruct both the arterial and venous systems (Fig. 4.5). Typically, when a vein graft is utilized from the extremities, the presence of valves mandates that for arterial bridging, the graft is reversed to prevent high resistance to flow against the valves. With this in mind, a long vein graft is taken from the forearm ranging from 10 to 15 cm. The proximal end of the graft can be anastomosed to the ulnar digital artery proximal stump and the distal end of the vein graft can be anasto-

mosed to one or two of the digital and dorsal veins in an end-to-end or end-to-side fashion, thereby creating an arterial-venous loop [11]. Then, once the team is ready to replant the thumb, the first steps of osteosynthesis and tendon repairs are performed. The vein loop is passed dorsally either through a subcutaneous tunnel to the dorsal branch of the radial artery in the snuffbox or through a longitudinal access incision. The loop is then divided, and the corresponding arterial and venous repairs are performed. This effectively bridges a large zone of injury in degloving or crush injuries.

Vein grafting does not appear to have an adverse effect on the viability or rate of successful replantation [2, 5, 6, 12]. Instead, vein grafting offers several advantages including the ability to facilitate an anastomosis without tension, avoidance of excessive bone shortening to achieve adequate vessel length, and the ability to bypass the zone of injury. Volar distal forearm veins may best reapproximate the digital neurovascular caliber, and dorsal wrist veins may be better suited for bridging a more proximal segment or to establish arterial inflow outside of the zone of injury. Additionally, dorsal foot veins are an excellent caliber match and a second team can dissect them while the hand is being evaluated. In settings where donor vein graft is unavailable due to multiple sites of trauma or their prior destruction through medical or patient comorbidity (e.g., intravenous drug use, dialysis fistula creation, regional degloving trauma), vein transposition from the index finger may offer an efficient solution. The radial digital neurovascular bundle of the index finger is dissected through either midlateral or Bruner-type incisions from the distal interphalangeal joint distally to the common digital vessels in the palm proximally. The vein and/or artery are dissected free of the digital nerve, distally transected, and transposed to the ulnar border of the amputated thumb through midlateral exposures. The anastomosis is then completed using a dorsal vein on the amputated part and the proximal stump of the ulnar digital artery within the amputated piece [14].

Following the vascular repair, the digital nerves should be repaired with two to three epineurial stitches. If significant debridement or injury created a nerve gap, early or late reconstruction can be performed with a nerve conduit, autograft (posterior interosseous nerve, distal lateral antebrachial cutaneous nerve, or sural nerve), or allograft. The timing and use of any of these elements is at the discretion of the surgeon and the expected outcome of the replanted thumb, as a donor nerve can have a significant morbidity, and allograft/conduit constructs can be expensive, yet the best time for reconstruction is frequently at the time of injury.

Tissue Coverage

Split-thickness skin grafts or spare-part full-thickness skin grafts should be liberally used in the setting of severe tissue injury or loss. The hand and thumb will swell significantly in the postoperative period, so all incisions should be either approximated loosely, left open to close by wound contraction, or covered with a skin graft. The midlateral relaxing incisions on the proximal and distal thumb should *not* be closed. This is especially true over the dorsum of the replanted thumb where the fragile venous anastomosis frequently occurs. If any tension is apparent at this closure, a split-thickness skin graft should instead be applied over the wound and vessels. During the initial debridement, all frankly necrotic or nonviable segments should be removed, but aggressive skin debridement or trimming should be discouraged. This can further amplify the soft tissue deficit, and many times small skin bridges will remain viable or function as a full-thickness skin graft.

Lastly, in injuries that involve the first webspace, postoperative contracture and thumb adduction can be a difficult late complication to manage. Therefore, some type of external fixator should be placed between the distal first and second metacarpals with the thumb radially and palmarly abducted. This can be easily performed with heavy (0.062 in. diameter) Kirschner wires or a specific external fixation system to keep the webspace open during the postoperative period and prevent late contracture.

Postoperative Management

In those cases where arterial inflow and venous outflow is established and demonstrated to be sufficient in the operating room, postoperative failures are frequently related to three main microvascular complications: hematoma, arterial thrombosis, and venous thrombosis [15]. Compressive hematoma can be avoided by meticulous hemostasis and irrigation at the completion of the procedure and the use of passive drains if significant dead space or contamination is apparent. Arterial thrombosis is usually related to two main elements: technical failure at the site of arterial coaptation or poor flow through the anastomosis secondary to distal clot or venous thrombosis [15]. This emphasizes adequate debridement of nonviable sections of proximal and distal artery following the initial injury. Additionally, replanted thumbs that demonstrate postoperative changes of mottling, swelling, temperature drop, and immediate capillary refill may have signs suggestive of venous outflow obstruction or insufficiency [16]. Immediate return to the operating room can result in a high salvage rate if these problems are noted prior to frank venous and arterial obstruction and clot

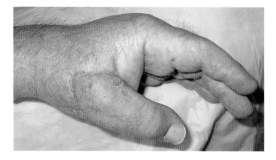

Fig. 4.6 Appearance and position of the hand of the patient with the avulsed thumb at follow-up

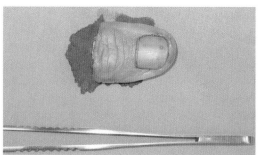

Fig. 4.7 A clean-cut amputation through the interphalangeal joint of the thumb. Distal, clean-cut injuries are frequently excellent candidates for replantation given the minimal tissue damage and crush following the injury

propagation throughout the capillary system of the digit [15].

The replanted thumb should be protected with a large dorsal and volar splint with an abundance of padding. The aim is to protect the part from disruption due to external abrasion or shear and not necessarily to position or guard the joints of the wrist and hand. Therefore, no pressure from the splint should be placed upon the dorsal thumb or the dorsoradial hand, so as not to compromise venous outflow. Additionally, the tip of the replanted digit should be visible or easily accessible within the dressing for postoperative monitoring. In our practice, the patient is typically discharged home on postoperative day 4 or 5 following a straightforward replantation in the same dressing that was placed in the operating room. Alternatively, the initial dressing may be removed within the first week, at which time hand therapy should be consulted for fabrication of a protective orthosis. If the initial dressing remains in place at the first visit in the office, usually 10–14 days after the initial trauma, a thermoplastic orthosis should be fabricated at that time. At this visit, stitches are typically removed, and the hand therapist begins gentle range of motion of the unaffected digits and wrist. Therapeutic exercises are initiated and will be tailored based upon the level of injury and quality of repair, as discussed further in Chap. 15. Finally, stabilizing Kirschner wires are removed at 6–8 weeks (Fig. 4.6).

A variety of postoperative measures may be utilized to verify the patency of the anastomosis and overall viability of the replanted part. Implantable Doppler devices can be utilized in the setting of a proximal vein graft to the radial artery or when the caliber of the artery and vein are sizeable enough that the presence of the probe would not cause compression due to edema or pedicle kinking.

External monitoring can include regimented checking of the vascular pedicle with a Doppler device, in addition to monitoring the temperature of the part [16]. Most commonly, capillary refill of the tip or the paronychial tissue adjacent to the nail bed is used to determine the viability of a part based on microvascular flow. Whenever in doubt, a small-gauge needle can be used to prick the distal tip of the replanted thumb to determine vascular flow, with the predominance of bright red arterial blood (as opposed to dark, congested venous blood) a sign of a healthy pedicle. However, frequent and unnecessary pricking of the digit should be avoided to avoid bacterial inoculation and stimulation of microvascular thrombosis.

In any event, if there are any changes in the parameters utilized to monitor the replanted thumb that cannot be explained by environmental or positional elements, an immediate operative exploration should be considered, if it is felt that something could be improved. If edema is felt to

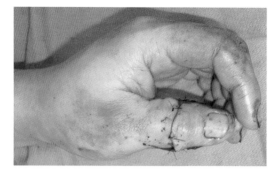

Fig. 4.8 Replantation of the thumb at the level of the interphalangeal joint using interosseous wiring for osteo-synthesis. Note the loosely closed incisions

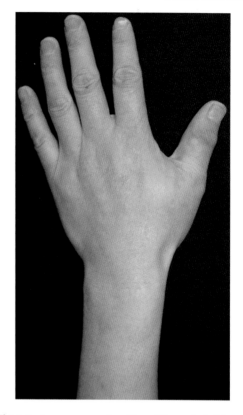

be compressing the pedicle, stitches may be removed at the bedside, but hematoma drainage and vascular pedicle inspection and revision should be performed in the operating room to maximize visualization and minimize ongoing deep tissue contamination.

Ultimately, functional success is based upon the ability of the surgeon to reconstruct the bony and soft tissues, as well as the patient's motivation and compliance with perioperative management and rehabilitative hand therapy [10, 17] (Figs. 4.7, 4.8, 4.9, and 4.10).

Fig. 4.9 Appearance and position of the replanted thumb in the patient with the interphalangeal joint-level amputation

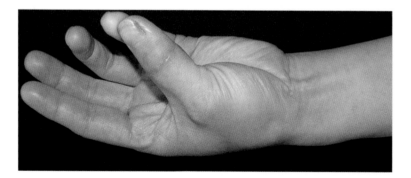

Fig. 4.10 Good range of motion and opposition of the thumb through the proximal joints, including the carpometacar-pal joint due to early hand therapy and prevention of stiffening

References

1. Goldner RD, Stevanovic MV, Nunley JA, Urbaniak JR. Digital replantation at the level of the distal interphalangeal joint and the distal phalanx. J Hand Surg Am. 1989;14(2 Pt 1):214–20.

2. Schlenker JD, Kleinert HE, Tsai TM. Methods and results of replantation following traumatic amputation of the thumb in sixty-four patients. J Hand Surg Am. 1980;5(1):63–70.

3. Emerson ET, Krizek TJ, Greenwald DP. Anatomy, physiology, and functional restoration of the thumb. Ann Plast Surg. 1996;36(2):180–91.

4. Rondinelli RD, Genovese E, Katz RT, Mayer TG, Mueller K, Ranavay M, Brigham CR (eds.). Guides to the Evaluation of Permanent Impairment. 6th ed. Chicago, IL: American Medical Association; 2008.

5. Sharma S, Lin S, Panozzo A, Tepper R, Friedman D. Thumb replantation: a retrospective review of 103 cases. Ann Plast Surg. 2005;55:352–6.

6. Janezic TF, Arnez ZM, Solinc M, Zaletel-Kragelj L. Functional results of 46 thumb replantations and revascularizations. Microsurgery. 1997;17:264–7.

7. Holmberg J, Arner M. Sixty five thumb replantations: a retrospective analysis of factors influencing survival. Scand J Plast Reconstr Surg Hand Surg. 1994;28:45–8.

8. Agarwal JP, Trovato MJ, Agarwal S, Hopkins PN, Brooks D, Buncke G. Selected outcomes of thumb replantation after isolated thumb amputation injury. J Hand Surg Am. 2010;35(9):1485–90.

9. Higgins JP. Ectopic banking of amputated parts: a clinical review. J Hand Surg Am. 2011;36(11):1868–76.

10. Goldner RD, Howson MP, Nunley JA, Fitch RD, Belding NR, Urbaniak JR. One hundred eleven thumb amputations: replantation vs revision. Microsurgery. 1990;11:243–50.

11. Wood MB. Finger and hand replantation: surgical technique. Hand Clin. 1992;8:397.

12. Ward WA, Tsai TM, Breidenbach W. Per primam thumb replantation for all patients with traumatic amputations. Clin Orthop Relat Res. 1991;266:90–5.

13. Muzaffar AR, Chao JJ, Friedrich JB. Posttraumatic thumb reconstruction. Plast Reconstr Surg. 2005;116(5):103e–22.

14. Rockwell WB, Haidenberg J, Foreman KB. Thumb replantation using arterial conduit graft and dorsal vein transposition. Plast Reconstr Surg. 2008;122(3):840–3.

15. Arakaki A, Tsai TM. Thumb replantation: survival factors and re-exploration in 122 cases. J Hand Surg Br. 1993;18(2):152–6.

16. Stirrat CR, Seaber AV, Urbaniak JR, Bright DS. Temperature monitoring in digital replantation. J Hand Surg Am. 1978;3(4):342–7.

17. Earley MJ, Watson JS. Twenty four thumb replantations. J Hand Surg Br. 1984;9(1):98–102.

Replantation of the Digits

5

Clifford Pereira and Kodi Azari

Any fool can cut off an arm or leg but it takes a surgeon to save one.

George C. Ross (1843–1892)

Introduction

Finger amputation demographics have remained constant in the United States [1]. The majority of injuries occur in men (5:1–6:1), with the average age being slightly less than 30 years. The commonest location of amputation injuries is either an industrial site (43 %) or the home (25 %) [2]. Machinery, in particular power saws, has been the dominant mechanism of injury with majority of injuries occurring between 6.00 AM and 6.00 PM. The dominant extremity is injured in 41 % cases with the index finger being the most common site of amputation [1, 2]. The socioeconomic and psychological impact of finger amputations however is immeasurable affecting not just individuals but entire families, especially if the amputee is a prime bread earner of the family.

C. Pereira, FRCS(Eng) (✉)
Department of Plastic and Reconstructive Surgery,
David Geffen School of Medicine at UCLA,
Los Angeles, CA, USA
e-mail: cpereira@mednet.ucla.edu

K. Azari, MD, FACS (✉)
Section of Reconstructive Transplantation,
Department of Orthopaedic Surgery
and Plastic Surgery, David Geffen School of
Medicine at UCLA, 10945 Le Conte Ave, Suite 3355,
Los Angeles, CA 90095, USA
e-mail: kazari@mednet.ucla.edu

Replantation of fingers represents the culmination of all the skills of a hand surgeon, from the precise repair of bony and tendinous injuries to the microsurgical anastomosis of artery, veins, and nerves. Since the first successful replant over 50 years ago by Malt and McKhan in 1962 of a 12-year-old boy's arm [3], technological advances and the use of the microscope have made replantation common practice. The goals of replantation remain the same, to restore circulation and regain sufficient function and sensation of the amputated part so as to allow utilitarian rehabilitation and expeditious return of patients back to near pre-injury functionality. Management should also be individually targeted to the patient's occupation, hobbies, and overall health. It is however imperative to distinguish between vascular survival and functional success. Functional success requires restoration of skeletal stability, joint mobility, power, and sensibility. In that regard not all amputees will benefit from replantation, necessitating strict selection criteria to optimize functional result. As Dr. Littler stated, "The result of vessel anastomosis is dramatic and signals survival – but it is only the beginning, for other less urgently required structures must be restored functionally if the initial success is to extend beyond the mere retention of a parasitic member" [4]. The surgeon must make the final

A.N. Salyapongse et al. (eds.), *Extremity Replantation: A Comprehensive Clinical Guide*,
DOI 10.1007/978-1-4899-7516-4_5, © Springer Science+Business Media New York 2015

decision to proceed with replantation keeping in mind the importance of avoiding secondary amputations that are very poorly tolerated by both patient and surgeon. This chapter discusses the indications, contraindications, pre- and post-operative care, and intraoperative technique involved in replantation of fingers. Replantation of the thumb and rehabilitation protocols will be discussed in subsequent chapters.

Definitions and Classifications

Amputations can be classified into complete or incomplete based upon whether or not a connection exists between the distal segment and proximal stump. Incomplete amputations can be either viable or nonviable depending on whether or not the distal segment maintains a sufficient blood supply. Incomplete viable amputations do not warrant additional microvascular anastomosis, whereas incomplete nonviable amputations necessitate microvascular reconstruction. Replantations can thus be defined as the reattachment of a completely amputated body part, whereas revascularization can be defined as the reattachment of an incomplete nonviable amputation where vessel reconstruction is necessary to maintain viability (Fig. 5.1a, b).

Amputations can also be classified based on mechanism of injury, such as guillotine, crush, avulsion, or a combination of any of these. Guillotine amputations are sharp injuries with no damage of tissues away from the site of amputation. Crush amputations are blunt crushing injuries with damage of tissues beyond the site of amputation, but not usually far from the site of amputation. Avulsion amputations are distraction or torsion injuries resulting in damage of tissues at variable distances from the site of amputation. Stretching of nerves and vessels usually leads to longitudinally transmitted injury along the structures, resulting in a worse prognosis. Amputations from a combination of the abovementioned mechanisms can also obviously occur. Ring avulsion injuries represent a type of combination injury wherein the predominant injury is avulsion along significant length of the finger resulting in a myriad of scenarios necessitating revascularization, soft tissue coverage, and even replantation [5].

Patient Selection

The decision to replant a severed digit is complex and influenced by a multitude of factors including mechanism of injury, level of injury, and ischemia time. Just as important are patient specific factors such as hand dominance, professional or personal needs/skills, comorbidities, and expectations. The indications and contraindications for replantation of digits are summarized in Tables 5.1 and 5.2.

Injury-Related Factors

The type of injury is the most important factor in determining the survival rate and functional outcome [6, 7]. Clean-cut guillotine type

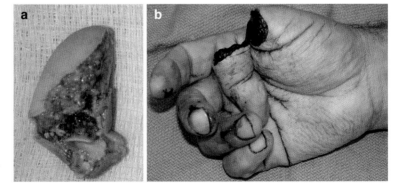

Fig. 5.1 (**a, b**) Difference between replantation and revascularization. (**a**) Represents a complete amputation requiring replantation. (**b**) Represents an incomplete nonviable amputation requiring microvascular anastomosis to maintain viability

Table 5.1 Indications for replantation

Absolute indications

Thumb

Multiple digits

Any amputation in a child

Amputation at level of palm, wrist, or forearm

Relative indications

Individual finger amputations

  (a) Distal to FDS insertion

  (b) At the level of distal phalanx

Ring avulsion injury – type II or IIIA injuries

Table 5.2 Contraindications for replantation

Relative contraindications

Zone 2 single-finger amputations

Severely crushed and mangled parts

Avulsion injuries with red-line or ribbon sign

Multiple level injuries

Mentally unstable patients

Absolute contraindications

Associated life-threatening injuries

Preexisting comorbidities that preclude a prolonged and complex operation

Table 5.3 Prioritization of fingers in multi-digit replants

1. Thumb – to restore prehensile function
2. Small and/or ring finger – to restore grip
3. Index and/or middle finger – to restore pinch grip

amputations have a very high success rate (99.5 %) and should be attempted, whereas extensively crushed and avulsion amputations have poor survival rate (crush amputations 33.3 %, avulsion amputations 78.6 %) and must be approached with caution.

Avulsion injuries associated with the "red-line sign" or the "ribbon sign" are poor prognostic indicators for replantation since they denote severe traction injuries to the neurovascular bundle. The red-line sign consists of small hematomas seen in the skin along the course of the neurovascular bundle caused by disruption of small branches to the skin. This in turn leads to intimal tears to the digital vessels and often makes replantation unsuccessful due to non-reflow from intimal injuries or disruption of skin-feeding branches from the digital artery. The ribbon sign is indicative of severe traction and torsion to a vessel resulting in a vessel that resembles a ribbon that has been stretched and curled on a gift-wrapping. If ribboning has occurred proximal to the trifurcation of the digital artery, which occurs at the distal interphalan-

geal joint, vein grafting proximal and distal to the zone can salvage the finger. However, involvement of the trifurcation bilaterally cannot be bypassed with a vein graft and is essentially a non-replantable injury.

Although level of injury has no bearing to the survival rate of replants, it does affect functional outcomes [7]. Good functional results are achieved with replantation of fingers with amputations distal to the FDS insertion, or at the palm, wrist, and distal forearm. Less functional recovery is expected with replants within zone 2 of the fingers since they result in stiffness and weakened grip strength that provide little or no functional benefit and often result in significant delays in return to work.

All thumbs should get first priority in replantation regardless of level of amputation or mechanism of injury [8]. This is because thumbs are responsible for 40 % of the hand function and important for prehensile abilities. In fact in multidigit amputations, if the thumb cannot be replanted, the least damaged finger should be replanted in the place of the thumb [9]. If the thumb is intact or replantable, the ring and small finger should be replanted to restore grip. Next the index and/or middle finger is replanted to restore pinch grip. See Table 5.3.

Digits lack muscle and hence are more tolerant to ischemia than other body part amputations. The permitted duration of warm ischemia is up to 12 h (compared to 6 h for a major limb). Cooling can prolong the ischemia time to up to 24 h. Reports of successful replantation after longer ischemia times have been reported for up to 94 h of cold ischemia [10].

Patient-Related Factors

Any amputation at any level and any mechanism of injury in children is an indication for replantation. Children have a tremendous recuperative ability with a good functional result. Similarly all healthy young adults with minimal comorbidities are good candidates for replants. Elderly patients may have significant cardiovascular and respiratory comorbidities that preclude a long operation. Furthermore, diseases that affect small vessels such as atherosclerosis, connective tissue disorders, autoimmune diseases, and diabetes mellitus can directly affect replantation success rates [11]. Joint stiffness, poor nerve regeneration, peripheral vascular disease, and coordination problems with poor recuperative abilities are additional inhibitory factors for good functional outcomes in elderly digital replants. That said, functional results are not entirely dependent on patient age and amputation level [12], and elderly replant candidates should be treated on a case-by-case basis. Replantation success rates are 2.3 times higher in female compared to male patients [6]. This however probably reflects the severity of injuries sustained by male patients. Alcohol does not affect replantation success rates [6]; however, personal habits such as smoking and caffeine consumption can affect microvascular patency. Nonsmokers have an 11.8 times greater rate of replant survival than smokers [6]. This is attributed to the vasoconstrictive properties of nicotine. Patients should be strongly advised to quit smoking completely after replantation. Some authors recommend no smoking be permitted within the very vicinity of a fresh replant [6].

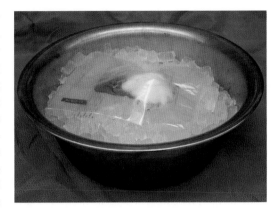

Fig. 5.2 Care of amputated part

intermediate teams, until the replant team is evaluating the patient [13].

Even if the part is not deemed replantable at the scene or at the local hospital, it should be preserved, since it can provide valuable tissue for reconstruction as a spare part. Hence the amputated part should be preserved by irrigating with normal saline to remove any contamination by foreign material, wrapped in a saline-moistened gauze and placed in a sealed plastic bag, which is placed in an ice container with an ice pack or ice cubes in water (1:4 proportion). The part should NOT be immersed in saline or water, since this causes cobwebbing of the intima as demonstrated by Urbaniak et al. [14]. The part should also NOT be placed directly on ice since this can result in a frostbite injury to the vessels [14] (Fig. 5.2).

Prehospital Care

The patient should be stabilized using standard ATLS protocols and transported to the nearest replantation center. They should be kept warm, and intravenous fluids should be commenced if possible.

The proximal stump should be wrapped in a compressive dressing and elevated. Bleeding vessels should not be blindly clamped as this may damage recipient vessels for replantation. If possible a picture of the part and the proximal stump should be taken before dressings are applied, so as to prevent the need to remove dressings repeatedly to be evaluated by ER personnel or

Preoperative Evaluation

Once the call is received for replantation, the surgeon needs to start assembling the appropriate personnel and equipment for the procedure. The operating room staff is notified so they can allocate the necessary equipment for the surgery. In the emergency room, the patient should undergo basic trauma survey for stabilization, fluid resuscitation, and detection of other life-threatening injuries. The patient should be warmed to prevent hypothermia, and appropriate pain medications should be administered. Tetanus prophylaxis should be determined and updated as required. Prophylactic broad-spectrum antibiotics should be commenced to cover *Staphylococcus aureus*, *Streptococcus*, and *Clostridium perfringens* [13]. Radiographic evaluation of the amputated part and proximal stump should be performed to determine the extent of the skeletal damage. Standard anteroposterior and lateral views should be obtained in the ER. The proximal stump and the amputated part should be photographed by the replant team for documentation. Informed consent should be taken after discussing with the patient and the family regarding the pros and cons of the procedure, length of the procedure, length of hospital stay, length of rehabilitation, realistic expectations for successful replantation, recovery of sensation, mobility, and function.

Intraoperative Technique

General Principles

Once the decision has been made to proceed with replantation, the surgeon needs to have the mindset that he/she is going to do the best to make it a successful outcome. Any lingering doubts about whether the effort is worthwhile or a half-hearted effort of going to the operating room just to take a look is doomed to failure and will make the surgeon entertain an easier amputation option. The goal of the surgery is to do emergently what would be difficult or impossible to do later. The use of "spare parts" from a non-salvageable finger for salvage of another finger is a prime example of this principle. Another guiding principle is the "one-stage treatment with early mobilization" [15]. This advocates a stable fixation, tension-free vascular repair, and skin closure, so as to allow rehabilitation as early as the first week following surgery to minimize tendon adhesions and joint stiffness.

Shortening of the bone within reason is done to reduce the risk of septic nonunion and to allow primary tension-free repair of vessels, nerves, tendons, and skin. As a rule it is better to trim more of the bone of the amputated part rather than the proximal stump so as to preserve length on the proximal stump in case the replant fails. All structures should be repaired primarily and tension-free if possible. When this is impossible,

Table 5.4 Sequence of repairs in finger replantation

1. Preparation of amputated part
2. Preparation of proximal stump
3. Bone shortening and stabilization
4. Extensor tendon repair
5. Flexor tendon repair
6. Digital artery
7. Dorsal veins
8. Nerve coaptation
9. Skin closure/coverage

nerve or tendon grafts should be employed. If tissue loss is too great and neither of these options are available, plans for staged reconstruction (i.e., tendon transfers) should be considered. The usual sequence of repair of structures is: bone shortening and stabilization, extensor and flexor tendon repair, arterial anastomosis, venous anastomosis, nerve coaptation, and skin coverage [16]. See Table 5.4.

Once in the operating room, the patient is placed on the operating table with proper pressure point padding. Warming blankets are placed and the ambient temperature of the operating room is kept warm to prevent hypothermia and vasospasm during the procedure. A urinary catheter is placed for accurate fluid status assessment and in preparation for a long procedure. An axillary block is placed with an indwelling catheter for intraoperative and postoperative pain control. A two-team approach is usually best, with one team preparing the proximal segment and the other the amputated segment. For multiple digit replants, it is better to take a structure-by-structure approach rather than one digit at a time. A tally sheet of injured and repaired structures helps decrease the incidence of errors and frustrations (Fig. 5.3).

Preparation of the Amputated Part

Preparation of the amputated part can be initiated on a back table under sterile conditions in the operating room long before the patient is brought to the operating room and while the patient is being anesthetized. We recommend stabilizing the segment on a tongue depressor as shown in Fig. 5.4, to facilitate dissection under

Fig. 5.3 Tally sheet of injured structures and repaired structures

	Thumb	Index	Middle	Ring	Small
Bone					
FDS					
FDP					
Extensor Tendon					
Artery					
Vein 1					
Vein 2					
R. Digital N.					
U. Digital N.				·	

Fig. 5.4 Stabilization of amputated segment on tongue depressor platform

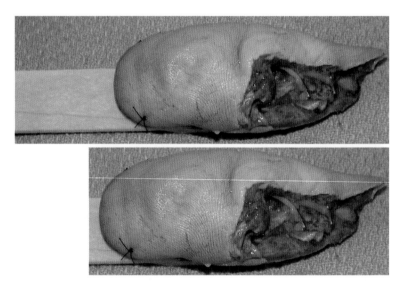

the microscope. If the part is grossly contaminated, it is irrigated with copious normal saline and foreign bodies removed. The neurovascular structures are exposed with bilateral mid-axial incisions (Fig. 5.5). Dorsal incisions may be needed to expose dorsal veins. The digital vessels and nerves are dissected and tagged with 9-0 nylon sutures or microclips. Digital vessels are assessed for signs of intimal damage (e.g., telescope, cobwebs, ribbon sign, terminal thrombosis). The lumen is irrigated with heparinized saline. The edges are freshened and need for vein grafts is assessed. If the need for a vein graft is indicated, harvesting a vein graft before bone fixation will help minimize warm ischemia time (Fig. 5.6). Half modified Kessler sutures (also known as the Tajima suture technique) are placed on the extensor and flexor tendons [17]. Bone shortening of up to 5–10 mm may be needed for tension-free vessel and nerve repair and is best performed with an oscillating saw. Excessive shortening is to be avoided, since most replants require vein grafts for tensionless repair unless the amputation is clean and sharp [18]. If the amputation destroys a substantial portion of the joint, the articular surface is removed to prepare for joint fusion. Retrograde K-wires or intraosseous wires are then placed through the bone on the amputated part.

Fig. 5.5 Mid-axial incisions to expose neurovascular bundle

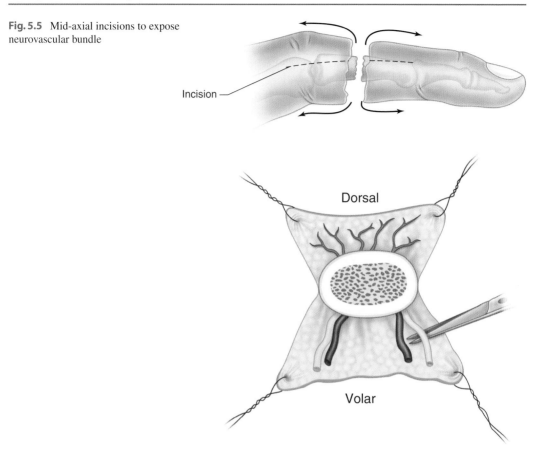

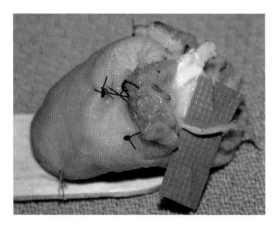

Fig. 5.6 Harvesting a vein graft, if deemed necessary, should be done before bone fixation to save warm ischemia time

incisions are similarly used on the proximal stump, instead of volar Bruner incisions, since the zigzag Bruner incisions would compromise amputation stump skin viability should the replant fail. Neurovascular structures are identified, dissected, and tagged with 9-0 nylon sutures or microclips. Finding and tagging the flexor and extensor tendons with half modified Kessler core sutures is best done before bone fixation since tendon exposure is easier (Fig. 5.7). Before exsanguination, the volar wrist veins are marked out, since volar wrist veins and dorsal foot veins are similar in caliber to digital vessels (Fig. 5.8) [18]. This saves time later if vein grafts are needed.

Preparation of the Proximal Stump

The digital stump is likewise irrigated and debrided back to healthy tissue. Mid-axial

Bone Fixation

Bone fixation should be performed by the most easy and quick method with good anatomic reduction while providing adequate stability and protection for vascular and nerve repairs in the short term and minimizing tendon adhesions and joint stiffness in the long run. Numerous techniques can be used for fracture fixation during replantation such as Kirschner wires (K-wires), cerclage wires with or without K-wires, lag screws, intramedullary headless differential pitch screws, and miniplates (Figs. 5.9 and 5.10) [19]. It is important while using any of these techniques to protect the soft tissues from iatrogenic damage during bone fixation, for example, soft tissue being caught on the drill or K-wires or while trimming bone with the oscillating saw. A technique we find useful is the Esmarch tissue protector: a piece of the Esmarch is used with a central hole to allow just the bone to protrude, thus isolating the bone from surrounding soft tissues (Fig. 5.11).

A single K-wire can be placed to initially fix the fracture, so that the distal segment can be rotated if needed during anastomosis. A second K-wire can be inserted at the end of the procedure to overcome rotational forces. K-wires are expeditious and simple to place; however, they have a higher nonunion rate (21 %) in cases of fracture communition [19]. In such cases intraosseous cerclage 90-90 wires can be placed, where two intraosseous wires are placed perpendicular to each other (Fig. 5.9). For juxta-articular fractures, intraosseous wires with K-wire fixation or tension-band wiring with K-wire (also known as Lister technique, Fig. 5.10) can provide adequate fixation [20]. Four-hole miniplates are best suited for transverse shaft fractures and provide rigid fixation allowing early mobilization. However, they require periosteal stripping for application, which can devitalize bone. External fixation is reserved for severely contaminated amputations. Ultimately the choice of bone fixation is individualized based on configuration and injury. Classically used bone fixation techniques based on level of amputation are summarized in Table 5.5.

Tendon Repair

Extensor tendons are repaired by tying the previously placed half modified Kessler sutures as mentioned in the above sections. In zone 1 and 2, a conventional U-stitch using 4-0 nylon suture can be used. The repair is protected with a temporary blocking pin for DIPJ, which is also used to fix the underlying fracture. If the DIPJ is to be

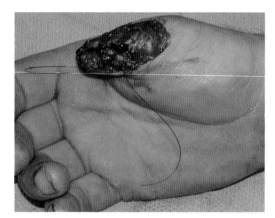

Fig. 5.7 Tagging flexor tendons prior to bony stabilization is easier due to easy tendon exposure

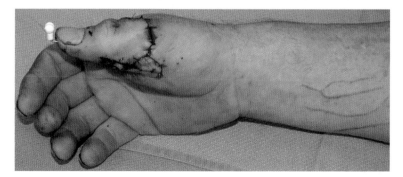

Fig. 5.8 Mapping of volar veins early saves time later if vein grafts are required

Fig. 5.9 Intraosseous 90-90 cerclage wire placement for fracture fixation

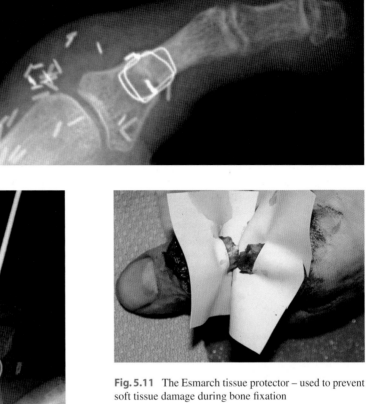

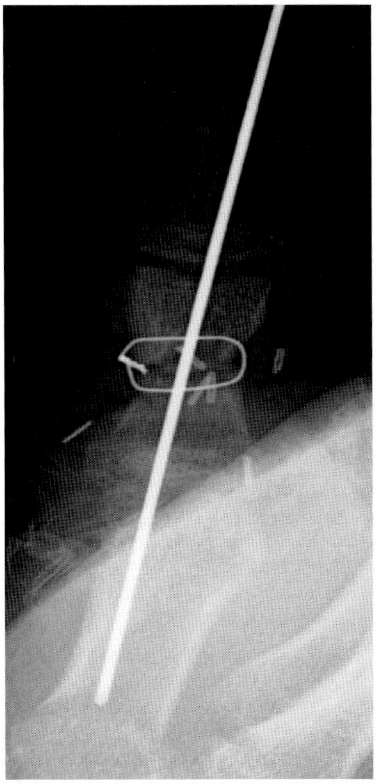

Fig. 5.11 The Esmarch tissue protector – used to prevent soft tissue damage during bone fixation

Fig. 5.10 Lister technique: K-wire with tension-band wiring to reduce juxta-articular fractures

fused, the tendon is not repaired. In extensor tendon zones 3–5 as well as in the case of PIPJ fusion, the lateral bands need to be repaired in addition to recover active DIPJ mobility.

Finger motion equals replant success. Hence, flexor tendon repair is of paramount importance for replant success. Flexor tendons are repaired by tying the previously placed half modified Kessler core sutures (Tajima technique) in the proximal and distal segment [17]. This is followed by precise 6-0 prolene epitendinous sutures to strengthen the repair (Fig. 5.12).

In zone 1, since an axial pin is temporarily placed to block the DIPJ, the FDP is repaired using a pullout 4-0 nylon suture supported on the nail and not a bone anchor suture since this would hinder the pinning. In zone 2, the FDP is repaired, while the FDS is either sacrificed or only a single slip of FDS is repaired to allow unobstructed FDP excursion in the flexor sheath. In zone 3, both tendons are always repaired.

Arterial Repair

Before arterial anastomosis is commenced, it is imperative that the tourniquet be let down to evaluate for proximal flow. Anastomosis should not be attempted until spurting pulsatile proximal arterial

Table 5.5 Classically used bone fixation techniques based on level of amputation

Amputation level	Fixation technique
Trans P3	Crossed K-wires
DIPJ	Arthrodesis with crossed K-wires/90-90 wires
P2 neck	Crossed K-wires with axial pin blocking DIPJ
P2 shaft	Crossed K-wires
PIPJ	Arthrodesis with tension-band wiring/crossed K-wires/90-90 wires
P1 neck	Crossed K-wires without PIPJ blocking
P1 shaft	Crossed K-wires

P3 distal phalanx, *DIPJ* distal interphalangeal joint, *P2* middle phalanx, *PIPJ* proximal interphalangeal joint, *P1* proximal phalanx

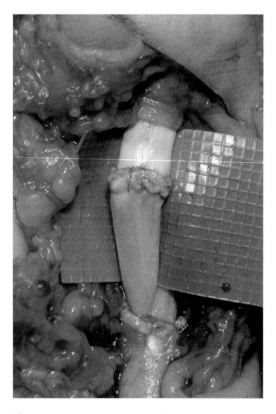

Fig. 5.12 Flexor tendon repair with Kessler core sutures and 6-0 prolene epitendinous sutures

flow is evident. If proximal flow is poor, the artery is examined under the microscope under 30× magnification. The lumen is checked for intralu-minal thrombus which can be cleared with hepa-rin flushes. The proximal artery is resected to healthy intima and dissected proximally to relieve tension (Figs. 5.6 and 5.13a, b). The artery is gen-tly flushed with papaverine (1:20 dilution). The general condition of the patient is checked to rule out and correct problems that can induce periph-eral vasoconstriction such as hypothermia, hypo-tension, hypovolemia, and acidosis.

Once proximal pulsatile flow is established, a double microvascular clamp is applied to approx-imate the two ends which should be sutured in a standard fashion using six to eight 9-0 nylon interrupted sutures for watertight closure. Beyond the DIPJ, four to six 10-0 or 11-0 sutures are suf-ficient. It must be reemphasized that anastomosis must be performed without any tension. If this is not possible, have a low threshold for vein graft-ing. For digital arteries, superficial axial veins of the forearm are suitable. The vein graft must be reversed (turned 180°) to respect the direction of flow.

Both digital arteries must be repaired if possi-ble to increase the chance of replant success. Equally important, repairing both digital arteries leads to improved sensory recovery [21]. However, if both digital arteries have large defects, it is not necessary to perform a double bypass.

Arterial shift can be performed to reconstruct one of the digital arteries wherein a normal artery from an adjacent finger is sacrificed and trans-ferred to the injured digit to revascularize the dis-tal segment. Alternatively one of the digital arteries in the injured finger can be crossed over to the other side of the same finger (Fig. 5.14). Sacrificing an artery from an adjacent normal fin-ger comes at a price to the normal finger, i.e., cold intolerance as well as scarring from the har-vest. This should only be considered in excep-tional circumstances such as a three-digit hand or in a child, with no alternative.

Venous Repair

Venous repair is the most difficult and problem-atic part of replant survival due to a low flow

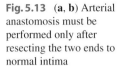

Fig. 5.13 (**a**, **b**) Arterial anastomosis must be performed only after resecting the two ends to normal intima

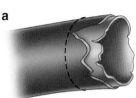

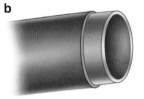

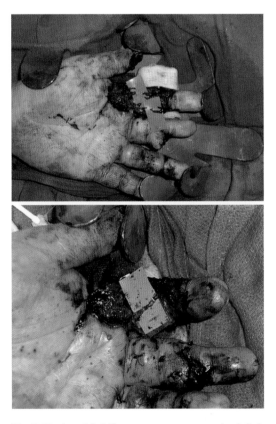

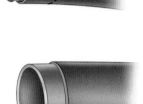

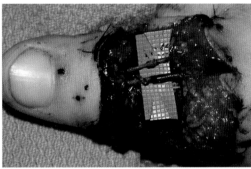

Fig. 5.15 Two veins must be repaired for every artery repaired

Fig. 5.14 Arterial shift – can anastomose proximal digital artery from one side to opposite side distal digital artery. Advantage is that this is quicker and easier than vein graft

system that can cause increased clot formation and thinner walls that are tougher to repair and more susceptible to compression. As a general rule, two veins must be repaired for each artery repaired (Fig. 5.15). Some authors recommend repair of veins before arteries since they are technically demanding and therefore better done when the surgeon is less fatigued. Also if done before the artery, there is lesser blood loss and a bloodless field is maintained [22, 23]. The other school of thought is to repair veins after the artery. The advantages are early revascularization and easier detection of the most functional veins recognized by their robust backflow. Repairing the artery first with confirmed inflow and outflow confirms a salvageable digit. If the veins are repaired first and no inflow occurs after subsequent arterial anastomosis, the surgeon has wasted time on a non-salvageable replant.

If veins cannot be repaired, several tricks can be used to prevent venous congestion. Look for

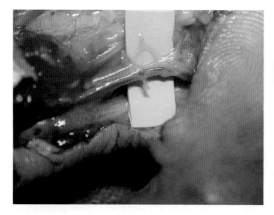

Fig. 5.16 If venous repair not possible, try volar veins

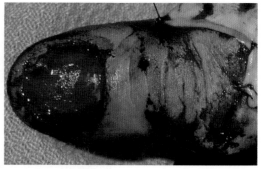

Fig. 5.18 Nail plate removal with scraping of nail matrix with cotton applicator and application of heparin-soaked gauze can allow venous egress and prevent venous congestion

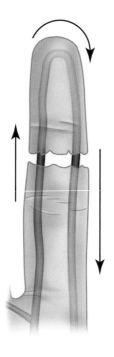

Fig. 5.17 If venous repair not possible, creation of an AV fistula by anastomosing of distal digital artery to proximal vein is performed

volar veins that can be utilized (Fig. 5.16). Provided it has backflow, one of the distal digital arteries can be anastomosed to a proximal vein to create an arteriovenous fistula (Fig. 5.17). The nail plate can be removed and the raw nail bed scraped with a cotton applicator every 1–2 h with application of heparin-soaked gauze to allow venous egress (Fig. 5.18). This can also be achieved via a stab incision on the para-ungual

area and dripping heparinized saline solution at the incision site to maintain external bleeding. Finally, medical-grade leeches may be placed on the finger every 15–30 min. Leeches attach to the finger and secrete hidurin – a local anticoagulant that allows bleeding from the distal segment, thereby preventing congestion. Leeches become engorged in 15–30 min and fall off. Application of leeches to the desired part of the finger is tricky. Leeches can be guided to the engorged part of the finger by either pinpricking the finger or placing a drop of D50 on the site. Another useful trick is to remove a plunger from a 3 cc syringe and stuff it with Xeroform™ gauze (Covidien, Dublin, Ireland). The leech is scooped into the back end of the syringe and the syringe is upturned on to the engorged finger. Leeches have an aversion to Xeroform™ and move toward the finger (Fig. 5.19). Leech therapy may be required for 5–7 days. Patients should be covered for infections with *Aeromonas hydrophila* from leeches, with ciprofloxacin.

Nerve Repair

Nerve coaptation is performed after vessel repair. Nerve ends, if jagged, are trimmed with a fresh 15 blade on a tongue depressor. If primary repair can be performed without tension, epineural suturing is performed with a 9-0 or 10-0 nylon suture with a cutting edge needle. The suture snap test is done to ensure that the repair

Fig. 5.19 Leech guidance to engorged finger using Xeroform-stuffed syringe

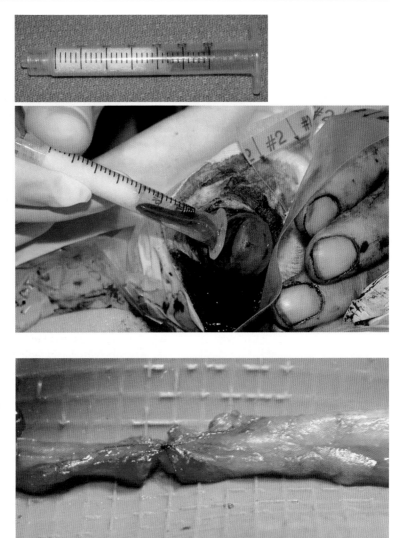

Fig. 5.20 Single suture test – a single 9-0 or 10-0 nylon suture should hold without snapping. If it snaps, the repair is under tension and should not be done

Fig. 5.21 Vein conduit for tensionless nerve repair

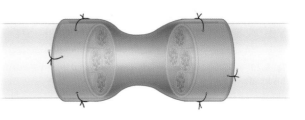

is not under tension (Fig. 5.20). If the suture snaps, the repair is under tension and a nerve conduit such as a vein or polyglycolic acid nerve tubes should be used (Figs. 5.21 and 5.22). If the nerve gap is significant, primary nerve grafts can be performed using either the posterior interos-seous nerve (PIN) or the medial antebrachial cutaneous nerve [24]. The PIN is preferred over the medial antebrachial nerve because this avoids a donor sensory deficit. In multi-digit amputations, digital nerves from discarded dig-its can be used.

Fig. 5.22 Nerve tube for tensionless nerve repair

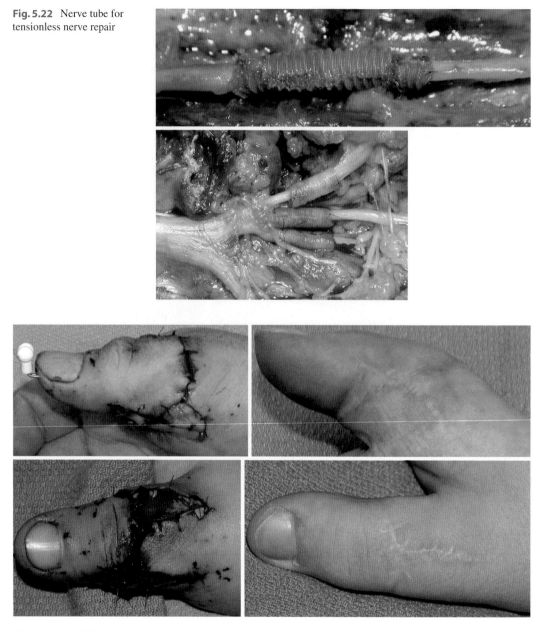

Fig. 5.23 Acellular dermal matrix can be placed over vascularized beds to cover less critical areas and aid in skin closure after a digital replant

Skin Closure and Dressings

Skin closure and application of dressings are important at the end of a replant, and attention to detail is essential as errors are common at the end of a lengthy procedure. For instance, tight sutures or dressings can cause vascular compression, venous congestion, and ultimately replant failure. Injury of an artery or vein with the suture needle is not uncommon. Meticulous hemostasis must be ensured prior to closure. The skin should be closed loosely with special care taken to prevent tension over vessels. Vital structures such as vessels and nerves must be covered to prevent desiccation. Skin grafts can be used to cover less important areas to allow tensionless closure of more important area overlying vessels or nerve repairs. Acellular dermal matrix can also be used to cover a vascularized bed and aid in closure (Fig. 5.23). A detailed description of local skin flaps is beyond the scope of this chapter; however, flaps such as the adipofascial turnover flap or flag flap can be considered. These local flaps have the added advantage of being venous carriers or providing further vein drainage.

Wounds should be covered with strips of Xeroform™ or petroleum gauze. Care must be taken to make sure that the strips are not continuous in a circumferential manner. The hand is immobilized with a volar splint and bulky dressings that extend above the elbow to prevent slippage. The entire upper extremity is wrapped in a Bair Hugger™ (3M, St. Paul, MN), with the replanted finger elevated and tip exposed for monitoring.

Postoperative Care

Postoperatively patients are admitted to a monitored bed for the initial 48–72 h for one-to-one nursing and close monitoring of the replanted digit. Patients can expect to be in hospital for 5–7 days after replantation. The replanted finger is closely monitored for arterial inflow or venous outflow problems. Early expeditious re-exploration is imperative for finger salvage.

Clinical monitoring is by far the most reliable method currently available. Color of the finger, capillary refill, temperature, and warmth are monitored on an hourly basis. Pallor indicates arterial inflow problems, whereas a brisk capillary refill or frank congestion indicates venous outflow problems. Other monitoring techniques include hourly arterial Doppler signals. Temperature probes and/or pulse oximetry probes can be used as adjuncts with a control probe on a healthy finger for more objective monitoring. Other sensitive techniques, including transcutaneous oxygen measurements, laser Doppler flowmetry, fluorescein perfusion, and Vioptix, have been utilized and but have not been found to be as reliable as clinical monitoring.

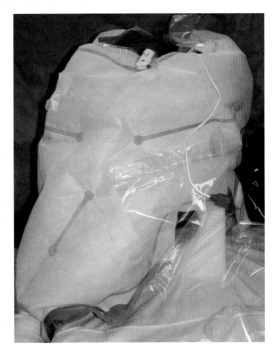

Fig. 5.24 Replanted finger is warmed by wrapping entire upper extremity with a Bair Hugger

Patient's room is warmed and cool drafts avoided. The upper extremity is wrapped in a Bair Hugger™ around upper extremity to avoid vasospasm (Fig. 5.24). The upper extremity is elevated to the level of the heart to minimize edema without compromising arterial or venous flow. The dressing is not changed for 4–5 days, unless excessive bleeding occurs. Dried blood soaked dressings can form a "blood cast" that can constrict circulation. Patient is kept on complete bed rest for at least 48–72 h followed by ambulation based on patient's course, personality, and desires under occupational therapist/physical therapist guidance. Smoking and caffeine are prohibited, and this should be part of the preoperative understanding with the patient.

Pharmacological support is continued for the entire hospitalization and includes adequate pain control, antibiotic coverage, and anticoagulation. Pain control can be achieved with either axillary block or patient controlled analgesia. An axillary catheter with administration of bupivacaine (5 ml of 0.25 % every 6–8 h) is preferred for its superior pain control as well as sympathetic blockade for vasodilation. Broad-spectrum antibiotics (second-generation cephalosporin) should be given intravenously for 5 days followed by oral cephalosporin for another 3–5 days.

Anticoagulation is a controversial subject [25–27]. As a general rule if amputation was clean-cut and anastomoses were technically easy, heparin is not indicated. Patients may be commenced on aspirin (325 mg/day) and low-molecular-weight Heparin (LWMH) at prophylactic doses or dextran 40 for 5 days is recommended. In case of crush or avulsion injuries or cases where the anastomoses were technically difficult or blood flow after anastomoses was tenuous, heparin is commenced at 1,000 U/h and continued for up to 5–7 days. Heparin dosage is titrated based on the activated partial thromboplastin time and maintained at 1.5 times normal. Heparin is used only for amputations distal to the wrist. Chlorpromazine (Thorazine) can be commenced as a sedative and peripheral vasodilator for 5 days at the dose of 0.3 mg/kg three times a day for 5 days.

Conclusion

Replantation tends to be one of the most difficult procedures in hand surgery due to high technical demand, a less than optimal tissue condition, a long operative time, usually at a suboptimal time (end of a long day, late at night into the early hours of the morning). Despite these demanding conditions, replantation surgery tends to be the most rewarding, especially when the indications are clear. There is so much to gain with very little for the patient to lose. Successful replants can restore hand function that is difficult to match by any secondary reconstructive procedures. The current success rate for digit replantation is about 85 % in a tertiary center and can be improved by better education for transport of the amputated part and expedited referral to a high-volume replant center. None the less, clear surgical indications must be respected to avoid functional failure, which can be disconcerting to both patient and surgeon.

References

1. Chung KC, Kowalski CP, Walters MR. Finger replantation in the United States: rates and resource use from the 1996 Healthcare Cost and Utilization Project. J Hand Surg (Am). 2000;25A:1038–42.
2. Goldner RD, Fitch RD, Nunley JA, Aitken MS, Urbaniak JR. Demographics and replantation surgery. Orthop Clin N Am. 1981;12:909–13.
3. Malt RA, McKhann CF. Replantation of severed arms. JAMA. 1964;189(82):618.
4. Littler JW. On making a thumb: one hundred years of surgical effort. J Hand Surg. 1976;1:35–51.
5. Urbaniak JR, Evans JP, Bright DS. Microvascular management of ring avulsion injuries. J Hand Surg. 1981;6A:25–30.
6. Dec W. A meta-analysis of success rates for digit replantation. Tech Hand Upper Ext Surg. 2006;10:124–9.
7. Waikakul S, Sakkarnkosol S, Vanadurongwan V, Un-nanuntana A. Results of 1018 digital replantations in 552 patients. Injury. 2000;31:33–40.
8. Soucacos PN, Beris AE, Malizos KN, Touliatos AS. Bilateral thumb amputation. Microsurgery. 1994;15:454–8.
9. Soucacos PN. Indications and selection for digital amputations and replantation. J Hand Surg. 2001;101:184–92.
10. Wei FC, Chen HC, Chuang CC. Three successful digital replantation in a patient after 84, 86, 94 hours cold ischemia time. Plast Reconstr Surg. 1988;82:346–50.
11. Heistein JB, Cook PA. Factors affecting composite graft survival in digital tip amputations. Ann Plast Surg. 2003;50:299–303.
12. Unglaub F, Demir E, Von Reim R, Van Schoonhoven J, Hahn P. Long-term functional and subjective results of thumb replantation. Microsurgery. 2006;26:552–6.
13. Lloyd MS, Teo TC, Pickford MA, Arnstein PM. Preoperative management of the amputated limb. Emerg Med J. 2005;22:478–80.
14. Su WF, Chen LE, Seaber AV, Urbaniak JR, Su WF, Chen LE, Seaber AV, Urbaniak JR. The effect of exposure time on microsurgical anastomoses of experimentally crushed arteries. Int Angiol. 1995;14(3):243–7.
15. Michon J, Merie M, Foucher G. Complex injury of the hand: one-stage treatment with early mobilization. Chirurgie. 1977;103:956–64.
16. Soucacos PN. Indications and selection for digital amputation and replantation. J Hand Surg. 2001;26B:572–81.
17. Tajima T. History, current status, and aspects of hand surgery in Japan. Clin Orthop Relat Res. 1984;184:41–9.
18. Chung KC, Alderman AK. Replantation of the upper extremity: indications and outcomes. J Am Soc Surg Hand. 2002;2:78–94.

19. Beris AE, Lykissas MG, Korompillias AV, Mitsionis GI, Vekris MD, Kostas-Agnantis IP. Digit and hand replant. Arch Orthop Trauma Surg. 2010;130:1141–7.
20. Sud V, Freeland AE. Skeletal fixation in digital replantation. Microsurgery. 2002;22:165–71.
21. Piquet M, Obert L, Laveaux C, Sarlieve P, Vidal C, Tropet Y. Influence of palmar digital artery patency on nervous recovery in palmar digital nerve lesions. Chir Main. 2010;29:94–9.
22. Chow JA, Bilos ZJ, Chunprapaph B. Thirty thumb replantations. Plast Reconstr Surg. 1979;64:626–30.
23. Dell PC, Seaber AV, Urbaniak JR. The effect of systemic acidosis on perfusion of replanted extremities. J Hand Surg Am. 1980;5:433–42.
24. Nunley JA, Ugino MR, Goldner RD. Use of the anterior branch of the medial antebrachial cutaneous nerve as a graft for the repair of defects of the digital nerve. J Bone Joint Surg Am. 1989;71:563–7.
25. Han SK, Lee BI, Kim WK. Topical and systemic anticoagulation in the treatment of absent or compromised venous outflow in replanted fingertips. J Hand Surg Am. 2000;25(4):659–67.
26. Pderson WC. Replantation. Plast Reconstr Surg. 2001;107:823–41.
27. Conrad MH, Adams Jr WP. Pharmacologic optimization of microsurgery in the new millennium. Plast Reconstr Surg. 2001;108:2088–96.

Replantation at the Level of the Radiocarpal Joint

6

Mauricio Kuri, Andrew Watt, and Gregory M. Buncke

Introduction

Upper extremity amputations can have a devastating effect on a person's quality of life [1, 2]. The social and psychological effects are also catastrophic [3, 4]. Malt and McKhann performed the first arm replant in 1962, and over the last 50 years, surgical technique, operative management, transportation of the part, patient selection, and postoperative care have evolved dramatically [5–10] The success rate for successful upper extremity replantation at microsurgical centers is over 90 %; nevertheless, success often depends on several factors such as amputation level, mechanism of injury, patient comorbidities, age, and surgical expertise [11, 12]. Overall, upper extremity replantation has shown superior functional and aesthetic results compared to revision amputation and prosthesis [8, 9, 13, 14].

In general, with the exception of transmetacarpal amputations, distal upper limb amputations tend to be more favorable than proximal upper limb amputations [15, 16]. Transmetacarpal amputations tend to have a poor functional outcome due to the damage of the intrinsic musculature of the hand [17, 18]. Frequently, these patients develop contractures, intrinsic minus postures, poor grip strength, and no return of pinch function.

Transcarpal and radiocarpal amputations present a distinct set of challenges for the replant surgeon. While there are no motor units at the level of the wrist, skeletal fixation can be challenging. Factors making replantation outcomes at this level more optimistic include preservation of proximal perfusion to the forearm musculature, the ability to perform primary repair of the tendons, and preservation of motor units for the hand [10]. In addition, radiocarpal amputations allow the surgeon the option to perform wrist arthrodesis, proximal row carpectomy (PRC), or shortening the radius accompanied by a Darrach procedure [19]. We tend to favor PRC or arthrodesis, because both methods shorten the bone and allow for primary repair of nerves, tendons, arteries, and veins. Furthermore, shortening the bone allows for a tension-free closure and soft tissue repair. All of these particularities of replantation at the carpus level contribute to the generally excellent postoperative function and recovery [11, 12, 20].

This chapter will focus on transcarpal amputations, encompassing the preoperative planning, surgical workup, technique, and postoperative care. We will address the goals of care and challenges of dealing with the wrist joint, addressing specifically different ways to approach the skeletal fixation to achieve primary repair of all structures.

M. Kuri, MD • A. Watt, MD
G.M. Buncke, MD (✉)
Division of Microsurgery, The Buncke Medical Clinic, San Francisco, CA, USA
e-mail: drmkuri@gmail.com; Ajwatt50@gmail.com; gbuncke@buncke.org

A.N. Salyapongse et al. (eds.), *Extremity Replantation: A Comprehensive Clinical Guide*,
DOI 10.1007/978-1-4899-7516-4_6, © Springer Science+Business Media New York 2015

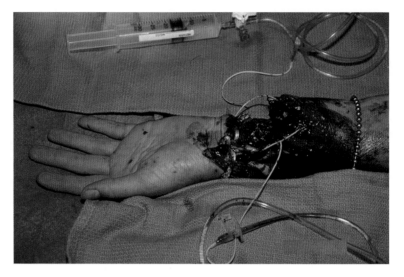

Fig. 6.1 Use of T shunt in a distal forearm amputation, during osteosynthesis, to minimize ischemia time

Initial Assessment

The general approach to extremity amputation has been well-covered earlier (see Chaps. 5 and 6). A few differences apply specifically to amputation at the carpal or radiocarpal level. Clinical examination of the amputated segment will allow identification of injured or lost cartilage surfaces of the carpal bones or distal radius. X-ray evaluation of the wrist and the amputated part can confirm the residual carpal bones and identify fractures of the radius or ulna that may preclude anatomic reconstruction; this will give the surgeon an idea of the zone of injury and how to address the bony fixation. When the initial evaluating team is not the same as the team that will provide definitive management, photo documentation of the part and amputation stump should be obtained. This is important in that we routinely communicate with transferring facilities with digital media [21]. Knowing the amputation level, extent of the injury, condition of the amputated part, ischemic time, and geographic location, the microsurgical team can have an operative plan ahead of the patient's arrival. The combination of the x-ray images and clinical photos can facilitate preparing appropriate fixation systems depending on whether anatomic reconstruction or arthrodesis will be performed. In addition, if the digitally sent picture

demonstrates a badly crushed or mangled part and the patient is not a candidate for replantation, the revision amputation can be performed at the transferring facility.

As a general rule, amputations proximal to the wrist ideally should have a warm ischemia times of less than 6–8 h, whereas distal to the wrist around 10–12 h [22, 23]. However, wrist level amputations have only intrinsic musculature, and, under appropriate conditions, we have replanted patients with cold ischemia times up to 12 h. There have even been reports of hand replants up to 54 h [24]. It is unclear how the prolonged cold ischemia time distal to the wrist affects replant survival and functionality. To our knowledge, transcarpal amputations have definitively more tolerance to cold ischemia times than the more proximal forearm amputations. Given this, if the part has been ischemic for close to 6 h, we may use a shunt to perfuse the part prior to the bony fixation; while we do not routinely use shunts for transcarpal amputation, we have found them useful in more proximal levels of amputation (Fig. 6.1). Shunts should not be placed by the transferring facility as this may delay transfer or even worse may lead to exsanguination if the shunt malfunctions during transport.

As mentioned above, x-rays are an extremely important part of the initial evaluation of the

Fig. 6.2 (**a**, **b**) Case example of patient who had an avulsion/crush injury by a pistachio conveyor belt. Although the near amputation is through the forearm, the zone of injury extends to the distal carpal bones

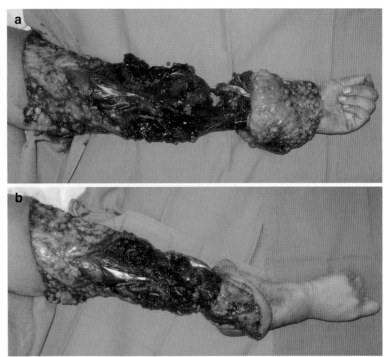

patient. All transferring facilities should obtain x-rays of the amputated part, as well as the stump and the joint proximal. Traction, crush, and degloving injuries can be particularly deceptive and the zone of injury might involve a joint more proximal to the actual amputation (Fig. 6.2a, b). This is particularly important during the microsurgical reconstruction, since intimal injury can be overlooked and compromise the replantation.

Upon arrival to the microsurgical center, the patient is again thoroughly evaluated. X-rays images are reviewed and full set of laboratory values ordered which include chemistry, complete blood counts, coagulation studies, blood type, liver function tests, and type and cross for four units of PRBCs. It is important to have a detailed discussion with the patient regarding the risks and benefits of the procedure including length of hospital stay, blood transfusions, anticoagulation therapies, rehabilitation, expected outcomes, and secondary surgeries. Motivation and intelligence are two factors that will positively influence replant outcomes [12].

Technical Aspects of the Replantation and Operative Sequence

Operative Sequence

After the patient has been stabilized, prior to transfer to the operating suite, the part is taken to the operating room for inspection and tagging of all the structures (Fig. 6.3a, b). Upper arm and forearm replants are routinely performed with two teams (Fig. 6.4). One team performs the debridement and tagging of the amputated part, while the other team does the same on the patient's arm. The sequence of events is summarized below in a stepwise fashion (some exceptions made depending on ischemia time):

1. Preparing the part
2. Aggressive debridement and stump preparation
3. Bony fixation
4. Flexor tendon repairs
5. Nerve and artery repairs
6. Extensor tendon repair
7. Vein repair

Fig. 6.3 (**a, b**) The amputated parts are taken back to the operating room and are tagged and inspected

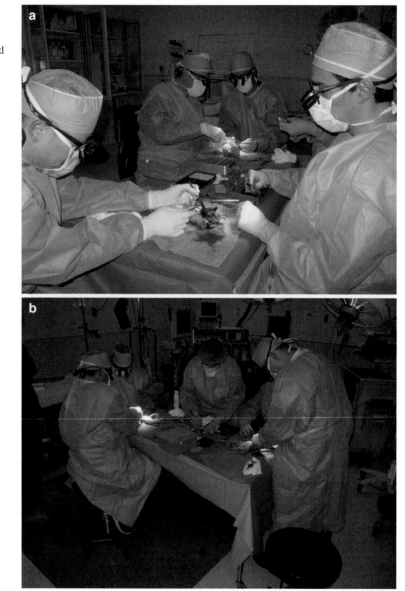

Fig. 6.3 (**a, b**) The amputated parts are taken back to the operating room and are tagged and inspected

Preparing the Part

We start by inspecting the part for any debris or foreign bodies. The part is washed thoroughly with soap and water; all debris is removed and the part is then prepped with Betadine solution. During the preparation of the part, we prefer to place the hand flat on a chilled iced container. Prior to tagging the structures, we inspect the part and debride all the nonviable skin and subcutaneous tissues. Tendons are trimmed to healthy

appearing substance and we reserve debriding the nerves and arteries until microscopic magnification is in place so that appropriate inspection of the intima and nerve fibers is performed.

By this time, the surgeon should have in mind a surgical plan for the bony fixation. If the mechanism of injury is through the proximal row, we perform the PRC of the part on the tagging table. If the proximal and distal rows are injured, restoration of a functional radiocarpal joint will be impossible, so we remove the proximal row and

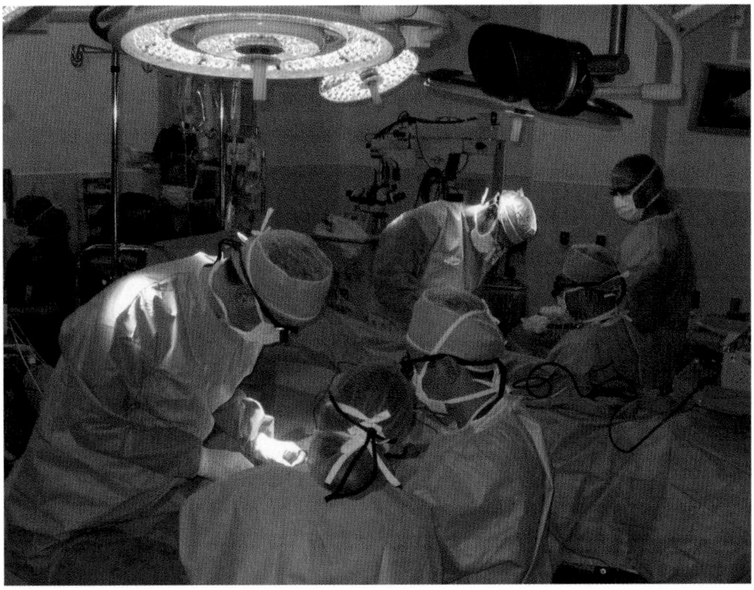

Fig. 6.4 Two-team approach working simultaneously on a bilateral forearm amputation

save the bone for bone grafting to help with wrist arthrodesis.

The part is carefully inspected for injuries. We normally test all the flexor tendons to make sure they are gliding properly and under fluoroscopy rule out any other bony injuries. If fractures or dislocations exist in the amputated part, K-wire fixation is performed prior to tagging the structures. We start volarly by opening the carpal tunnel and Guyon's canal. The median and ulnar nerve are identified and neurolyzed. The flexor tendons are identified and a DOLLS (double-opposing, locking-loop suture)-type suture with 4-0 FiberWire is placed on all the FDS and FDP distal stumps [25]. Then the radial artery and ulnar artery are identified and released appropriately to ensure a tension-free repair.

The hand is then turned dorsally and exposure to the extensor tendons is done taking into consideration the venous drainage of the wrist. The two major draining veins are the cephalic and the basilic veins that drain the metacarpal venous plexus (Fig. 6.5). The exposure to the dorsum is usually done in an H-type pattern, being conservative with the skin incisions (Fig. 6.6a, b). The draining veins are identified and clipped as downstream as possible to preserve length. The extensor tendons are dissected free just enough to ensure an appropriate repair.

In anticipation of swelling associated with ischemia and reperfusion of the intrinsic muscles, the compartments of the hand are released. Two dorsal incisions (approximately 2 cm each) are made on the second and fourth compartment and the fascia is released. However, the surgeon should not disrupt the dorsal venous drainage when releasing the dorsal compartments. Similarly, the thenar and hypothenar compartments are released volarly. Lastly, the superficial branch of the radial nerve is identified and tagged. The part is then handed off to the sterile table (Fig. 6.7).

Debridement of Non-vital Tissue

Simultaneously, the patient is prepped and draped with a nonsterile tourniquet in place, and the second team begins debriding the forearm stump. Depending on the extent of injury, the thigh and leg are prepped as well for possible vein, skin, or tendon grafting. Nonviable skin, subcutaneous tissue, tendons, and muscle are inspected and debrided appropriately. Important decisions are made while this process is taking place; the surgeon must determine at this time the viability of the radiocarpal joint and decide if the joint is appropriate for a proximal row carpectomy,

Fig. 6.5 Dorsal drainage venous system

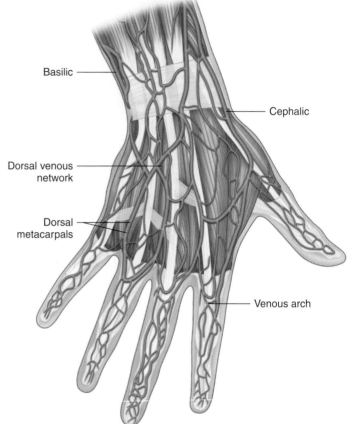

Basilic

Cephalic

Dorsal venous
network

Dorsal
metacarpals

Venous arch

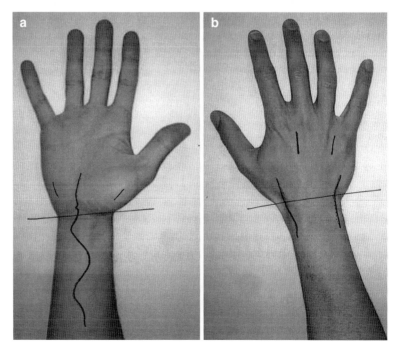

Fig. 6.6 (**a**, **b**) Volar and
dorsal approach of transcarpal amputation. While
releasing the dorsal
compartment, it is important
to protect and preserve the
venous drainage. Volarly, the
carpal tunnel and Guyon's
canal are released.
Proximally, both forearm
compartments are released as
well

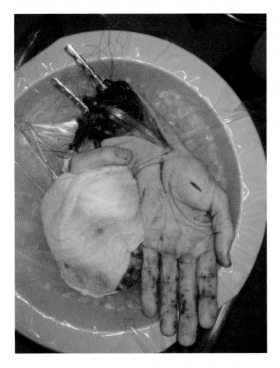

Fig. 6.7 Bilateral upper extremity replantation: the parts are kept on ice until the forearm team is ready for osteosynthesis and revascularization. Notice that the parts already have the plates and k-wires and are ready for bony fixation

arthrodesis, or radial shortening. The motor units are inspected and the zone of injury assessed. This will determine if vein grafts, nerve grafts, or tendon grafts will be needed. Specifically, we tend to address each soft tissue compartment separately. The skin is inspected and surgical release of compartments is planned so that vital structures are covered. In addition, if there is a soft tissue deficit, and the patient might need microvascular transplant down the road, we plan our incisions so that the vascular anastomoses are protected. When available, healthy skin and subcutaneous coverage is limited, we prefer to prioritize this coverage to vessels and nerves, leaving muscle and tendon to coverage with skin grafts or dressing changes. When no good coverage is available, we have skin grafted over vessels and nerves as a temporizing measure to protect them from desiccation.

Depending on the pattern of injury, we extend our incisions proximally after the debridement is performed, usually in an H pattern. The forearm fascia is released and the structures inspected and tagged appropriately in a similar fashion as the part. The flexor tendons are tenolyzed and separated individually to match the distal targets. We start by tagging the deeper structures such as the FDP and move volarly to the FDS. The radial artery and ulnar artery are identified and tagged. The ulnar nerve and median nerve are neurolyzed and tagged. Dorsally the extensor tendons are identified and the accompanying draining veins are tagged. Usually the cephalic vein is sufficient for transcarpal replants, but the carpus has several proximal appropriate targets. As in the case of the amputated hand, it is important to release the forearm fascia to account for postoperative swelling.

Bony Fixation

Technically, transcarpal replants are relatively straightforward. The vessels are larger, the carpal venous drainage is constant, and the muscle units are excluded from the zone of injury. The tendinous repairs are performed primarily and the functional results are excellent [10, 12, 14, 26]. However, in order to achieve a tension-free repair without the use of nerve or vein grafts as well as to prevent tight tendon repairs, bone shortening must be address in a systematic fashion. Bony fixation is dependent on the mechanism of injury through the carpus itself. As outlined previously, the bone is addressed in three different ways: (a) proximal row carpectomy, (b) wrist arthrodesis, and (c) radial and ulnar shortening or Darrach procedure for the ulna assuming carpus is intact.

Bony fixation is determined by the mechanism of injury and the quality of the carpal bones. The decision to perform an arthrodesis versus a proximal row carpectomy is primarily dependent on the integrity of the distal row and the lunate facet. If there is bony injury to the any of the bones of the distal row, we inspect the carpal bones and if possible perform open reduction and internal fixation of the damage bones to preserve the distal row and attempt wrist salvage with a PRC. If, however, there is comminution or intracarpal instability or the injury is extensive, we proceed with arthrodesis. Unfortunately, few radiocarpal amputations are clean through the joint and have an intact capitate-lunate joint; nevertheless an attempt to preserve motion to the wrist should be a priority.

If the mechanism of injury is through the proximal and distal carpus, we remove the proximal carpus and perform a wrist arthrodesis. We use the proximal carpus as bone graft and shorten the wrist by 2–3 cm. If more bone graft is needed, we used iliac crest as a donor site. Arthrodesis with a dorsally placed plate offers the greatest stability and lowest chance for nonunion. Plates specifically designed for this are readily available, with the most common employing a slight bend at the level of arthrodesis that allows positioning of the wrist in roughly 20–30° of extension. Proximally, the plat should be positioned along the centerline of the radius, typically along the floor of the fourth compartment. Removal of Lister's tubercle and contouring of a slight trough in the dorsal aspect of the distal radius can facilitate accurate placement and alignment of the plate. If a straight plate is employed, contouring of the distal radius is not necessary. When dissecting the middle finger metacarpal for distal plate placement, the venous drainage must be preserved and protected if the drainage is through the carpal circulation.

The second option is to perform a proximal row carpectomy (Fig. 6.8a–n). The decision can be made while inspecting the part, and the carpectomy should be performed simultaneous with debridement of the stump. Important for obtaining a good outcome, the proximal capitate and lunate fossa should be relatively uninjured. Postoperatively, the wrist motion in this group of patients is excellent [14, 27]. Temporary fixation is performed with a pair of 0.062 k-wires through the radiocarpal joint capturing the lunate fossa and capitate as well as the scaphoid fossa and trapezium. A third k-wire is place through the ulna to the hamate. Routinely, we perform radial styloidectomy to prevent impingement with the distal row. The radial styloidectomy can be performed with a rongeur or an osteotome prior to the bony fixation of the part.

The third option is to shorten the radius more proximally and perform a distal resection of the ulna, the so-called Darrach procedure. This option is not routinely performed but has been reported when the amputation is through the radiocarpal joint and the integrity of the proximal and distal carpal rows is intact [19]. Alternatively, if the TFCC is intact, ulnar and radial shortening preserving the radiocarpal joint as well as the TFCC can be performed, and 0.062 K-wires are used for fixation since the proximity of the joint precludes volar plate fixation (Fig. 6.9a–r).

Flexor Tendon Repair

The tendons are inspected, and depending on the quality of the tendons, we make the decision to repair both FDS and FDP or use FDS as tendon grafts for FDPs. Prior to placing the sutures, the tendon must be trimmed appropriately to healthy tendon substance. Some authors advocate FDS resection and just repairing FDP tendons [14]; however, at this level of amputation, both FDS and FDP should be repaired since results at this level are excellent [12]. We use a double loop locking suture technique, placing the knot in the substance of the tendon. It is a four-strand repair, and in our experience, we have encountered only a handful of postoperative tendon ruptures. The repair should proceed from deep to superficial, starting with the FDP moving volarly to the FDS. We rarely use tendon grafts in this area, since shortening the carpus provides enough length for primary repair; however, the FDS from the index through the small can be used if needed.

Vessels and Nerves

Once the appropriate tension has been established by repairing the volar flexors, we turn our attention to the nerves. However, depending on ischemia time, we may modify the order of repair. If the part has been ischemic for several hours, we may only repair, the FCR, FCU, or FDPs to set the wrist tension, and turn our attention to the arteries. We always repair both arteries. If the

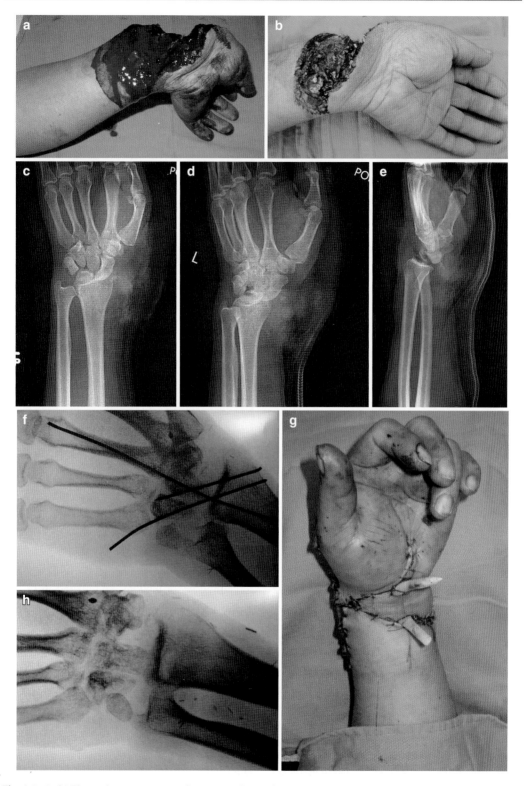

Fig. 6.8 (**a**, **b**) Figure shows a near-complete amputation through the radiocarpal joint. The proximal row was damaged, as well as the radio carpal ligaments. (**c–e**) Radiographs of the patient show radial and volar translation of the carpus. (**f**) After proximal row carpectomy and fixation. (**g**) All volar and dorsal structures were repaired; venous outflow was preserve by an ulnar skin bridge. (**h**) After removal of k-wires, 8 weeks. (**i–n**) 10 months after surgery, after flexor tenolysis

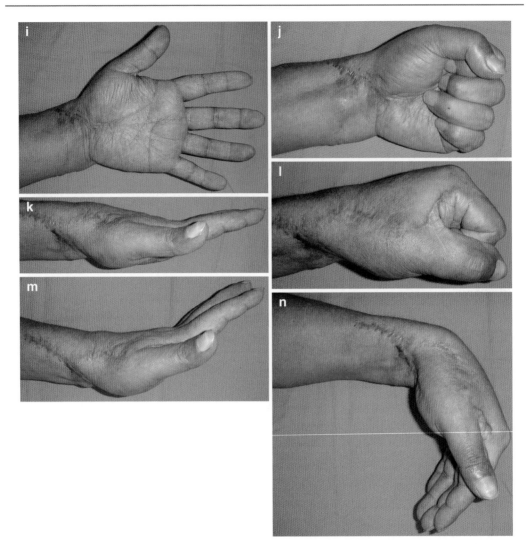

Fig. 6.8 (continued)

arteries are under any tension, we use the contralateral forearm veins or dorsal veins of the foot for vein grafting. As we proceed to perform the first anastomosis, the patient is started on a dextran drip (low molecular weight dextran) at 25 cc/h. Once the arterial repairs are performed, and prior to releasing the tourniquet, we ensure the patient has blood available. On average we use 4 units of blood per transcarpal replant. Upon release of the tourniquet, we allow for 5 min of venous bleeding to clear potential toxic concentrations of potassium as well as lactic acid [28]. During this time, we finish the repair of the median and ulnar nerves. Similarly, the any

remaining flexor tendons are repaired. Although primary tensionless repair is the gold standard, if there is a nerve gap that would impede a tension-free repair, we use allografts for combined sensory or motor nerves. As discussed in Chap. 3, emerging literature shows that nerve conduits provide at least equal return of motor and sensory function [29, 30]. Using allografts in the setting of traumatic amputations provides several advantages: (a) shortens intraoperative and ischemia time, (b) reduces the morbidity of the donor site, and (c) does not eliminate the possibility of autograft harvest in the future. On the other hand, the main disadvantage for allograft use is cost [31].

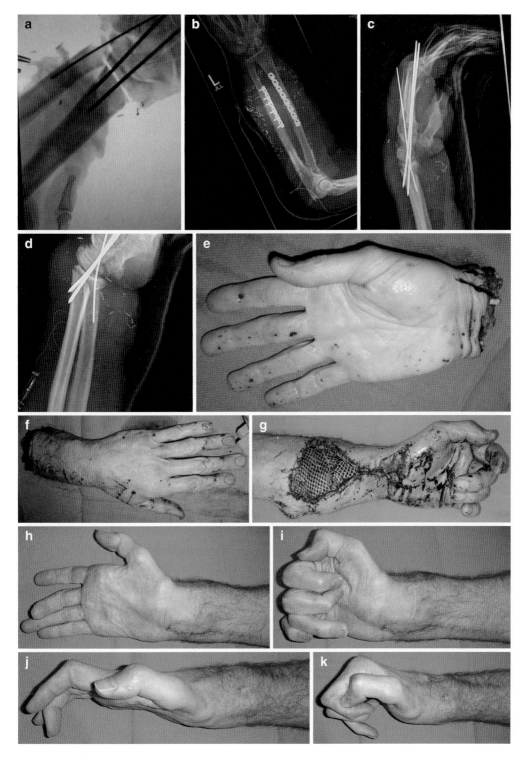

Fig. 6.9 Patient with bilateral forearm amputation, the left hand through mid-forearm, and the right hand distal forearm, just proximal to the distal radio ulnar joint. (**a–d**) Radiographs of the patient, note that the right hand amputation is proximal to the DRUJ; therefore, we shortened both the radius and ulnar proximal to the joint. (**e, f**) Right and left hands. (**g**) The wounds were loosely closed with skin flaps and skin grafts, allowing for postoperative swelling to occur. (**h–l**) Right hand after tenolysis. (**m–r**) Left hand after tenolysis. Both achieve two-point discrimination and full range of motion except the right hand had limited supination but full pronation

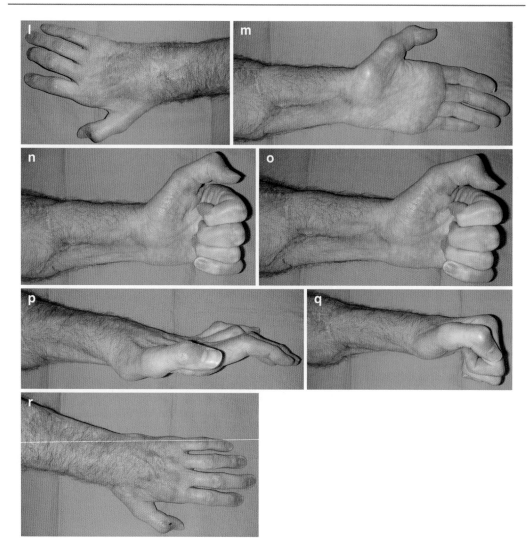

Fig. 6.9 (continued)

Dorsal Tendon Repairs

The dorsal tendon repairs are performed with 4-0 Ethibond suture in a figure of eight fashion. The proximal targets, which were tagged previously, can be secured with 25-gauge needles to relieve some of the tension. If there is tendon missing or the injury pattern is oblique, the tendons can be tenodesed together with healthy motor units. If the zone of injury is wide and there is segmental tendon loss, depending on the mechanism of injury, we may elect to perform tendon grafting acutely or delay the grafting as a second-stage reconstruction. The ECU and ECR are repaired in a similar fashion as the flexor tendons with a 4-strand repair.

Veins

Routinely, we used the cephalic vein as our outflow; however, we prefer to also use a second carpal vein when available. At the wrist, the veins tend to be 3–4 mm in size, and after several minutes of bleeding, the veins can be selected based on how well they drain. The anastomosis is routinely performed with 8-0 nylon suture. For transcarpal amputations, we always repair the veins last. Performing the anastomosis with draining blood is technically more difficult, but it has twofold advantage, (a) it allows the blood to drain the toxic metabolites and (b) it gives the surgeon the opportunity to visualize and inspect the draining veins. Frequently, postoperative swelling precludes primary closure of all incisions. If there is not enough soft tissue coverage, we use split-thickness skin grafts for coverage. When grafts are placed over muscle, this may provide definitive closure; as mentioned above, coverage of vital structures, such as vessels and nerves, may require a secondary free tissue transfer for definitive coverage. This, however, should be performed after confirmation of survival of the replantation.

Postoperative Care and Monitoring

After the replant is completed, the wound is covered with a nonadherent, loosely wrapped dressing to avoid constriction or pressure on the anastomoses and a long-arm splint with the wrist in neutral (or slight extension, if an arthrodesis has been performed). Postoperative monitoring and maintenance of vascular patency follow guidelines addressed in Chap. 8. In contrast to more distal amputations, however, transcarpal replants tend to have larger veins that can be monitored with an implantable Doppler. Although clinical examination by monitoring color and capillary refill as well as arterial pencil Doppler represents the gold standard for monitoring, placement of an implantable Doppler facilitates nursing care and provides instant feedback.

Complications

Complications related to anastomotic flow occur usually in the first 48 h, although longer times have been reported [6]. If perfusion is compromised, the first step is to remove the dressings and evaluate the hand. The suture line is inspected for any tension or compression on the anastomosis. If there is suspicion that the artery or vein are occluded, the patient should be taken back to the

operating room for exploration. Often times if the venous outflow is occluded, the dressings are saturated with blood, because smaller unclipped draining veins and skin edges bleed to relieve congestion. The hand will appear congested and will have increased turgor. On the other hand, if the artery is occluded, the hand will be pale and will have very slow capillary refill. Once the patient is in the operating room, if either of the anastomoses has occluded, we tend to use interposition grafts and start heparin drip with goal therapy of PTT at 40–60. At this point in time, the hand is usually more swollen and primary closure should be avoided, and we tend to temporarily cover open areas with skin grafts. After swelling subsides, the patient is evaluated for the possibility of soft tissue coverage. Stable soft tissue cover is essential since many patients will require secondary extensor and flexor tenolysis. Most soft tissue reconstruction with microvascular transplants occurs during the primary hospitalization after necessary debridement of devitalized soft tissue occurs.

Conclusion

Literature reports on isolated functional wrist and proximal hand-level replantation results are limited. Reports of upper extremity replantation are usually combined with replantation at other levels [1, 2, 32–34]. However, if independently evaluated, wrist replantations can achieve high functional results and excellent patient satisfaction [8, 10, 12]. There are no long-term functional results for PRC in the setting of transcarpal replantations; however, PRC in the setting of arthritis has long-term durable and reliable results [27, 35, 36]. Wrist arthrodesis is an alternative option that has been described for injuries occurring through both proximal and distal rows [2, 26].

The main challenge of replantation through the wrist is how address the bony framework. Once the decision is made to perform a PRC or arthrodesis, the same algorithm applies as other upper extremity replants. Bony shortening whether through a PRC or arthrodesis provides the opportunity for primary neural and vessel repair. One of the most critical factors after a replant is neural regeneration, thus at this level, performing primary nerve repairs is critical; therefore, PRC offers not only the advantages of a functional wrist joint but the benefits of bony shortening and primary repair of vessels, nerves, and tendons.

References

1. Larson JV, Kung TA, Cederna PS, Sears ED, Urbanchek MG, Langhals NB. Clinical factors associated with replantation after traumatic major upper extremity amputation. Plast Reconstr Surg. 2013; 132(4):911–9.
2. Vanstraelen P, Papini RPG, Sykes PJ, Milling MAP. The functional results of hand replantation: the Chepstow experience. J Hand Surg. 1993;18B:556–64.
3. Tamai S. Twenty years' experience of limb replantation – review of 293 upper extremity replants. J Hand Surg Am. 1982;7:549–56.
4. Freeland AE, Psonak R. Traumatic below-elbow amputations. Orthopedics. 2007;30(2):120–6.
5. Malt RA, McKhann CF. Replantation of severed arms. JAMA. 1964;189:716–20.
6. Buncke HJ. Replantation surgery. In: Buncke HJ, editor. Microsurgery transplantation and replantation: an atlas text. Philadelphia: Lea & Febiger; 1991. p. 594–633.
7. Beris AE, Soucacos PN, Malizos KN, Mitsionis GJ, Soucacos PK. Major limb replantation in children. Microsurgery. 1994;15:474–8.
8. Graham B, Adkins P, Tsai TM, Firrell J, Breidenbach WC. Major replantation versus revision amputation and prosthetic fitting in the upper extremity: a late functional outcomes study. J Hand Surg Am. 1998; 23(5):783–91.
9. Ipsen T, Lundkvist L, Barfred T, Pless J. Principles of evaluation and results in microsurgical treatment of major limb amputations: a follow-up study of 26 consecutive cases 1978–1987. Scand J Plast Reconstr Hand Surg. 1990;24:75–80.
10. Meyer VE. Hand amputations proximal but close to the wrist joint: prime candidates for reattachment (long-term functional results). J Hand Surg. 1985;10A: 989–91.
11. Meyer VE. Upper extremity replantation – a review. Eur Surg. 2003;35:167–73.
12. Buncke G. Replantation and revascularization. In: Mathes S, editor. Plastic surgery: the hand and the upper limb part I. Philadelphia: Elsevier; 2006.
13. Dagum AB, Slesarenko Y, Winston L, Tottenham V. Long term outcome of replantation of proximal-third amputated arm: a worthwhile endeavor. Tech Hand Up Extrem Surg. 2007;11:231–5.
14. Hoang NT. Hand replantations following complete amputations at the wrist joint: first experiences in Hanoi, Vietnam. J Hand Surg Br. 2006;31(1):9–17.
15. Patradul A, Ngarmukos C, Parkpian V. Major limb replantation: a Thai experience. Ann Acad Med Singapore. 1995;24(4 Suppl):82–8.
16. Laing TA, Cassell O, O'Donovan D, Eadie P. Long term functional results from major limb replantations. J Plast Reconstr Aesthet Surg. 2012;65(7):931–4.
17. Zhong-Wei C, Meyer VE, Kleinert HE, Beasley RW. Present indications and contraindications for replantation as reflected by long-term functional results. Orthop Clin North Am. 1981;12(4):849–70.
18. Russell RC, O'Brien BM, Morrison WA, Pamamull G, MacLeod A. The late functional results of upper limb revascularization and replantation. J Hand Surg Am. 1984;9(5):623–33.
19. Jones NF. Replantation in the upper extremity. In: Charles T, editor. Grabb and smith. Philadelphia: Lippincott Williams & Wilkins; 2006. Ch 91.
20. Woo SH, Lee YK, Lee HH, Park JK, Kim JY, Dhawan V. Hand replantation with proximal row carpectomy. Hand (N Y). 2009;4(1):55–61.
21. Buntic RF, Siko PP, Buncke GM, Ruebeck D, Kind GM, Buncke HJ. Using the internet for rapid exchange of photographs and X-ray images to evaluate potential extremity replantation candidates. J Trauma. 1997;43:342–4.
22. Gold AH, Lee GW. Upper extremity replantation: current concepts and patient selection. J Trauma. 1981;21:551–7.
23. Goldner RD, Nunley JA. Replantation proximal to the wrist. Hand Clin. 1992;8:413–25.
24. VanderWilde RS, Wood MB, Zu ZG. Hand replantation after 54 hours of cold ischemia: a case report. J Hand Surg Am. 1992;17:217–20.
25. Lee H. Double loop locking suture: a technique of tendon repair for early active mobilization. Part II: clinical experience. J Hand Surg Am. 1990;15(6):953–8.
26. Hanel DP, Chin SH. Wrist level and proximal-upper extremity replantation. Hand Clin. 2007;23(1):13–21.
27. Croog AS, Stern PJ. Proximal row carpectomy for advanced Kien- bock's disease: average 10-year follow-up. J Hand Surg Am. 2008;33:1122–30.
28. Hicks TE, Boswick Jr JA, Solomons CC. The effects of perfusion on an amputated extremity. J Trauma. 1980;20:632–48.
29. Cho MS, Rinker BD, Weber RV, Chao JD, Ingari JV, Brooks D, Buncke GM. Functional outcome following nerve repair in the upper extremity using processed nerve allograft. J Hand Surg Am. 2012;37(11): 2340–9.
30. Brooks DN, Weber RV, Chao JD, Rinker BD, Zoldos J, Robichaux MR, Ruggeri SB, Anderson KA, Bonatz EE, Wisotsky SM, Cho MS, Wilson C, Cooper EO, Ingari JV, Safa B, Parrett BM, Buncke GM. Processed nerve allografts for peripheral

nerve reconstruction: a multicenter study of utilization and outcomes in sensory, mixed, and motor nerve reconstructions. Microsurgery. 2012;32(1):1–14.

31. Ducic I, Fu R, Iorio ML. Innovative treatment of peripheral nerve injuries: combined reconstructive concepts. Ann Plast Surg. 2012;68(2):180–7.

32. Sugun TS, Ozaksar K, Ada S, Kul F, Ozerkan F, Kaplan I, Ademohlu Y, Kayalar M, Bal E, Toros T, Bora A. Long-term results of major upper extremity replantations. Acta Orthop Traumatol Turc. 2009;43(3):206–13.

33. Scheker LR, Chesher SP, Netscher DT, Julliard KN, O'Neill WL. Functional results of dynamic splinting after transmetacarpal, wrist, and distal forearm replantation. J Hand Surg. 1995;20B:584–90.

34. Chow JA, Bilos ZJ, Chunprapath B, Hui P. Forearm replantation—long-term functional results. Ann Plast Surg. 1983;10:15–23.

35. Imbriglia JE, Broudy AS, Hagberg WC, et al. Proximal row carpectomy: clinical evaluation. J Hand Surg Am. 1990;15:426–30.

36. Richou J, Chuinard C, Moineau G, Hanouz N, Hu W, Le Nen D. Proximal row carpectomy: long-term results. Chir Main. 2010;29(1):10–5.

Replantation of the Forearm or Arm

7

Michael Waters and Brian J. Harley

Introduction

Amputations and near amputations of the upper extremity at the level of the forearm and arm are uncommon injuries outside of wartime and major disasters. Amputations proximal to the carpal bones are commonly referred to as major upper extremity amputations. This terminology stems from fundamental differences between distal (carpal bones and below) and proximal amputations with regard to the typical mechanism of injury, differences in anatomy within the forearm and arm, and most importantly, different healing/regenerative potential of the proximal anatomy. In distal amputations, limited muscle mass in the amputated stump allows for prolonged ischemia times without myonecrosis and therefore more predictable results. Neurologic recovery is also more predictable in distal injuries owing to decreased regenerative distance to end organs as well as the significantly fewer number of innervated structures requiring reinnervation [1]. When taking all of these factors into consideration, it is not surprising that the increased complexity of treatment of major upper extremity amputations portends a much more unpredictable result as well as a higher rate of systemic complications.

Major amputations of the upper extremity exist on a continuum, from complex open fractures with extensive soft tissue damage (termed "near amputations") to complete transection of all structures of the extremity. Near amputations are a more common injury overall and are also more commonly a salvageable injury than complete amputations [2]. Near amputations are distinguished by some "functional continuity" between the proximal and distal segments. The continuous segment is typically a portion of the skin, muscle, and/or nerve that preserves some degree of venous return despite arterial insufficiency. They tend to have higher rates of functionality [3]. Regardless of the completeness of the amputation, the functional outcome of any amputated or near-amputated major upper extremity is typically dependent upon the quantity of intact tissue, the quality of repair possible, and the regenerative potential of the repaired nerves. As a general rule, as the level of amputation moves proximally, expected functional return decreases [4].

Reduced functional outcomes are also directly related to the increased energy necessary to produce proximal amputations. Owing to the much stronger skeletal structures as well as a more substantial soft tissue envelope, amputations through the forearm, elbow, or arm require a much higher level of energy than distal amputations and infrequently occur as a result of a sharp

M. Waters, MD • B.J. Harley, MD, FRCSC (✉)
Department of Orthopedic Surgery,
SUNY Upstate Medical University,
Syracuse, NY, USA
e-mail: Mike.s.waters@gmail.com;
harleyb@upstate.edu

A.N. Salyapongse et al. (eds.), *Extremity Replantation: A Comprehensive Clinical Guide*,
DOI 10.1007/978-1-4899-7516-4_7, © Springer Science+Business Media New York 2015

mechanism. Riding lawnmowers and boat propellers are examples of machines that have sufficient energy to cause "sharp" amputations, but the high revolutions associated with these mechanisms typically result in amputations that are segmental in nature and therefore typically not salvageable. Industrial and farming accidents are more common causes of major upper extremity amputations that tend to result in a single distal segment. Typically, the victim's clothing is pulled into powerful machinery such as a machine press, power take-off, or auger. These may be salvageable, but as the amputation is more the result of crushing and/or avulsion, the end result is a larger zone of injury. This necessitates extensive debridement and bone shortening on either side before replantation can be considered. Soft tissue contamination with both organic and inorganic material in these industrial/farmyard accidents can necessitate extensive debridement of otherwise healthy margins. Decreased function is therefore typically accepted in order to reduce the risk of infection and prolonged inflammation [5].

A patient's overall health both pre- and post-injury is also key in distinguishing treatment. Distal amputations are frequently isolated injuries and rarely life threatening, which means that the majority of patients can be considered for replantation. In contrast, major limb amputations are often associated with significant trauma and concomitant injuries. Patients often have had large volumes of blood loss, and additional loss is expected intra- and occasionally postoperatively. Physiologically, they can be acidotic and/or coagulopathic. Attention to volume status and appropriate resuscitation are therefore critical. Although the exact likelihood of simultaneous thoracic, abdominal, and head fractures or other injuries is not fully defined, they are much more likely and must be addressed prior to replantation [4, 6].

Once a patient with a major upper extremity amputation has been cleared for surgery, the same basic replantation principles apply as for distal replantation with regard to restoring anatomy. However, there are some significant differences between proximal and distal replantation surgery. These include debridement procedures, urgency of arterial restoration, fasciotomies for expected compartment syndrome, and the likelihood of complementary soft tissue coverage/secondary procedures in the first week after reattachment. The extent of surgical debridement is usually more extensive and time consuming and not uncommonly, significant necessary bone shortening. Timely intervention is needed to prevent ischemic muscular necrosis, and this may require an alteration from the standard distal replantation sequence. Temporary arterial bypass shunting is frequently performed to allow for more rapid arterial inflow resulting in restoration of aerobic metabolism and drainage of toxic metabolites. Fasciotomies will be required in almost all instances of major limb replantation, and the patient will also require at least one return to the operating room for additional exploration and debridement after demarcation has occurred. Finally, as the amputation site moves proximal, the surgeon and patient must understand that multiple reconstructive surgeries will likely be required to provide some combination of final soft tissue closure and/or coverage, identify and eradicate foci of deep infection, revise fixation, release scars, graft, or transfer nerves, or improve function.

Initial Evaluation

Timely, expeditious, and thorough evaluation of a patient presenting with a major upper limb amputation is critical. Full ATLS guidelines should be followed and other serious injuries ruled out before replantation can be considered. In the setting of a major trauma, assistance of a trauma surgery team is often helpful to expedite the evaluation and provide clarity with this aspect. A rapid secondary survey should be performed in an attempt to identify other potential injuries or sights of pain. A simultaneous thorough history by the replantation surgery team is necessary. Pertinent history includes determining the mechanism and energy of the injury as well as time from injury and method of storage of the amputated part. An assessment of potential contamination with organic material, standing water, or other contaminants should be done. The first responders may need to be specifically questioned in this regard. The patient's overall physical health and comorbidities should be identified by direct questioning or via family conference in the setting of an unconscious/unresponsive patient. General activity level, employment, and demands of the extremity should be ascertained.

A detailed examination of the proximal stump may not be possible until the patient is in the operating theater due to ongoing bleeding/bandages and tourniquets, but the distal segment should be quickly examined before returning it to a cold environment. In addition to confirming the level of amputation, the extent of the injury to all structures including the skin, skeletal elements, muscles and tendons, and neurovascular structures should be noted. Radiographic imaging of the proximal and distal segments is done. This aids in evaluation of the bony and/or articular injury and helps in preoperative planning for fixation options and needed bone shortening. Careful attention must be paid to the physical examination and radiographs of the distal segment of the amputated part, as segmental injuries can be missed. Worst of all, significant morbidity to a patient could occur if replantation of a nonviable amputation is initiated.

As part of the primary and secondary surveys, ascertainment of the patient's volume status is of critical importance. The vast majority of major upper limb amputation patients have experienced significant blood loss prior to arrival at the treating facility. Appropriate volume resuscitation through large-bore peripheral and/or central lines should be initiated. In those patients who have lost significant volume, a growing body of evidence supports volume resuscitation with fresh frozen plasma and apheresis platelets in conjunction with packed red blood cells [7]. When large volumes of transfused products are required, many have advocated for a 1:1:1 ratio [8]. Foley catheter placement in the emergency department is also necessary to ascertain adequacy of volume resuscitation. Expected urine output of at least 30 ml/h is the goal. A lactic acid less than 2 mmol/L and a base deficit between −2 and 2 are other helpful parameters in judging end-organ hypoperfusion as the resuscitation progresses through the surgical and postoperative phases [9].

Intravenous antibiotics and tetanus prophylaxis should be administered in the emergency department. An antibiotic regimen similar to that used for open fractures is preferred. Intravenous (IV) cefazolin plus additional gram-negative coverage with an aminoglycoside is usually initiated taking into account possible allergies. Anaerobic coverage with penicillin or Flagyl® (Pfizer, NY, NY) is typically added with organic contamination.

If the amputated segment has not been cooled upon arrival or has been improperly packaged, then immediate attention should be paid to this once segment. After examination, like all amputated segments, the arm is best wrapped in damp saline-soaked gauze inside a plastic bag placed on ice until it can be brought expeditiously to the operating room [10]. An immersion technique has also been described, but with the possible risk of increased edema of musculature, we favor the wrapping technique [11]. Once it has been determined that a replantation is indicated and the patient is healthy enough to proceed, it is ideal for the amputated segment to be brought to the operating room simultaneously to the patient being fully stabilized. This facilitates preparation for replantation, including cleaning and debridement of the distal segment as well as identification and/or tagging of important structures.

Patient Selection

Since the first viable replantation performed in 1962 by Malt and McKhann [12], replantation surgery has progressed so that now replantation centers should expect 80–90 % viability rates [13–17]. While viability implies that a replantation was successful from a vascular standpoint, functional success is not implied. The most important decision in this regard is in whom to perform replantation. When considering replantation proximal to the wrist, this patient selection issue takes on even greater importance. The main considerations include both patient factors and injury-specific factors. Patient factors include the general pre- and post-injury health. Injury factors include ischemia time, mechanism of injury, degree of contamination, and level of the amputation [4, 18]. Other important factors include patient desires and expectations as well as economical considerations.

Replantation Versus Prosthesis

The first guiding principle regarding replantation of an upper limb should be utility of a replantation compared to revision amputation and prosthesis fitting. Limited data exist on the subject, but that available indicates that major replantation offers superior results. Graham et al. compared 22 major replantations (16 forearm or proximal) and found that the likelihood of achieving a good or excellent result was significantly improved with replantation. The relationship was maintained when matched for age and level of injury [19]. Peacock and Tsai compared the function of a 12-year-old bilateral transhumeral amputee with one replanted limb and one revision amputation and prosthesis. She had better range of motion and strength on the replanted side and preferred it for daily use [20]. Interestingly, Wright et al. questioned 135 patients with wrist or proximal prostheses and found that 39 of 42 patients with a below-elbow prosthesis used the prosthesis, while only 9 of 21 and 8 of 14 patients used their above-elbow or wrist disarticulation prostheses, respectively [21]. Recent advances in upper extremity prostheses such as individually powered fingers have improved their usability, but lack of sensation remains a significant challenge [22].

Patient Condition (Fig. 7.1a–d)

As previously mentioned, patient's presenting with proximal amputations are generally much more physiologically "sick" than those with distal amputations. Full ATLS guidelines must be followed, and other serious and life-threatening injuries must be ruled out or appropriately treated prior beginning replantation. As previously mentioned, blood loss is a significant concern, and it is not uncommon for the amputee to be in the advanced stages of hypovolemic shock [23]. Massive transfusions may be required.

General patient health and comorbidities must therefore be given careful consideration. Pediatric patients, for example, are almost always excellent candidates for major replantation given their low rates of baseline comorbidities that are not significantly altered or made life threatening in the presence of hypovolemic shock as a result of the injury and subsequent surgeries. By comparison, an adult patient with significant comorbidities such as diabetes, coronary or peripheral vascular disease, or renal or hepatic impairment may not have the physiological capacity to endure further blood loss and the multiple secondary surgeries associated with major limb replantation. Generally speaking, elderly patients are poor candidates for major replantation surgeries for all of the reasons listed as well as the poor regenerative potential within the replanted limb.

Age itself is not an absolute determinant of replantation though. Replantation may be considered in a healthy elderly patient with a distal forearm amputation with reasonable expectation for some return of extrinsic finger muscle/tendon function and therefore an assistive hand. As discussed previously, almost any amputation should be considered for replantation in a healthy child [24–28]. Functional outcomes are bolstered by excellent musculoskeletal healing and nerve regeneration capabilities. Epiphyseal growth is generally retained but may be slowed, following replantation unless the amputation or debridement encroaches upon the physis [29–32]. Given that 80 % of humeral growth occurs at the proximal physis and the majority of forearm length occurs through the distal radial and ulnar growth plates, even direct injury to the elbow growth plates will result in limited long-term limb length inequality. In patients less than 10 years of age, excellent neuroregenerative capabilities will usually result in reasonable recovery of sensation. Loss of motion or function in denervated muscle is common. In patients over the age of 10, sensory return is less predictable, and motor function

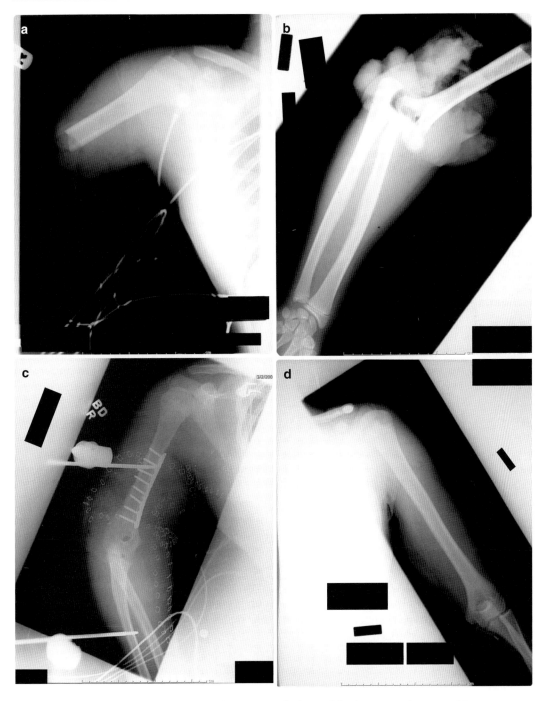

Fig. 7.1 (**a**) This transhumeral amputation with an associated elbow dislocation occurred as a result of an 11-year-old girl getting her sleeve caught in a manure spreader. (**b, c**) Despite the segmental injury and barnyard contamination, replantation was attempted as the patient's age was favorable and the limb arrived to the replant center on ice within 4 h of the injury. (**d**) A crude x-ray of the contralateral humerus is shown to allow for appreciation of the necessary shortening. While plate fixation was performed for humeral fixation, a spanning external fixator was temporarily used to stabilize the elbow joint. A pedicled latissimus flap was turned down to reconstruct the missing biceps/brachialis and also provide soft tissue coverage of the hardware. Ultimately the patient went on functional elbow range of motion and assist hand function but required a number of debridements for soft tissue infection, even up to 12 months following replantation

Table 7.1 Ischemic tolerance times by tissue

Muscle: 4 h
Nerve: 8 h
Fat: 13 h
Skin: 13 h
Bone: 4 days

Adapted with permission from Blaisdell [113]

in the hand is generally unexpected. Koul et al. presented the case of a 6-year-old girl who underwent bilateral proximal transhumeral replantations. At 23 months, she had regained sensation in both hands and only experienced denervation [33] of the left intrinsic requiring tendon transfers.

Ischemia Time

Ischemia time is especially critical when considering major limb replantation or revascularization. Of all the tissue found in the upper extremity, skeletal muscle is the least tolerant of ischemia. Experimental models have shown that skeletal muscle will tolerate 4 h of warm ischemia before myocyte death consistently begins [34–36]. At 6 h, near complete myocyte death is almost certain. The ability of muscle to survive to this extent seems to be linked to its ability to initially use glycogen and creatine phosphate as energy sources preferentially to adenosine triphosphate (ATP). However, once ATP depletion is initiated, myonecrosis occurs quickly [37]. Labbe et al. found that after 3, 4, and 5 h of ischemia, myonecrosis was 2, 30, and 90 %, respectively [38]. See Table 7.1 for ischemic tolerance by tissue type.

As a general rule, replantation of the forearm or arm should not be performed if the warm ischemia time is greater than 6 h. The extent of muscle necrosis beyond this point will preclude any reasonable expectation of functional recovery and, even more importantly, will expose the patient to the risk of metabolic and infectious complications implicit from the preservation of this nonviable tissue. Having an accurate time cutoff (as determined from the history) is vitally important because the clinical evaluation of ischemic necrosis can be unreliable as there is often

no gross evidence of myonecrosis until several hours after myocyte death. Laboratory findings have found that muscle necrosis initially occurs centrally with minimal peripheral involvement or clinical evidence in response to ischemia [38]. If the replantation is performed outside of this 6 h window, the near complete muscle necrosis will become clinically apparent within 24 h of the replantation and becomes an unnecessary major source of infection and/or vascular thrombosis. Infections can be severe and even life threatening resulting in sepsis or gas gangrene.

Determining whether a limb is warm ischemic versus cold ischemic is still a source of variability when deciding to proceed with a major limb replantation. There have been reports of successful major limb replantations beyond 6 h after amputation but only when the amputated limb has been significantly cooled for the majority of the avascular period. Tantry et al. reported on a series of 14 upper extremity replantations (2 wrist level and 12 proximal) that underwent replantation at an average of 12 h. Of these, nine limbs retained viable vascular status. Importantly, all limbs had less than 2 h of warm ischemia [39].

Preservation of Amputated Parts

In addition to constant adequate external cooling as described previously, perfusion of an amputated limb with cold physiologic solution coupled with adequate external cooling likely represents the most effective means to temporarily cool the amputated part both pre- and intraoperatively during the debridement phase. This can be accomplished with injection of cold (4 °C) heparinized Ringer's lactate or saline solution [18, 40] and external application of cold saline-soaked pads [40]. Perfusion with tissue preservation solutions such as University of Wisconsin (UW) or Euro-Collins (EC) solutions have also been used effectively both in animal experiments and clinically in preservation of amputated parts, although we have not had direct experience with these solutions [41–45]. When used, injection at 4 °C and 120 cm hydrostatic pressure has been found to be safe [42]. Once the part has been

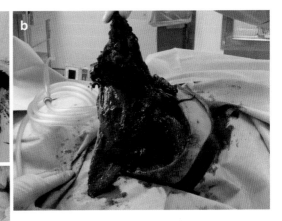

Fig. 7.2 (**a**) A high humeral complete avulsion-type amputation that was sustained after the 55-year-old farmer's arm was pulled into a hay bailer. Although the patient arrived between 2 and 3 h after amputation, the decision was not to replant given the patient's age, purely avulsion mechanism, proximal level of injury, and gross organic contamination. (**b**, **c**) Note the distal bone injury with varying levels of injury to the muscle, nerves, vessels, and skin proximally over a segment greater than 20 cm

injected and cleaned and appropriately tagged, it may be placed in refrigerator at 4 °C or packed appropriately in an ice-filled cooler if additional time is required.

Other proposed forms of tissue preservation include perfusion with heparinized arterial blood and storage in hyperbaric oxygen. Some limited data suggest that these may also have some efficacy [18, 46, 47].

Mechanism/Extent of Injury
(Fig. 7.2a–c)

Given the high-energy level required to produce a major limb amputation, many extremities are so mangled by the injury itself that the possibility of replantation is excluded. The degree of injury to both the amputated part and the proximal stump has been found to be good indicators for immediate- and long-term success of major replantation [48]. However, full assessment of the injury including the status of the distal microvasculature is oftentimes not possible until the operating room. Internal damage to the vasculature, both due to the amputation as well as ischemic damage, may render it impossible to successfully reperfuse the distal segment despite what appears to be an acceptable anastomosis, the "no reflow phenomenon."

Classically, there are three main mechanisms for amputation: guillotine, crush, and avulsion [4, 49]. Guillotine types are generally thought to be the most amenable to replantation given the typically smaller zone of injury and less extensive debridement required [13, 50, 51]. Most importantly, the nature of the injury does not typically avulse or stretch out the muscle units, nerves, and vessels during the course of the amputation. Unfortunately, most major proximal amputations

Table 7.2 Chuang classification for avulsion amputations based on neuromuscular level

Type I: Avulsion at or within the musculotendinous aponeurosis, remaining muscle functional and intact
Type II: Avulsion within the muscle bellies and distal to the neuromuscular junction, proximal muscle remains innervated
Type III: Avulsion within the muscle bellies and proximal to the neuromuscular junction, entire muscle is denervated
Type IV: Avulsion through the joint

Data from Chuang et al. [53]

are more frequently the result of a combination of all types, and often a predominance of the latter two mechanisms is typical. Given the heat involved with the machinery that causes many of these amputations, there is also a variable component of thermal injury. The resultant zone of thermal injury is often underappreciated in the early phase, much like burn surgery. This may result in significant loss of soft tissue coverage over vital structures a few days out from successful revascularization.

Crush type amputation injuries result in large zones of injury and irregular wounds. An avulsion component is sometimes present within the soft tissues as well, and these injuries are sometimes referred to as crush-avulsion injuries. Due to the large area of injured tissue, extensive debridement and significant shortening are generally required. However, when adequate, debridement is performed, and clean margins can be obtained; a crush injury can be converted to a guillotine type and does not necessarily preclude replantation or portend a poor functional outcome [5].

Avulsion injuries typically carry the worst prognosis with regard to replantation [4, 52]. Their poor prognosis is attributable to many factors. Tissues in avulsion injuries are torn as opposed to cut. The individual structures are usually disrupted at different levels, and the zone of injury extends over a long distance. Tendons are often torn from their muscular junction rendering them next to impossible to repair. Chuang et al. proposed a classification for avulsion amputations based not on bony level but rather on neuromuscular level [53] See Table 7.2. Several studies

have found this classification a useful predictor of functional level [53–55].

What this classification fails to address is that the neurovascular damage is usually extensive, and it is difficult to clinically assess the healthy margins of the damaged nerve and vascular tissues in the acute phase. Consequently, even after shortening the nerves and vessels, damaged tissues can easily be coapted together. This renders repaired vessels prone to thrombosis, and neurologic recovery is often compromised. If the decision is made to proceed with a replant in the setting of an avulsion type of injury, long interposition vascular grafts are typically indicated to bypass damaged vessel segments. When these long vascular grafts are performed, it is quite likely that distal perfusion can be restored, and there is typically initial optimism with the results. However, the critical perfusion of the muscle bellies in the intervening segmental zone that has been literally bypassed can be further compromised by this long vein graft and can result in a large area of secondary muscle necrosis. In the setting of an avulsion-type amputation, especially in a contaminated environment, successful replantation may simply be impossible, and as the level of injury ascends to the proximal forearm and above, it is generally in the patient's best interest to proceed directly with revision amputation and wound closure.

Level of Amputation

While the mechanism of amputation is the most important consideration when deciding whether to proceed with replantation, the level of amputation actually plays the most important role in determining functional prognosis. Generally, the more distal the level of the amputation, the better the anticipated functional outcomes after replantation [4, 17, 19, 52, 56]. In distal forearm amputations, outcomes are improved due to the ability to repair musculotendon units mostly through tendon, the level of injury occurring distal to the nerve end-plate innervation of the majority of the forearm musculature, a smaller distance required for nerve regeneration, the need to only repair the medial and ulnar nerves, and the injury occurring in an area of usually rapid bone healing [57, 58]. Successful reinnervation may be possible before end-organ atrophy has occurred.

The prognosis for proximal forearm amputations is more guarded primarily due to the loss of nervous innervation to an increasing number of musculotendon units [59]. Amputations through the elbow joint carry an even lower prognosis for return of clinical function to the hand. Elbow flexion and extension can be restored if the joint is stable, but injury to and potential subsequent degeneration of the joint compound the surrounding soft tissue injury. The result is frequently loss of range of motion. While revascularization of transhumeral amputations can be successfully accomplished, they carry an extremely guarded functional prognosis due to poor restoration of nerve function [16, 60]. Although the hand may regain protective sensation [16, 60], it is unusual that significant wrist and finger muscle function will return except in the setting of pediatric replantation [26]. However, if functional elbow flexion and extension can be achieved (with or without functional muscle transfers), there may be some utility if conversion to a below-elbow prosthesis can be achieved [18, 21]. Segmental amputations generally carry a poor prognosis and are relative contraindications to replantation. However, in select patients such as the pediatric population or those with clean, guillotine-type wounds, replantation may be considered [2, 61].

Surgical Treatment

Initial surgical treatment of the major upper limb replantations involves a thorough cleaning and debridement. When the patient arrives in the operating room, the affected arm and at least one leg should be prepped into the operative field. At the same time a critical inspection of the tissue is carried out and a rapid decision made as to whether replantation is a viable option. Meticulous debridement is critical and should be carried out under loupe magnification.

If possible, this should be performed under an appropriate tourniquet to minimize blood loss and facilitate the speed of the process. All devitalized, avascular muscle should be removed back to the tendinous junction, and fascial planes between the skin and muscle as well as between major muscle groups should be aggressively inspected for debris. Muscle adjacent to the amputation site is often severely injured and must be trimmed back a minimum of 1–2 cm. Bone shortening of an amputation is inevitable, and even with a guillotine-like wound, a minimum of 3 cm of total shortening is routine.

The importance of the debridement phase cannot be overstated. Major limb amputations are high-energy injuries that commonly result from highly contaminating mechanisms, and farm and industrial accidents are typical. Given the inherent risk of myonecrosis, infection is the most common and potentially devastating complication of major limb replantation. Replantation is aborted if the part cannot be debrided to a clean wound, the extent of damage is too severe, the ischemia time is prolonged, or the amputated part is not perfusable due to microvascular damage [62, 63]. Once the wound is converted to a clean, guillotine-type wound, tagging of neurovascular structures can be performed, and tendon ends can be sutured in preparation for repair. The bone ends are then approximated for appropriate fixation. During this process, it is advisable to perfuse the amputated part with 1 L or more of cold heparinized saline or ringer's lactate to flush out stationary blood and prime the vascular system. While UW solution can also be used for a complete amputation, it must not be used to perfuse an incomplete amputation as it is highly systemically toxic. UW solution must be completely flushed out of an amputated part prior to venous repair. Throughout the debridement, the intraoperative hypothermia should be maintained with bags of ice placed on the amputated part.

The foundation of major upper limb replantation is early revascularization. For this reason, once the decision to proceed with replantation is made, prompt vascular shunting (even prior to bone fixation) can be performed [64–67]. This can be performed directly from the proximal stump or with the use of the contralateral arm or femoral artery [68, 69]. If the amputation is incomplete and adequate venous drainage exists, then the vascular dilemma is less problematic as arterial shunting is all that is required. In complete amputations or incomplete injuries with inadequate venous return, venous shunting (after a delay of 10–15 min to allow for drainage of toxic metabolites) can be performed to help minimize blood loss [66]. Shunting may be performed with a large intravascular (IV) catheter, ventriculoperitoneal (VP) shunt, or Sundt's carotid shunt. Our experience is that this approach should be considered if the ischemia time is approaching 6 h for forearm amputations or 4 h for upper arm amputations.

If system limitations or geographic restrictions predict that the transport time of an injury of this type to a replant center will be prolonged (greater than 6 h), initial judicious debridement and vascular shunting may be best performed by the referring institution prior to transport if a vascular surgeon is available [63]. While temporary shunting may be the only way to get a major upper limb amputation to a replantation center within the ischemic window, great care must be taken when transporting after shunting. The shunts must be secured firmly, and the patient should be sent with several units of packed red blood cells for transport as continuous bleeding is expected and life-threatening exsanguination is a real possibility. Other authors have favored perfusing the limb with heparinized arterial blood when delay in transport is expected [18].

Once the amputation has been successfully debrided and the injury is deemed to be replantable, the sequence of repair of a major upper extremity amputation differs from digital- and hand-level replantations. There is no one definitive sequence of events that must be followed, but generally speaking, rapid reestablishment of arterial inflow is paramount. Once a decision is made whether to shunt based upon the guidelines set out above, a general, reasonable order for a replantation protocol is as follows:

1. Rapid bone shortening and stable fixation
2. Arterial repair
3. Venous repair
4. Muscle/tendon repair
5. Nerve repair if possible
6. Skin coverage and/or soft tissue coverage reconstruction

Bone Fixation/Shortening (Fig. 7.3a–e)

Bone should be shortened to remove contamination and comminution as well as allow for direct well-approximated bony apposition that allows for ease of fixation and reliable bone healing. Rapid but stable fixation that allows for early motion is key [70, 71]. We prefer to use plates when possible, and in adults, 3.5 mm dynamic compression plates (DCP) are preferred for the forearm and 4.5 mm DCP plates for the humerus. Pediatric patients will need more size appropriate fixation – and any combination of 2.0–4.5 mm compression plates can be appropriate for either forearm or humerus depending upon the size of the child. If the bone is tightly apposed transversely, then standard compression plating techniques are sufficient, whereas locking screws may be indicated for spanning type constructs if length preservation is required. In forearm amputations, resection of the distal ulna can be considered if the injury is too distal for shortening or too comminuted for repair. Creation of a one-bone forearm should also be considered if bone comminution precludes rapid and stable fixation of both forearm bones. In the very uncommon instance where there is an associated unstable elbow not amenable to internal fixation and ligament repair, a spanning external fixator could be used.

The amount of shortening should be judged critically before final fixation performed, and one should err on the side of slightly too much shortening rather than not enough. Proper shortening enables adequate debridement of the zone of injury and facilitates reapproximation of the musculotendinous units and neurovascular structures and sets up a higher likelihood of primary soft tissue approximation.

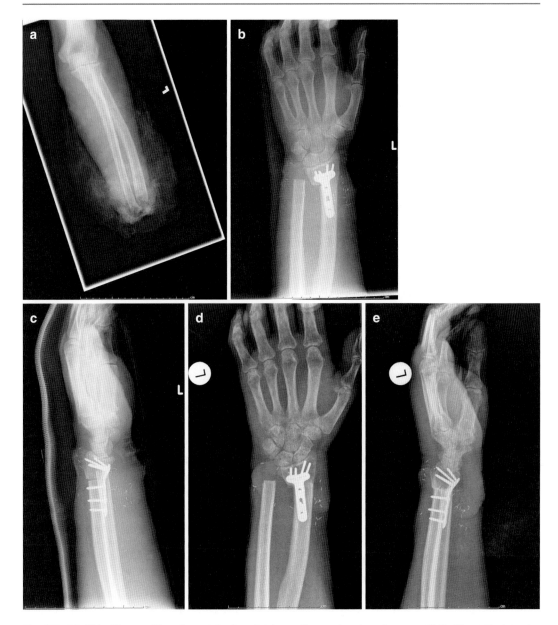

Fig. 7.3 (**a**) This 66-year-old male sustained a distal forearm amputation as a result of a radial arm saw with a resultant sharp mechanism and narrow zone of injury – primarily thermal. (**b**, **c**) Skeletal shortening and fixation were accomplished with volar plating of the distal radius and Darrach-type resection of the small portion of distal ulnar head that remained with the distal segment. (**d**, **e**) The replantation was successful in the short term, and the radius went on to unite uneventfully. The patient eventually achieved very strong flexion and extension of the fingers with a secondary tenolysis performed 6 months after index procedure. Sensory return to the hand was limited, and intrinsic motor function was absent. An extensor indicis opponensplasty was performed at the time of tenolysis to improve thumb function even though this tendon had been repaired at the time of amputation

Arterial Repair

Arteries must be debrided to healthy ends with no apparent intimal damage via inspection under magnification. This is best judged by testing the adherence of the intima to the muscularis layer. The microscope facilitates examination of the vessels, particularly below the elbow. Tensionless direct repair is preferable but often not possible, and interposition vein grafting should be performed as required. If two surgical teams are present, one team can rapidly harvest the saphenous vein, while the other team stabilizes the bone and freshens the arterial inflow. Saphenous vein harvested from above the knee works well as a size match for grafting of the brachial artery, while vein from the same system below the knee works well for the radial and/or ulnar arteries. Judging the appropriate length of a vein graft to inset into the arm can be tricky, especially when the graft crosses the elbow joint. As the arm and elbow are usually laying in extension during replantation, the arterial repair is usually performed in extension. This can result in the graft being subjected to kinking when the elbow is later flexed and the graft accordions on itself. In forearm amputations, one or both arteries may be repaired depending upon the quality and size of both vessels.

Venous Repair

Veins are repaired after a 10–15-min period of time has passed after arterial repair to allow for physiologic washout of the vascular system. At least two veins should be repaired, and three or more are ideal. Large cutaneous veins are generally easier to dissect and repair than the deep veins, which tend to be harder to dissect as they are thinner walled and more adherent to the surrounding deep muscle due to frequent branches. However, in some crush or avulsion injuries with skin compromise and/or loss, the venae comitantes may be the only repairable veins. Proximal to the wrist, these veins are usually of an adequate diameter to be repaired and do provide adequate drainage despite their smaller stature.

The artery can be unclamped during venous repair. Some surgeons will administer a systemic bolus of heparin at this point to help prevent thrombosis of the arterial repair, typically 2,500–3,000 units, although the necessity of this is unclear, and anastomosis patency seems more related to surgical technique [72, 73]. Additionally, if ischemia time has been prolonged or if extensive

muscle mass is present, a bolus of sodium bicarbonate prior to unclamping of the vein and return of acidic byproducts to the system circulation can be considered. This is typically given at a dose of 1 meq/kg body weight (usually 1.5–2 ampules) and is run in slowly over roughly 5 min prior to unclamping of the repaired vein.

Musculotendinous Repair

Repair is significantly easier in distal forearm guillotine-type amputations where the flexor and extensor tendons can be directly repaired. Repair is performed with the surgeons preferred method but should allow for early mobilization; we prefer a six-strand cruciate-type repair.

The flexor pollicis longus tendon is often the most compromised because of its very distal belly. If it is nonviable or not repairable, then transfer of the index profundus at the time of replant should be performed to restore this critical thumb function. The index profundus tendon can be sutured side to side to the middle finger in this scenario.

Amputations through the muscle bellies or at the musculotendinous junction more proximally in the forearm present a greater challenge. In this setting, the tendon is typically woven through any remaining proximal tendon and the muscle belly and secured with nonabsorbable suture. When this is not possible, the epimysium is reapproximated to try and reduce the gap in the muscle fibers, and a layered repair from deep to superficial is sometimes helpful to better align fibers and eliminate dead space that serves as a nidus for hematoma and/or infection. In some amputations where little to no functional return would be expected because of tendon or muscle loss in a given muscle or muscle group, tendon grafts or tendon transfers may be used for primary reconstruction, although one must be certain of the viability and preserved innervations of both the tendon to be transferred as well as the synergistic tendons remaining.

The biceps and triceps are generally easily approximated for amputations at the level of the elbow, but when the injury is more than 4–5 cm above the distal humerus, the tendons may not be repairable. In the higher-energy injuries typical of transhumeral level, significant loss of the muscle can represent both a functional as well as a wound closure problem. Oftentimes, a rotational muscle transfer utilizing the latissimus dorsi provides a healthy wound coverage solution, and the transferred tendon can even be inset and tensioned such that it can be functional to help restore elbow flexion or extension [74–77].

Nerve Repair

If a tensionless primary repair can be performed after bone shortening and trimming of the nerve ends back to what appears to be healthy margins, a primary epineural repair may be performed. After the nerves are trimmed back under the microscope, it is not uncommon that the gap between the nerves is not amenable to direct repair, and nerve grafts are required. Grafting is generally performed primarily with sural nerve grafts if the replantation appears stable and the wounds are able to be reapproximated over the graft. If the replant viability is questionable or the soft tissue coverage is uncertain, grafts can be performed at a later date. Delayed nerve grafting has the advantage of allowing one to determine that the limb can be successfully revascularized, decreasing the morbidity of an unnecessary nerve graft harvest. Additionally, a delay provides a situation wherein a healthy margin of the nerve can be better determined and one can ensure that nerve grafts can be inset against healthy fascicles proximal to the zone of injury. If delayed nerve repair is chosen, nerve ends should be tagged to facilitate identification at a later time.

Skin Coverage

Like muscles, skin edges should be debrided until healthy, bleeding edges are obtained. In extensive crush-avulsion injuries, large deficits may be the result, and in the early hours after the injury, definitive margins may be very difficult to determine. If skin edges cannot be directly apposed, the goal is for early, but not necessarily immediate, coverage. A combination of rotational or transposition skin flaps, pedicled muscle flaps, and skin grafts can be used to close wounds. Wounds should be allowed to drain and initially may either be left open or covered with a negative pressure device as long as neurovascular structures, especially vein grafts, are not exposed. In some instances, grafts may need to be placed or tunneled into extra-anatomic positions to facilitate soft tissue coverage. While, split-thickness skin grafts may be used to cover native vessels or nerve grafts, in no instances should skin graft be placed directly over vein grafts due to the risk of desiccation, thrombosis, or even rupture. Immediate rotational tissue transfer with the latissimus may be useful, and, occasionally, free tissue transfer is required.

Once the initial skin closure and coverage of vein or nerve grafts are performed, fasciotomies of the forearm are generally indicated for all major upper extremity limb replantations [5, 23].

All patients return to the operating room in 2–3 days for a repeat examination and debridements as necessary. In cases of severely contaminated wounds, two or more debridements may be required. Definitive wound closure of the fasciotomies can sometimes be accomplished with delayed primary closure, but split-thickness grafting is more typically utilized at this point once the viability of the underlying fasciotomy bed is ascertained.

Postoperative Care

Postoperatively, the patient is admitted to the intensive care unit for close monitoring of the flap, but this also serves the dual purpose of monitoring the patient for signs and symptoms of reperfusion syndrome. A Foley catheter is maintained, and urine output is monitored with a goal of 2.5 ml/kg/h [78]. Telemetry is necessary due to the concern for hyperkalemia. Serial lab work is performed to monitor for renal function, blood counts, and disseminated intravascular coagulation (DIC). Intravenous fluids and blood products are given as needed to maintain intravascular volume. The hematocrit should be kept between 20 and 25 at a minimum and higher if the patient has underlying cardiac risk factors. Intravenous antibiotics are given until the time of definitive wound closure.

The hand is kept elevated, and all standard efforts are made to reduce vasospasm. The room is kept warm, caffeine and nicotine are prohibited, and pain is controlled to the maximal extent possible. In cases of distal forearm replants, an indwelling proximal nerve catheter placed by an anesthesiologist may be utilized. In cases of significant patient anxiety, benzodiazepines are given.

Dressings should provide adequate padding and absorb drainage but should be kept sufficiently loose in order to prevent any obstruction to venous outflow. The dressing may be windowed to allow access for clinical checks as well as additional monitoring. Frequent dressing changes may be required as they become soiled, although dressings directly over skin grafts should simply be debulked and reinforced, rather than risking dislodgment of grafts with complete dressing changes in the first few days.

The method of immobilization varies depending on the level of the injury but typically consists of an above-elbow splint with the elbow at 70–80° and the wrist maintained in slight extension. Fingers can be splinted to prevent clawing by ensuring there is metacarpophalangeal joint flexion in the splint.

Clinical evaluation remains the standard for monitoring [79, 80]. Clinical checks are performed hourly by trained nurses for the first 2 post-operative days 1 and 2 by trained nurses. The replant is assessed for color, warmth, and cap refill if an area of skin is visible. Checks are changed to every 2 h on postoperative day 3 and then discontinued on postoperative day 4 or 5. If clinical suspicion for vessel compression exists, constricting dressings are removed. Intermittent sutures may also be removed to relieve pressure. Ultimately, if perfusion is compromised or even strongly suspected, the patient should return to the operating room immediately for examination under anesthesia. Revascularization will need to occur rapidly in order to save the replant, although a second hit

of anoxia may be more than the compromised limb can recover from and result in ultimate loss of the replant.

Several additional monitoring methods have been proposed for replants, including indwelling and handheld Doppler probes, surface temperature monitoring, laser Doppler, and near-infrared spectroscopy [80]. Most of these are commonly used for monitoring of microvascular anastomoses following free tissue transfer and may also be utilized in the replant setting. When skin overlying the cutaneous arteries is present, the area is marked for monitoring with a handheld Doppler. We routinely place an indwelling Doppler probe on the vein at a minimum and on the artery as well if the dressings prevent surface monitoring. Studies have indicated that an indwelling venous Doppler has a false-negative rate of 0 % and a false-positive rate of 6.7 % [81, 82].

Anticoagulation

Pre-, intra-, and postoperative anticoagulation is an area of great controversy for all replants, and major upper extremity injuries are no different [83–87]. We prefer to start patients on LMWH at deep vein thrombosis prophylaxis dosing and continue this throughout their hospitalization. We do not routinely use any other chemical anticoagulation specifically for the vascular anastomoses. While aspirin, heparin, low-molecular-weight heparin (LMWH), and dextran or a similar branched polysaccharide have all been described, many microvascular surgeons elect to use no pre-, intra-, or postoperative antithrombosis prophylaxis and report good results in a free flap population, and we use the same protocols for our free flaps and replants [87, 88].

Expectations

Outcomes after major upper limb replantation can be measured in a number of different ways. Despite early vascular viability, exceeding 90–95 %, the need for ultimate amputation after successful replantation may be delayed days or

Table 7.3 Chen classification for grading replantation functional outcomes

Grade	Functional level
I	Ability to resume previous work with critical contribution from the replanted part
	Collective range of joint motion exceeds 60 % of normal, including the joint just proximal to the amputation
	Nearly complete sensory recovery with minimal cold intolerance
	Muscle power grade 4 or 5
II	Able to resume work but not original employment
	Range of joint motion exceeds 40 %
	Nearly complete sensory recovery in median and ulnar nerve distributions without severe cold intolerance
	Muscle power grade 3 or 4
III	Able to perform activities of daily living independently
	Range of motion exceeds 30 %
	Poor but useful sensory recovery (example only protective sensation recovered)
	Muscle power grade 3
IV	Tissue survival without useful functional recovery

Adapted with permission from Zhong-Wei et al. [4]

even weeks due to the time necessary for myonecrosis and/or secondary infection to stabilize, and so initial optimism should be tempered in all discussions with patients. A thorough discussion with the patient and family about how reattaching the arm does not guarantee that the structures within the arm will work again is critical to laying a realistic expectation of what can actually be accomplished in the long term.

Functional outcome is never complete and remains largely unpredictable [5, 53, 60, 89–91]. However, the main three factors influencing this are level of injury, ischemia time, and extent of wound damage, including near amputation versus complete amputation. Other factors include age, patient condition, type of vessel and nerve repair required, extent of bone shortening, and wound contamination among others. In 1981, Chen proposed a classification for grading replantation functional outcomes that has now become the outcome reporting standard in the literature [4]. The classification incorporates four main factors: return to work, range of motion, sensation, and strength. See Table 7.3.

Gulgonen and Ozer reported on nine patients, including four distal arm and elbow disarticulations, with a minimum of 15 years follow-up. All patients regained protective sensation. As expected, the forearm replantations regained more grip and pinch strength. No patient advanced a Chen grade after 5 years from surgery, but cold intolerance did improve up to 12 years from surgery [55].

In his classic 1981 article, Chen noted that functional recovery rapidly and progressively diminishes as the level of amputation moves proximally up the arm [4]. Battison et al. found in a series of 52 forearm, elbow, and arm replants that 75 % of their forearm replants achieved Chen grade I or II while only 33 % of their elbow and arm replants obtained this same level [5]. Hierner et al. reported on 65 patients and observed a "functional extremity" (Chen I or II) in 58, 30, and 25 % with distal forearm, proximal forearm, and upper arm replantation, respectively [91]. Yaffe et al. observed that functional recovery in their patients was closely linked to Chuang's classification relating the amputation site to the level of innervation. The injuries that occurred distal to the innervations of the extrinsics all did good or excellent, while only four of the nine replantations performed proximal to the neuromuscular interface did good with no excellent results [56].

Complications

Most complications related to major upper extremity replantations and near-amputation reconstructions are merely extensions of the injury. Deep infections are not infrequent despite attention to detail during debridement and must be treated with additional surgical debridement, antibiotics, and occasionally free tissue coverage. When treated appropriately, salvage of the replant is frequently possible [92, 93]. Other complications include non-septic soft tissue necrosis, nonunion, unrecognized brachial plexus palsies, stiffness, sensory deficits, and even complex regional pain syndrome.

Reperfusion Injury

Reperfusion injury is a complication that is specific to major limb replantation and consists of both local and systemic components [39]. Locally, reactive oxygen species and other inflammatory breakdown products of ischemic cells produce an inflammatory response with reperfusion. This is both predictable and unavoidable in all replantations of this nature, and some propagation of the tissue injury is expected as a result. This is partly responsible for the significant swelling and edema observed clinically in the replanted limb within the first 4–6 h after reperfusion. Extension of endothelial damage causes arterial vasoconstriction and intravascular thrombosis and may result in propagation of the no reflow phenomenon [94].

The systemic effects of reperfusion after major limb replantation have been known since the first years following the first major limb replant [95]. These include hypotension, acidosis, hyperkalemia, myoglobinuria, disseminated intravascular coagulation, and end-organ failure. Greater than 4 h of warm ischemia in any major muscle mass is a risk factor for systemic reperfusion injury, and the risk increases with the duration of ischemia [39, 96, 97]. The systemic aspect of the reperfusion injury can be severe and can threaten both the limb and life [98–101]. Clinically, reperfusion syndrome can manifest as fever and altered mental status. A severe systemic inflammatory response can lead to widespread endothelial damage and significant third spacing. In this situation, under resuscitation results in end-organ hypoperfusion and acute renal failure, while over-resuscitation can often lead to pulmonary edema. Studies have found that the main cause of mortality due to reperfusion syndrome is cardiopulmonary. Cardiac dysfunction has also been reported.

Numerous treatments including antioxidants, antithrombotics, hyperbaric oxygen, and post-reperfusion hypothermia among others have been proposed in the treatment of ischemia-reperfusion injury [102–104], but currently the mainstay of treatment is supportive care in an intensive care unit with adequate volume resuscitation. Ultimately, if the clinical picture is sufficiently severe or does not resolve with supportive measures, reamputation is necessary [75, 101].

Secondary Procedures

Secondary procedures after successful replantation surgery at the level of the proximal forearm, elbow, or above are generally the rule and not the exception. Chew and Tsai had an average of 3.1 additional procedures in their series of 34 viable wrist and proximal replantations [18]. As Sabapathy [105] describes it, these are of two varieties. The first is to correct soft tissue contracture or joint stiffness. The second is function enhancing procedures including tendon transfers, tendon or nerve repair, or selective arthrodesis.

Common secondary procedures include tendon transfers, tenolysis, neurolysis, capsular releases, nerve grafting, skin grafting, flap coverage, and functional muscle transfers (free or rotational) and are discussed further in Chap. 14.

Special Considerations

Temporary Ectopic Replantation

Temporary ectopic replantation has been used both as a means to primarily delay definitive orthotopic replantation and to salvage prior replantations complicated by infection. Wang et al. replanted two complex forearm amputations to the contralateral upper extremity to allow for treatment of critical injuries and soft tissue improvement [106]. Chernofsky and Sauer temporarily replanted a midforearm amputation to the abdominal wall with successful orthotopic replantation at 11 weeks [107]. Cavadas et al. reported the case of a transhumeral amputation that was initially orthotopically replanted at roughly 6 h of warm ischemia time. Subsequent infection at the replantation site failed multiple debridements. At 5 days postoperatively, the arm was transferred to the thigh via a superficial femoral artery-greater saphenous vein arteriovenous fistula. Orthotopic replantation was performed 9 days later using the retained vein graft with ultimate functional outcome of Chen grade III [108].

Crossover Limb Replantation

In the rare setting of bilateral amputation in which the extent of the proximal and distal injuries precludes orthotopic replantation yet a replantable wound exists proximally on one side and distally on the contralateral limb, crossover limb replantation may be considered. This is particularly true when the amputation on one side occurs proximally and distally on the other. This allows the surgeon to cleanly revise the amputation to the needed level based on the contralateral proximal stump. Most reports have involved crossover at the level of the forearm [109–111], but Oscelik et al. do report a case of crossover replantation at the transhumeral level combined with functional latissimus dorsi transposition, achieving a Chen grade III functional outcome. The patient ultimately declined a revision amputation with conversion to a below-elbow prosthesis as he was capable of using the arm for basic daily activities [112].

References

1. White JC. Nerve regeneration after replantation of severed arms. Ann Surg. 1969;170(5):715–9.
2. Russell RC, O'Brien BM, Morrison WA, Pamamull G, MacLeod A. The late functional results of upper limb revascularization and replantation. J Hand Surg Am. 1984;9(5):623–33.
3. Blomgren I, Blomqvist G, Ejeskar A, Fogdestam I, Volkman R, Edshage S. Hand function after replantation or revascularization of upper extremity injuries. A follow-up study of 21 cases operated on 1979–1985 in Goteborg. Scand J Plast Reconstr Surg Hand Surg. 1988;22(1):93–101.
4. Zhong-Wei C, Meyer VE, Kleinert HE, Beasley RW. Present indications and contraindications for replantation as reflected by long-term functional results. Orthop Clin North Am. 1981;12(4):849–70.
5. Battiston B, Tos P, Clemente A, Pontini I. Actualities in big segments replantation surgery. J Plast Reconstr Aesthet Surg. 2007;60(7):849–55.
6. Omoke NI, Chukwu CO, Madubueze CC, Egwu AN. Traumatic extremity amputation in a Nigerian setting: patterns and challenges of care. Int Orthop. 2012; 36(3):613–8.
7. Neal MD, Marsh A, Marino R, Kautza B, Raval JS, Forsythe RM, et al. Massive transfusion: an evidence-based review of recent developments. Arch Surg. 2012;147(6):563–71.
8. Cushing M, Shaz BH. Blood transfusion in trauma patients: unresolved questions. Minerva Anestesiol. 2011;77(3):349–59.
9. Porter JM, Ivatury RR. In search of the optimal end points of resuscitation in trauma patients: a review. J Trauma. 1998;44(5):908–14.
10. Morgan RF, Reisman NR, Curtis RM. Preservation of upper extremity devascularizations and amputations for replantation. Am Surg. 1982;48(9):481–3.
11. VanGiesen PJ, Seaber AV, Urbaniak JR. Storage of amputated parts prior to replantation–an experimental study with rabbit ears. J Hand Surg Am. 1983;8(1):60–5.
12. Malt RA, McKhann C. Replantation of severed arms. JAMA. 1964;189:716–22.
13. Axelrod TS, Buchler U. Severe complex injuries to the upper extremity: revascularization and replantation. J Hand Surg Am. 1991;16(4):574–84.
14. Leclere FM, Mathys L, Juon B, Franz T, Unglaub F, Vogelin E. Macroreplantations of the upper extremity: a series of 11 patients. Arch Orthop Trauma Surg. 2012;132(12):1797–805.
15. Tamai S. Twenty years' experience of limb replantation-review of 293 upper extremity replants. J Hand Surg Am. 1982;7:549–56.
16. Wood MB, Cooney WP. Above elbow limb replantation: functional results. J Hand Surg Am. 1986;11: 682–7.
17. Malt RA, Remensnyder JP, Harris WH. Long-term utility of replanted arms. Ann Surg. 1972;176(3):334–42.
18. Chew WY, Tsai TM. Major upper limb replantation. Hand Clin. 2001;17(3):395–410, viii.
19. Graham B, Adkins P, Tsai TM, Firrell J, Breidenbach WC. Major replantation versus revision amputation and prosthetic fitting in the upper extremity: a late functional outcomes study. J Hand Surg Am. 1998;23(5):783–91.
20. Peacock K, Tsai TM. Comparison of functional results of replantation versus prosthesis in a patient with bilateral arm amputation. Clin Orthop Relat Res. 1987;214:153–9.
21. Wright TW, Hagen AD, Wood MB. Prosthetic usage in major upper extremity amputations. J Hand Surg Am. 1995;20(4):619–22.
22. Zlotolow DA, Kozin SH. Advances in upper extremity prosthetics. Hand Clin. 2012;28(4):587–93.
23. Goldner RD, Nunley JA. Replantation proximal to the wrist. Hand Clin. 1992;8(3):413–25.
24. Beris AE, Soucacos PN, Malizos KN, Mitsionis GJ, Soucacos PK. Major limb replantation in children. Microsurgery. 1994;15(7):474–8.

25. Zuker RM, Stevenson JH. Proximal upper limb replantation in children. J Trauma. 1988;28(4):544–7.
26. Daigle JP, Kleinert JM. Major limb replantation in children. Microsurgery. 1991;12(3):221–31.
27. Sood R, Bentz ML, Shestak KC, Browne Jr EZ. Extremity replantation. Surg Clin North Am. 1991;71(2):317–29.
28. Shenaq SM, Dinh TA. Pediatric microsurgery. Replantation, revascularization, and obstetric brachial plexus palsy. Clin Plast Surg. 1990;17(1):77–83.
29. Demiri E, Bakhach J, Tsakoniatis N, Martin D, Baudet J. Bone growth after replantation in children. J Reconstr Microsurg. 1995;11(2):113–22; discussion 122–3.
30. Nunley JA, Spiegl PV, Goldner RD, Urbaniak JR. Longitudinal epiphyseal growth after replantation and transplantation in children. J Hand Surg Am. 1987;12(2):274–9.
31. Kropfl A, Gasperschitz F, Niederwieser B, Primavesi C, Hertz H. Epiphyseal growth after replantation in childhood. Handchir Mikrochir Plast Chir. 1994;26(4):194–9.
32. Raimondi PL, Petrolati M, Delaria G. Replantation of large segments in children. Hand Clin. 2000;16(4):547–61.
33. Koul AR, Cyriac A, Khaleel VM, Vinodan K. Bilateral high upper limb replantation in a child. Plast Reconstr Surg. 2004;113(6):1734–8; discussion 1739–41.
34. Sabido F, Milazzo VJ, Hobson 2nd RW, Duran WN. Skeletal muscle ischemia-reperfusion injury: a review of endothelial cell-leukocyte interactions. J Invest Surg. 1994;7(1):39–47.
35. Strock PE, Majno G. Microvascular changes in acutely ischemic rat muscle. Surg Gynecol Obstet. 1969;129(6):1213–24.
36. Eckert P, Schnackerz K. Ischemic tolerance of human skeletal muscle. Ann Plast Surg. 1991;26(1):77–84.
37. Eisenhardt HJ, Isselhard W, Prangenberg G, Pichlmaier H, Klein PJ. Energy metabolism and histomorphological findings in replanted rat hind limbs using various conservation methods. Microsurgery. 1984;5(2):61–9.
38. Labbe R, Lindsay T, Walker PM. The extent and distribution of skeletal muscle necrosis after graded periods of complete ischemia. J Vasc Surg. 1987;6(2):152–7.
39. Tantry TP, Kadam D, Shenoy SP, Bhandary S, Adappa KK. Perioperative evaluation and outcomes of major limb replantations with ischemia periods of more than 6 hours. J Reconstr Microsurg. 2013;29(3):165–72.
40. Rosen HM, Slivjak MJ, McBrearty FX. The role of perfusion washout in limb revascularization procedures. Plast Reconstr Surg. 1987;80(4):595–605.
41. Hicks TE, Boswick Jr JA, Solomons CC. The effects of perfusion on an amputated extremity. J Trauma. 1980;20(8):632–48.
42. Kour AK, Phone MH, Chia J, Pho RW. A preliminary report of tissue preservation with University of Wisconsin cold storage solution in major limb replantation. Ann Acad Med Singapore. 1995;24(4 Suppl):37–41.
43. Yokoyama K, Kimura M, Itoman M. Rat whole-limb viability after cold immersion using University of Wisconsin and Euro-Collins solutions. Transplantation. 1996;62(7):884–8.
44. Norden MA, Rao VK, Southard JH. Improved preservation of rat hindlimbs with the University of Wisconsin solution and butanedione monoxime. Plast Reconstr Surg. 1997;100(4):957–65.
45. Tsuchida T, Kato T, Yamaga M, Ikebe K, Oniki Y, Irie H, et al. Effect of perfusion during ischemia on skeletal muscle. J Surg Res. 2001;101(2):238–41.
46. Shimizu H, Tsai TM, Firrell JC. Effect of ischemia and three different perfusion solutions on the rabbit epiphyseal growth plate. Microsurgery. 1995;16(9):639–45.
47. Edwards RJ, Im MJ, Hoopes JE. Effects of hyperbaric oxygen preservation on rat limb replantation: a preliminary report. Ann Plast Surg. 1991;27(1):31–5.
48. Waikakul S, Vanadurongwan V, Unnanuntana A. Prognostic factors for major limb re-implantation at both immediate and long-term follow-up. J Bone Joint Surg Br. 1998;80(6):1024–30.
49. Trautwein LC, Smith DG, Rivara FP. Pediatric amputation injuries: etiology, cost, and outcome. J Trauma. 1996;41(5):831–8.
50. Ipsen T, Lundkvist L, Barfred T, Pless J. Principles of evaluation and results in microsurgical treatment of major limb amputations. A follow-up study of 26 consecutive cases 1978–1987. Scand J Plast Reconstr Surg Hand Surg. 1990;24(1):75–80.
51. Patradul A, Ngarmukos C, Parkpian V. Major limb replantation: a Thai experience. Ann Acad Med Singapore. 1995;24(4 Suppl):82–8.
52. Atzei A, Pignatti M, Maria Baldrighi C, Maranzano M, Cugola L. Long-term results of replantation of the proximal forearm following avulsion amputation. Microsurgery. 2005;25(4):293–8.
53. Chuang DC, Lai JB, Cheng SL, Jain V, Lin CH, Chen HC. Traction avulsion amputation of the major upper limb: a proposed new classification, guidelines for acute management, and strategies for secondary reconstruction. Plast Reconstr Surg. 2001;108(6):1624–38.
54. Gulgonen A, Ozer K. Long-term results of major upper extremity replantations. J Hand Surg Eur Vol. 2012;37(3):225–32.
55. Yaffe B, Hutt D, Yaniv Y, Engel J. Major upper extremity replantations. J Hand Microsurg. 2009;1(2):63–7.
56. Kleinert HE, Jablon M, Tsai TM. An overview of replantation and results of 347 replants in 245 patients. J Trauma. 1980;20(5):390–8.
57. Meyer VE. Hand amputations proximal but close to the wrist joint: prime candidates for reattachment (long-term functional results). Hand Surg Am. 1985;10(6 Pt 2):989–91.

58. Visnjic MM, Kovacevic PT, Paunkovic LM, Milenkovic SS. Single centre experience of the upper limb replantation and revascularisation. Folia Med (Plovdiv). 2004;46(4):32–6.

59. Dagum AB, Slesarenko Y, Winston L, Tottenham V. Long-term outcome of replantation of proximal-third amputated arm: a worthwhile endeavor. Tech Hand Up Extrem Surg. 2007;11(4): 231–5.

60. Chen Z, Zhang J. Replantation of severed limbs: current status and prospects. Chin Med J (Engl). 1999;112(10):914–7.

61. Yousif NJ, Muoneke V, Sanger JR, Matloub HS. Hand replantation following three-level amputation: a case report. J Hand Surg Am. 1992;17(2):220–5.

62. Hanel DP, Chin SH. Wrist level and proximal-upper extremity replantation. Hand Clin. 2007;23(1): 13–21.

63. Godina M. Early microsurgical reconstruction of complex trauma of the extremities. Plast Reconstr Surg. 1986;78(3):285–92.

64. Nunley JA, Koman LA, Urbaniak JR. Arterial shunting as an adjunct to major limb revascularization. Ann Surg. 1981;193(3):271–3.

65. Davins M, Llagostera S, Lamas C, Lopez S. Role of temporary arterial shunt in the reimplantation of a traumatic above-elbow amputation. Vascular. 2007; 15(3):176–8.

66. Weinstein MH, Golding AL. Temporary external shunt bypass in the traumatically amputated upper extremity. J Trauma. 1975;15(10):912–5.

67. Cavadas PC, Landin L, Ibanez J. Temporary catheter perfusion and artery-last sequence of repair in macroreplantations. J Plast Reconstr Aesthet Surg. 2009;62(10):1321–5.

68. Lee JW, Pan SC, Lin YT, Chiu HY. Cross-limb vascular shunting as an auxiliary to major limb revascularisation. Br J Plast Surg. 2002;55(5):438–40.

69. Lee YC, Pan SC, Shieh SJ. Temporary femoral-radial arterial shunting for arm replantation. J Trauma. 2011;70(4):1002–4.

70. Tupper JW. Techniques of bone fixation and clinical experience in replanted extremities. Clin Orthop Relat Res. 1978;133:165–8.

71. Ikuta Y. Method of bone fixation in reattachment of amputations in the upper extremities. Clin Orthop Relat Res. 1978;133:169–78.

72. Chen CM, Ashjian P, Disa JJ, Cordeiro PG, Pusic AL, Mehrara BJ. Is the use of intraoperative heparin safe? Plast Reconstr Surg. 2008;121(3):49e–53.

73. Rumbolo PM, Cooley BC, Hanel DP, Gould JS. Comparison of the influence of intraluminal irrigation solutions on free flap survival. Microsurgery. 1992;13(1):45–7.

74. Schoeller T, Wechselberger G, Hussl H, Huemer GM. Functional transposition of the latissimus dorsi muscle for biceps reconstruction after upper arm replantation. J Plast Reconstr Aesthet Surg. 2007;60(7): 755–9.

75. Parmaksizoglu F, Beyzadeoglu T. Functional latissimus dorsi island pedicle musculocutaneous flap to restore elbow flexion in replantation or revascularisation of above-elbow amputations. Handchir Mikrochir Plast Chir. 2003;35(1):51–6.

76. Haas F, Hubmer M, Koch H, Scharnagl E. Immediate functional transfer of the latissimus dorsi myocutaneous island flap for reestablishment of elbow flexion in upper arm replantation: two clinical cases. J Trauma. 2004;57(6):1347–50.

77. Mordick 2nd TG, Britton EN, Brantigan C. Pedicled latissimus dorsi transfer for immediate soft-tissue coverage and elbow flexion. Plast Reconstr Surg. 1997;99(6):1742–4.

78. Wijayaratna SB, Suraweera HJ, Lamawansa MD, Mudalige SP, Esufali ST, Goonasekera CD. Postoperative critical care and outcomes of limb replantation: experience in a developing country. Injury. 2008;39(2):203–8.

79. Bakri K, Moran SL. Monitoring for upper-extremity free flaps and replantations. J Hand Surg Am. 2008; 33(10):1905–8.

80. Sabapathy SR, Venkatramani H, Bharathi RR, Bhardwaj P. Replantation surgery. J Hand Surg Am. 2011;36(6):1104–10.

81. Rosenberg JJ, Fornage BD, Chevray PM. Monitoring buried free flaps: limitations of the implantable Doppler and use of color duplex sonography as a confirmatory test. Plast Reconstr Surg. 2006;118(1): 109–13; discussion 114–5.

82. Smit JM, Whitaker IS, Liss AG, Audolfsson T, Kildal M, Acosta R. Post operative monitoring of microvascular breast reconstructions using the implantable Cook-Swartz doppler system: a study of 145 probes & technical discussion. J Plast Reconstr Aesthet Surg. 2009;62(10):1286–92.

83. Levin LS, Cooper EO. Clinical use of anticoagulants following replantation surgery. J Hand Surg Am. 2008;33(8):1437–9.

84. Askari M, Fisher C, Weniger FG, Bidic S, Lee WP. Anticoagulation therapy in microsurgery: a review. J Hand Surg Am. 2006;31(5):836–46.

85. Ashjian P, Chen CM, Pusic A, Disa JJ, Cordeiro PG, Mehrara BJ. The effect of postoperative anticoagulation on microvascular thrombosis. Ann Plast Surg. 2007;59(1):36–9; discussion 39–40.

86. Xipoleas G, Levine E, Silver L, Koch RM, Taub PJ. A survey of microvascular protocols for lower-extremity free tissue transfer I: perioperative anticoagulation. Ann Plast Surg. 2007;59(3):311–5.

87. Buncke GM, Buncke HJ, Kind GM, et al. Replantation. In: Achauer BM, editor. Plastic surgery: indications, operations, and outcomes. St. Louis: Mosby; 2000. p. 2131–47.

88. Veravuthipakorn L, Veravuthipakorn A. Microsurgical free flap and replantation without antithrombotic agents. J Med Assoc Thai. 2004;87(6):665–9.

89. Daoutis NK, Gerostathopoulos N, Efstathopoulos D, Misitzis D, Bouchlis G, Anagnostou S. Major

amputation of the upper extremity. Functional results after replantation/revascularization in 47 cases. Acta Orthop Scand Suppl. 1995;264:7–8.

90. Hierner R, Berger A, Brenner P. Considerations on the management of subtotal and total macro-amputation of the upper extremity. Unfallchirurg. 1998;101(3): 184–92.

91. Sugun TS, Ozaksar K, Ada S, Kul F, Ozerkan F, Kaplan I, et al. Long-term results of major upper extremity replantations. Acta Orthop Traumatol Turc. 2009;43(3):206–13.

92. Datiashvili RO, Chichkin VG. Flap transfer for complications of major limb replantation. Ann Plast Surg. 1993;31(4):327–30.

93. Cavadas PC. Salvage of replanted upper extremities with major soft-tissue complications. J Plast Reconstr Aesthet Surg. 2007;60(7):769–75.

94. al-Qattan MM. Ischaemia-reperfusion injury. Implications for the hand surgeon. J Hand Surg Br. 1998;23(5):570–3.

95. Nabseth DC, Mayer RF, Deterling Jr RA. Experimental basis of limb replantation. Adv Surg. 1966;2:35–57.

96. Steinau H. Major limb replantation and postischemia syndrome: investigation of acute ischemia-induced myopathy and reperfusion injury. New York: The University of California/Springer; 1988.

97. Shin CS, Han JU, Kim JL, Schenarts PJ, Traber LD, Hawkins H, et al. Heparin attenuated neutrophil infiltration but did not affect renal injury induced by ischemia reperfusion. Yonsei Med J. 1997;38(3):133–41.

98. McNeill IF, Wilson JS. The problems of limb replacement. Br J Surg. 1970;57(5):365–77.

99. Hales P, Pullen D. Hypotension and bleeding diathesis following attempted arm replantation. Anaesth Intensive Care. 1982;10(4):359–61.

100. McCutcheon C, Hennessy B. Systemic reperfusion injury during arm replantation requiring intraoperative amputation. Anaesth Intensive Care. 2002;30(1): 71–3.

101. Khalil AA, Aziz FA, Hall JC. Reperfusion injury. Plast Reconstr Surg. 2006;117(3):1024–33.

102. Wang WZ, Baynosa RC, Zamboni WA. Update on ischemia-reperfusion injury for the plastic surgeon: 2011. Plast Reconstr Surg. 2011;128(6):685e–92.

103. Salgado CJ, Jamali AA, Ortiz JA, Cho JJ, Battista V, Mardini S, et al. Effects of hyperbaric oxygen on the replanted extremity subjected to prolonged warm ischaemia. J Plast Reconstr Aesthet Surg. 2010; 63(3):532–7.

104. Mowlavi A, Neumeister MW, Wilhelmi BJ, Song YH, Suchy H, Russell RC. Local hypothermia during early reperfusion protects skeletal muscle from ischemia-reperfusion injury. Plast Reconstr Surg. 2003;111(1):242–50.

105. Sabapathy SR, Venkatramani H, Bharathi RR, Dheenadhayalan J, Bhat VR, Rajasekaran S. Technical considerations and functional outcome of 22 major replantations (The BSSH Douglas Lamb Lecture, 2005). J Hand Surg Eur Vol. 2007;32(5): 488–501.

106. Wang JN, Tong ZH, Zhang TH, Wang SY, Zhang HQ, Zhao GQ, et al. Salvage of amputated upper extremities with temporary ectopic implantation followed by replantation at a second stage. J Reconstr Microsurg. 2006;22(1):15–20.

107. Chernofsky MA, Sauer PF. Temporary ectopic implantation. J Hand Surg Am. 1990;15(6):910–4.

108. Cavadas PC, Landin L, Navarro-Monzones A, Soler-Nomdedeu S. Salvage of impending replant failure by temporary ectopic replantation: a case report. J Hand Surg Am. 2006;31(3):463–7.

109. Reagan DS, Reagan JM. Emergency cross-arm transfer. Plast Reconstr Surg. 2000;106(3):648–52.

110. Holmes WJ, Williams A, Everitt KJ, Kay SP, Bourke G. Cross-over limb replantation: a case report. J Plast Reconstr Aesthet Surg. 2013;66(10):1428–31.

111. Liang K, Zhong G, Yin J, Xiang Z, Cen S, Huang F. Cross-arm replantation for traumatic bilateral upper extremity amputations: a case report. Arch Orthop Trauma Surg. 2011;131(2):157–61.

112. Ozcelik IB, Mersa B, Kabakas F, Sacak B, Kuvat SV. Crossover replantation as a salvage procedure following bilateral transhumeral upper limb amputation: a case report. Arch Orthop Trauma Surg. 2011;131(4):567–72.

113. Blaisdell FW. The pathophysiology of skeletal muscle ischemia and the reperfusion syndrome: a review. Cardiovasc Surg. 2002;10(6):620–30.

Optimizing Vascular Patency in Replantation

8

Andrew D. Navarrete and Michael L. Bentz

Introduction

In replantation surgery, the artery and the vein are most often anastomosed following repair of the other injured structures. Once the decision to replant an amputated part is made, the earliest, most critical factor in both the short- and long-term success of such an operation is vascular patency. A perfectly performed bony fixation and tendon repair will not result in recovery of function if perfusion is not reestablished and maintained. Replantation success rates are approximately 75–80 %, while free tissue transfer enjoys a survival rate which has improved in recent years, with most large series demonstrating success rates of approximately 96–98 % (range 90–100 %), depending upon the flap type and clinical situation [1, 2]. In this chapter, strategies to optimize outcomes ranging from preoperative measures to postoperative management and salvage are discussed.

Microsurgical Strategies

A full review of basic microsurgical techniques is not within the intended scope of this text and is readily available elsewhere. Rather, we will focus on approaches and techniques that are unique or pertinent in replantation. A more comprehensive review of such specific strategies is further available within chapters in this text that discuss varying levels of amputation.

Back Table Preparation

Once a patient who has sustained an amputation arrives in the emergency department and once evaluation of the patient, mechanism of injury, and the amputated part reveal a situation in which a replantation is indicated, there is often a significant delay before the patient arrives in the operating room. This is due to trauma evaluation, stabilization of other injuries, resuscitation, preoperative checklists, and organization of operating room staff, equipment, and room preparation.

Once the operative team has set operating room preparation in motion, efficiency is maximized if a back table can be prepared with microsurgical instruments and a microscope. The surgeon can then transport the amputated part to the operating room ahead of the patient, without the need for a scrub tech or other support.

A.D. Navarrete, MD • M.L. Bentz, MD (✉)
Division of Plastic Surgery, University of Wisconsin
Hospital and Clinics, Madison, WI, USA
e-mail: navarrete.md@uwalumni.com;
bentz@surgery.wisc.edu

A.N. Salyapongse et al. (eds.), *Extremity Replantation: A Comprehensive Clinical Guide*,
DOI 10.1007/978-1-4899-7516-4_8, © Springer Science+Business Media New York 2015

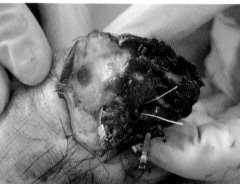

Fig. 8.1 An example of tagging pertinent structures in a thumb replant. Here, silver/gold clamps are utilized to mark arteries and black clamps to mark dorsal veins. A stitch is placed in the flexor tendon. A similar tagging strategy is begun on the amputated part prior to the patient's arrival to the operating room to expedite the replantation process. Bony fixation can be placed on the amputated part and nerves identified during this process as well

Evaluation of the amputated part can commence, and suitability for replantation can be confirmed. Half or more of the necessary preparation for repair can be performed prior to the patient's arrival to the operating room.

Bony fixation can be placed on the distal amputated part, whether this is in the form of Kirschner wires in the case of digital amputation or plates and screws in more proximal amputations. Definitive sutures can be placed in tendons, such that half of the tendon repairs have been performed. Fine suture tags mark epineurium or nerves to be repaired. Vessels are dissected far enough to evaluate for signs of trauma and resected back to uninjured intima. Atraumatic vessel clamps are placed on arteries and veins. Should vein grafts be anticipated, the distal anastomosis can be performed. An example of this preparation on a proximal thumb amputation is seen in Fig. 8.1. If two surgeons or surgical teams are available, this work can continue after the patient arrives, further minimizing ischemic time, especially in the context of multi-digit amputation or more proximal amputation which includes muscle distal to the level of amputation.

Vein Grafting/Venous Flaps

Vein Grafting

Given that there is often a significant zone of vascular injury associated with amputations, interposition vein grafts are often necessary to reconstruct vessel loss from injury or debridement. Bony shortening can be an option to avoid such grafting, but the amount of shortening tolerated is dependent upon the level of injury. Concern has arisen historically that two anastomoses "in sequence" may be at higher risk of complication or thrombosis. However, when faced with the option of placing a single anastomosis under tension (or not debriding questionably damaged vessel) versus a vein graft, vein grafts provide superior outcomes. No difference in patency rates have been found retrospectively in cases necessitating vein grafts versus those that do not, whether the grafts are used for arterial or venous reconstruction or both [3].

In any case where the possible need for vein grafts is anticipated, a suitable donor site should be prepped into the sterile field. In the case of a digital, hand, or distal forearm amputation, the most optimal donor site is the ipsilateral forearm. An upper arm tourniquet should be placed and inflated above arterial pressure without exsanguinating so as to fill the veins for visualization. Marking pens are used to draw marks of varying diameter, coinciding with the diameter of the visible superficial veins. Particular attention is paid to branching points, which may be useful in certain situations, such as reconstructing the branching of the palmar arch or simultaneously reconstructing both radial and ulnar digital arteries.

To optimally match the length and diameter, the deficit to be grafted should be measured and a similar length of in situ graft harvested. If the graft is harvested, anastomosed either proximally or distally, and trimmed, and the second anastomosis performed; a significant difference in length, typically redundant, may be noted. All vein grafts should be reversed when utilized for arterial reconstruction, since even very small diameter veins have valves allowing one way flow, which can be present over any length of

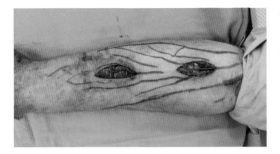

Fig. 8.2 When the need for vein grafts is anticipated, an upper arm tourniquet inflated prior to prepping and draping and without exsanguinating allows the identification of forearm superficial veins of various sizes. Varying widths of marks can be used to identify relative vessel diameters, and particular attention is paid to branching patterns which can decrease the number of necessary anastomoses when harvested

graft. If the vein can easily be flushed with heparinized saline in an in situ anterograde fashion, however, this may not be necessary.

A microvascular technique that is unique to vein grafting (or other situations where one vessel is highly mobile but rotating the vessels is difficult) is the "flipping" technique. In the case of the first anastomosis, whether proximal or distal, the anterior wall of the anastomosis is performed, and the free vessel flipped over the opposite to expose the back wall for completion of the anastomosis. The second anastomosis of the vein graft is performed utilizing standard techniques.

Venous Flaps

Venous flow through flaps can be utilized when there is a need for both vascular reconstruction and soft tissue coverage. Leaving vascular repairs uncovered or tenuously covered leads to likely desiccation, thrombosis, or leak. Venous flaps can be designed with a network of superficial veins with overlying subcutaneous fat and skin. By marking the superficial venous plexus preoperatively as described above (Fig. 8.2), the necessary veins, branching pattern, and skin paddle size can be found and utilized. The physiology that allows venous flaps to survive is not completely understood. Smaller, more distal grafts in the extremity have the advantage of a more complex venous network, multiple supplying and

draining vessels, and fewer valves. This makes the volar wrist, dorsal hand, and dorsal foot reasonable donor sites that can often be closed primarily.

Intra- and Postoperative Pharmacology

The overall physiology in the setting of amputation is pro-thrombotic. Catecholamines are abundant in the circulation, related to the stress of the traumatic injury, anesthesia, and postoperative pain and anxiety. Vessel walls are damaged not only at the site of amputation but also within the zone of injury due to stretch or crush. Platelets and the clotting cascade become activated as a result. Anticoagulant drugs can be indicated during replantation and during the postoperative course. The available literature is reviewed in the following sections. Beneficial effects such medications impart include decreasing platelet function, increasing blood flow or decreasing viscosity, and counteracting the effects of thrombin on platelets and fibrinogen [4].

The use of the majority of these drugs is not based on significant evidence. Much of their use is based on experience, and the way they are used in practice, in some cases, is not supported by available laboratory data. Complicating the available laboratory generated data is the view of many researchers that rodent veins have a unique capability to recanalize once thrombosed. Clinical data and outcomes are further clouded by the fact that most studies are performed utilizing multiple anticoagulant medications concordantly, and any number of combination regimens have been shown to have benefit. That being said, the reported favorable outcomes in the literature substantiate their use. The risks and benefits of each medication should be considered when designing a regimen for use in a specific surgeon's practice.

Heparin

Heparin is used in many forms in replantation and microsurgery. It is used topically as heparinized saline irrigation intraoperatively and intravenously prior to anastomosis, as well as a postoperatively as an intravenous drip or subcutaneously for prophylactic anticoagulation. Its actions and effects on clotting are many. When used topically or intravenously, it binds to damaged endothelium, reversing the loss of normal negative charge. By doing so, platelet aggregation is inhibited. Heparin also decreases fibrinogen activity while decreasing blood viscosity. The clotting cascade is impaired at multiple points, clinically measured by a prolongation of the activated partial thromboplastin time (PTT), with a twofold prolongation considered therapeutic anticoagulation. The most significant effect on the clotting cascade is in activating antithrombin, which accelerates antithrombin's inhibition of thrombin and factor Xa. The multiple actions of heparin make it the most utilized anticoagulant drug in microsurgery [5]. Given heparin's interaction with plasma proteins, however, its dose-response curve is unpredictable, and activity levels must be followed clinically (PTT) to assess therapeutic level when used as a continuous drip. A continuous drip offers the flexibility of turning therapy on and off as needed based upon clinical circumstance, i.e., turning the drip off in the setting of bleeding.

Laboratory evidence supports the use of heparin intraoperatively. In a model of venous crush injury in the rat femoral vein, topical heparin yielded a 93 and 87 % patency rate at 1 h and 7 days post-anastomosis, compared to the use of saline irrigation, with a patency rate of 13 and 7 % at the same time points [6]. In a similar model of rat femoral artery crush, topical heparin and low-molecular-weight heparin (enoxaparin) both showed a significant improvement in patency rate at 1 and 7 days over saline and streptokinase [7]. The use of topical heparin is experimentally supported as an irrigant during the course of microvascular anastomosis, especially in the setting of crush injury.

Heparin use has also been substantiated in the case of post-replantation arterial thrombosis and venous insufficiency. Clinically, an 85 % overall survival rate was seen in a series of 13 replanted digits when 2,500–5,000 units of heparin was administered intravenously shortly after the development of arterial thrombosis. The same authors experimentally noted the intravenous bolus of heparin to affect the balance of coagulation and fibrinolysis, tipping the process in favor of fibrinolysis and increasing the recanalization rate [8]. In cases where a venous anastomosis could not be performed or when venous thrombosis occurs, an overall survival rate of 76 and 64 % has been shown, respectively. The approach utilizes a combination of external bleeding by paraungual incision and heparinized saline topical drip and intravenous heparin drip [9]. The use of intravenous heparin at the time of identification of arterial or venous thrombosis does not obviate the need for a return to the operating room for revision of anastomosis but can be used in the interim prior to returning to the operating room.

An intravenous bolus of heparin (40 units/kg) is typically given either prior to clamping and division of vessels in microsurgery or prior to release of clamps and reperfusion in replantation. This theoretically protects the anastomoses from a thrombotic tendency related to intimal damage, adventitial or foreign body (suture) exposure, or stasis related to vascular clamping. The use of heparin is not without possible complications, namely, the risk of bleeding or heparin-induced thrombocytopenia (HIT) and an antibody-mediated activation of platelet activity resulting in significant platelet consumption and thrombosis.

Low-Molecular-Weight Heparin (LMWH)

Low-molecular-weight heparins are derived from unfractionated heparin through hydrolysis into shorter polysaccharide fragments. These smaller molecules have been shown to have the same effect in inhibiting factor Xa but a weaker effect on thrombin. Enoxaparin and dalteparin are the two most commonly utilized and are once- or twice-daily dosed subcutaneously. LMWH has proven clinically useful due to its higher bioavailability, longer half-life, and steady dose-response relationship as compared to heparin. Because of this, prophylactic and therapeutic dosages are better defined, and laboratory values do not need to be followed to assess therapy. LMWH has less of an effect on PTT than heparin for a similar degree of anticoagulation. If clinically warranted, activity can be assessed by obtaining an anti-factor Xa assay.

Beyond the above advantages over heparin, it has also been shown to have similar anti-thrombotic effect, but no significant increase in bleeding complications [10, 11]. LMWH also has a significantly lower risk of heparin-induced thrombocytopenia. Due to the reliable dosing, it can be administered on an outpatient basis, which is a useful entity in either extending therapy or decreasing duration of hospitalization. Due to these advantages, we typically use subcutaneous LMWH postoperatively as an inpatient following free tissue transfer and replantation.

Acetylsalicylic Acid (Aspirin)

The antithrombotic activity of aspirin occurs via the irreversible inhibition of cyclooxygenase, an enzyme which acts to break arachidonic acid down to produce prostaglandins and thromboxane. This blocks thromboxane's action as a potent vasoconstrictor and activator of platelet aggregation. Beyond this, aspirin has been shown to decrease thrombin production at the site of a vascular injury [12]. Given these and other downstream effects, aspirin has been shown to experimentally decrease thrombosis in rat models of microvascular injury, although the effect is less than that of heparin [13].

Multiple studies have examined the timing (pre-, intra-, and postoperative) and dosage of aspirin, mainly in rat models. In order to avoid complications both intraoperatively (bleeding) and longer term (systemic effects), the general recommendation has been to initiate low-dose aspirin therapy immediately postoperatively and return to routine general health recommendations for cardiovascular protection by 2–4 weeks postoperatively. The optimal dose has been shown to be approximately 3 mg/kg/day, which allows a decrease in thromboxane production while not

significantly decreasing the protective effect of prostaglandin synthesis by endothelium [14]. We routinely utilize aspirin 325 mg rectally in the postanesthesia care unit, followed by daily low-dose therapy for a period of 1 month.

Dextran

Dextran has a unique combination of effects that impart antithrombotic properties. Dextrans are polysaccharides synthesized by *Leuconostoc mesenteroides streptococcus* from sucrose. Dextran both reduces the activity of platelets and causes an increase in blood volume while decreasing viscosity. Dextran binds to platelets, erythrocytes, and endothelium, causing them to become electronegative and reducing aggregation and activation of platelets, which are further inhibited by dextran decreasing von Willebrand factor. When platelets do become activated, their distribution in the thrombus is more organized and diffuse, allowing thrombolysis to be a more orderly and efficient process [5]. Dextran has been utilized for its action as an osmotic agent in the setting of hypovolemia. This osmotic action increases blood volume and decreases blood viscosity, two properties that have shown to be beneficial in promoting vascular patency.

Dextrans come as varying size compounds, with the most commonly utilized being dextran-40 (molecular weight 40 k daltons). This is important, as at this molecular size, approximately 70 % is excreted by the kidneys in 24 h, with the remaining staying in the bloodstream for multiple days, prolonging both the beneficial and potentially harmful effects [15]. In a prospective, randomized study of head and neck microvascular reconstruction, Disa et al. showed that the use of dextran for 48 or 120 h had no clinical benefit over aspirin for 120 h postoperatively [16]. However, in this study, the rate of systemic complications compared to aspirin was 3.9 times higher with 48 h of infusion and 7.2 times higher at 120 h of infusion.

Serious, well-documented complications have been the consequence of the use of dextran. These include anaphylaxis, acute pulmonary edema, adult respiratory distress syndrome, cerebral edema, acute renal failure, and congestive heart failure. Despite the multiple mechanisms of action in decreasing thrombotic complications in microsurgery, these complications, in addition to the lack of definite clinical benefit, have made dextran fall out of favor with microvascular surgeons.

Papaverine

Papaverine is an opium alkaloid antispasmodic drug found in the opium poppy. Its pharmacologic uses include relieving spasm of the gastrointestinal tract, bile ducts, and ureter. In the vasculature, it is a smooth muscle relaxant, where applications include the therapy of subarachnoid hemorrhage in the cerebral vasculature and coronary artery disease in the internal mammary vessels during coronary artery bypass grafting. When used topically (30 mg/mL) directly on vessels during the course of a microvascular anastomosis, vasodilation and relief of vasospasm are seen [17].

In a rabbit model following microvascular anastomosis of the carotid artery, a significant increase in blood flow was seen following topical administration of papaverine. An added effect was noted with the use of papaverine in combination with either 2 or 20 % lidocaine. In an in vitro model, papaverine showed a dose-dependent reversal of the effect of norepinephrine [17].

Lidocaine

Lidocaine is a commonly used anesthetic that acts as a stabilizer of cell membranes. Its mechanism of action on the vasculature has not been fully elucidated, but varying responses are seen based on the concentration utilized [18]. In the study that investigated the effect of papaverine, 2 % lidocaine caused augmented constriction of in vitro vessels pretreated with norepinephrine, while 20 % lidocaine reversed the norepinephrine effect. In the rabbit carotid artery model, 2 % lidocaine did not alter blood flow through anastomosed vessels, while 20 % lidocaine caused a significant increase in blood flow. It should be noted that prior studies of mechanical ischemia demonstrated initial vasodilation followed by a prolonged period of rebound vasoconstriction

[19]; this effect was not seen in the above study following microvascular anastomosis with higher concentration of lidocaine.

The clinical use of 4 % lidocaine is common in microsurgery. The available literature supports the use of higher doses of lidocaine as a topical agent to promote vasodilation. While low-dose lidocaine does not relieve vasospasm, high-dose lidocaine (16–20 %) exerts high osmotic pressure and may damage vessel walls [20], not to mention the theoretical concern for systemic toxicity. Thus, the optimal concentration of lidocaine for use in microsurgery is 10 %.

Fibrinolytic Agents

Intra-arterial injections of urokinase, streptokinase, and tissue plasminogen activator (t-PA) have been utilized in the management of failing free tissue transfers or replantations due to thrombosis. Typically, t-PA is utilized in the case of a technically sound anastomosis without flow or when clot is noted at the anastomosis. In this case, it is assumed that distal embolization has occurred into the free flap or amputated part. Local use at recommended doses has been utilized safely without life-threatening bleeding complications being encountered, with many "saves" noted in the microsurgery literature [21].

Hirudin

Hirudin is a natural polypeptide of small size (7 kDa) produced by the leech *Hirudo medicinalis*. It is a natural direct thrombin inhibitor, without the additional effects seen with other anticoagulant medications. Recombinant forms, lepirudin and desirudin, have been produced with use as systemic anticoagulants in the setting of heparin-induced thrombocytopenia [22]. Hirudin's use in replantation is limited to the use of leeches in the setting of venous insufficiency and rarely in the case of a patient with HIT.

Other Medications

Pain, anxiety, nausea, hypertension, and hypotension all have detrimental effects on the dynamics of microvascular blood flow in replantation and free tissue transfer. Routine postoperative care will prophylax against and treat these factors.

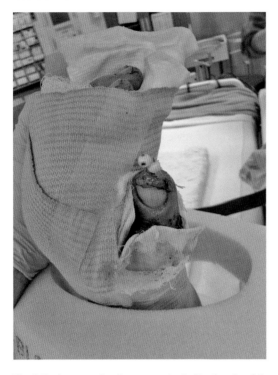

Fig. 8.3 An example of postoperative bulky dressing following thumb replantation, with caution to avoid compression of the replanted part. Elevation is provided by placement in a Carter block pillow

Postoperative Care and Monitoring

Postoperative Care

A critical aspect of postoperative care in extremity replantation is the avoidance of vasospasm. Many microsurgeons utilize routine postoperative strategies that are aimed at doing so. Dressings are soft, bulky, and non-circumferential to avoid compression (Fig. 8.3). These are typically left in place for the first 3–5 days, unless they are saturated, as dressing changes are often painful, anxiety-inducing events, and run the risk of mechanical damage to the replanted part. Warming of the patient's room to above 74° (for many surgeons, above 78°) can increase the temperature of the part by causing peripheral vasodilation as well as decreasing the cooling effect of the ambient air. While many microsurgeons dispute the effect of ambient temperature on free flaps, replanted extremities are uniquely exposed to room air, as compared to free

flaps on the body surface. More easily agreed upon is the fact that replanted parts are sensitive to acute changes in temperature and remain so for years, resulting acutely in vasospasm threatening perfusion and chronically in cold intolerance [23].

Patients must avoid ingestion of substances that can cause vasoconstriction. This includes caffeine, chocolate, and, most notably, nicotine. In a series of replantations performed at the Christine M. Kleinert Institute, a group of late failures were noted 2–3 weeks postoperatively. These coincided with a return to tobacco use. Smoking status was thought to be a contributor to early failure (0–3 days), but not causative [24]. Patients must be strongly counseled to avoid smoking upon discharge from the hospital given this risk.

It is necessary, both intraoperatively and postoperatively, to avoid physiologic responses leading to vasoconstriction, including hypovolemia, anemia, hypoxia, hyperoxia, hypoventilation, hyperventilation, and pain [25]. A balance of administration of isotonic fluids and blood products to maintain a hematocrit of 30 % will optimize viscosity and oxygen delivery. While vasopressors have been shown to be safe in breast and head and neck microsurgery, similar data has not been reported in replantation [26–28]. Vasopressors should be avoided in favor of fluid- and blood-based resuscitation when possible.

An indwelling brachial plexus blockade catheter has been shown to be effective in a number of ways. Although taking an average of 45 extra minutes preoperatively, a supraclavicular or axillary blockade catheter placement can be an effective method of intra- and postoperative pain control for 3–5 days. A continuous infusion of 0.125 % bupivacaine can help minimize pain and anxiety, as well as provide sympathetic blockade and subsequent decrease in vasospasm [29]. Utilization of a continuous brachial plexus blockade has shown a trend toward increase in surface temperature of the replanted part [30]. Smaller digital arteries are particularly prone to vasospasm, and thus, an indwelling catheter should be considered in both proximal and distal replantations. To be most effective, the catheter should be placed preoperatively to provide continuous sympatholytic effect and pain relief.

If a brachial plexus catheter was not placed preoperatively, a silicone catheter or ureteral stent can be inserted during the operation at the distal forearm level, adjacent to the median and/or ulnar nerve depending upon the site of the amputated part. Long-acting local anesthetics have been shown to impart a sympathetic block that resists vasospasm due to pain, anxiety, systemic, and environmental factors. Infusing a small amount (5 mL) of 0.25 % bupivacaine every 6–8 h has been shown to be effective [31].

Brachial plexus catheters and indwelling catheters near peripheral nerves are not utilized in all cases of extremity replantation. They are more commonly indicated in difficult situations with higher risk of replant failure. These include injuries with a significant crush or avulsion component, poor proximal flow prior to anastomosis, revision anastomoses, and in children.

Monitoring

Postoperative monitoring of a replanted digit or extremity has much in common with that of free tissue transfer. Early recognition of poor perfusion or vascular thrombosis, followed by expeditious nonoperative or operative intervention, allows the best chance for salvage of the replanted part. A reliable, well-trained, and experienced nursing staff is paramount in the postoperative care of these patients. Depending on local hospital policy and nurse staffing, the necessary frequent postoperative monitoring can feasibly and safely take place in either general, intermediate, or intensive care settings.

Clinical and research experience has shown that vascular thrombosis is most likely to occur in the first 12–24 h postoperatively, and the critical time for thrombosis occurrence is the first three postoperative days [24, 32]. Given this, many surgeons stop routine scheduled monitoring of the replanted part on the fourth postoperative day, depending upon the clinical situation. Late failure (beyond 7 days) is rare and is often attributed to factors such as a return to smoking, infection, or repeat mechanical trauma [33].

The ideal monitoring system in extremity replantation would need to fulfill a number of criteria. It would have to continuously monitor and quickly alert to changes in blood flow, deciphering

arterial versus venous insufficiency. Necessary would be the ability to monitor skin perfusion and flow through a range of vessel sizes. All of this would have to be done in a noninvasive, inexpensive, reliable fashion that can easily be interpreted by various members of the medical staff. A number of monitoring methods that are utilized clinically will be reviewed here, but no method has been able to fully supplant clinical evaluation by a trained and experienced clinician.

Clinical Evaluation

As noted above, the gold standard for assessment of perfusion of a free tissue transfer or replanted part is clinical evaluation by an experienced clinician. Key portions of the evaluation include tissue color, turgor, temperature, capillary refill, and bleeding. Assessing distally, a pale, flaccid, cool digit with slow or nonexistent capillary refill (greater than 3 s, examined and measured most easily at a lateral nail fold) and no bleeding on prick with a 22-guage needle would be consistent with a replant with an arterial inflow problem. A dark red or purple digit that is swollen, firm, and warm with brisk capillary refill (less than 1 s) that produces dark, brisk bleeding on needle prick would strongly suggest venous insufficiency.

The examination of a replanted part is often complicated by bulky dressings, by staining of the skin from the initial injury or from bleeding, or by removal of the nail plate. Clearly, the clinical evaluation is often not as obvious as the vignettes above, and more subtle changes in the examination must be noted early if a threatened replanted part is to be salvaged.

Surface Temperature

Surface temperature has been used clinically as an adjunct to clinical and other monitoring. A decrease in surface temperature as compared to a control area (uninjured digit or contralateral hand) of 1.8–3.0 °C [34, 35] has been found to be a significant change, as has the temperature of the replanted digits dropping below 30.0 °C [36]. Temperature monitoring was found to be 100 % sensitive and 61 % specific in identifying vascular compromise. When used in combination with clinical examination, a sensitivity of 100 % and specificity of 99 % was attained [35]. Pitfalls in temperature monitoring are changes in core and ambient temperature, inaccurate readings by recording device, and the retention of heat by dressings.

Handheld Doppler Ultrasonography

Handheld pencil Doppler (5–8 MHz) is a readily available and frequently utilized method of flap and replant monitoring. An audible arterial signal at or distal to the anastomosis is reassuring to clinicians and patient alike. The experienced examiner may be able to assess both the arterial and venous flow, depending on vessel size and spacing. That being said, subtle changes in phasicity and amplitude of the signal are difficult to realize for the inexperienced examiner. Despite venous thrombosis, an arterial signal can often remain for a significant period of time; thus, handheld Doppler is an adjunct to clinical examination.

Implantable Doppler

A number of implantable Doppler devices are commercially available. These can either be in the form of a silicon cuff that is secured around the blood vessel to be monitored or incorporated into a coupling device more typically used for venous anastomoses of adequate vessel diameter. Both types of device utilize a 20-MHz ultrasonic Doppler probe on a wire which exits the patient via an incision or stab wound and connects to a monitoring box. By monitoring the vein, information is obtained with regard to both arterial and venous flow, although a thrombosis cannot be localized by this data alone. Once the monitoring period is complete, the wire and probe can be removed from the cuff or coupler, which remain in situ.

With these implantable Doppler devices, salvage rates of 94.7–100 % have been shown in postoperative free flap monitoring, with all thrombotic events being recognized by the device [37, 38]. However, using these devices in small vessels is more difficult, and in proceeding more distally into the small vessels of the hand and digits, these types of monitoring devices become impractical. In our clinical use of coupler Dopplers in free flap reconstruction, the utility of directly monitoring the draining vein has been clear and has alerted our team to ongoing thrombosis or vessel kinking, but a number of drawbacks have been noted. These include the vessels becoming kinked or tethered by the associated wire and causing vascular compromise, as well as the probe pulling out of the device unintentionally and unbeknownst to the surgical team, thus complicating decision making.

Tissue Oximetry

The measurement of the level of oxygenated and deoxygenated hemoglobin in the microcirculation of the skin can be measured by a number of devices. Pulse oximetry is commonly used on hospitalized patients, typically placed on a finger. The device emits two wavelengths of light which pass through the fingertip and the changing absorbance of each wavelength is measured, allowing a determination of the percentage of hemoglobin in the oxyhemoglobin configuration. Real-time, constant measurements of tissue oxygenation allow easy assessment of perfusion. For a digital replant, placing this device on the finger would be cumbersome, risk injuring the replanted part, and obstruct clinical examination. For more proximal replants, a simple pulse oximeter may be useful in monitoring.

A more sophisticated method of measuring tissue oximetry utilizes near-infrared spectroscopy (NIRS). This device (by ViOptix, Fremont, CA) emits near-infrared light of wavelength 600–1,000 nm. The reflected spectrum is analyzed by a photodiode via a small probe placed on the skin surface. Oxyhemoglobin has two peaks in its extinction spectra, which decrease in amplitude and begin to merge within deoxygenation, allowing an indirect measurement of tissue perfusion. This was found to be reliable in a series of 64 replanted digits and correlated well with fluorescein monitoring and digit perfusion [39]. In practice, however, Buntic found the device numbers to vary widely and difficult to clinically correlate.

Fluorometry and Fluorescence Imaging

Classic fluorometry has been utilized in replant monitoring, in which 0.5–1.0 mg/kg of fluorescein is injected intravenously, and a handheld quantitative fluorometer was used simultaneously on the replanted part and a control area. The lack of rise in fluorescence at 10 min indicates arterial insufficiency, and a lack of a fall at 60 min correlates with venous insufficiency [39].

A more sophisticated, novel system (SPY Technology) utilizes indocyanine green intravenous injection with real-time monitoring, typically in the operating room, of both macro- and microcirculation. This has been utilized as part of a standardized protocol in artery-only fingertip replantation to assess the need for further therapy to augment venous outflow [40], but has not been evaluated for standard postoperative use in replantation.

Recommendations

At our institution, nursing staff on the plastic and reconstructive surgery ward have been well trained and are competent in the monitoring of free tissue transfers. Our typical postoperative monitoring of free flaps includes regular clinical and handheld Doppler examinations by nursing staff, supplemented with frequent checks by resident and attending staff. Monitoring by nursing staff takes place every 1 h for the first 24 h, every 2 h for the following 24 h, and every 4 h until discharge from the hospital.

Given the cumbersome nature of some of the more complex techniques noted above, we take a similar simple approach to monitoring replants. Clinical examination is supplemented by handheld Doppler. In cases where clinical examination is complicated (by tissue staining or drainage, e.g.), simple measures are added when the level of amputation allows. Given the sensitivity of clinical examination combined with temperature probe monitoring, as well as the small size and noninvasive nature of the monitor, this can be simply added. A pulse oximeter has utility in more proximal amputations where the monitor can be safely applied. In deciding upon a monitoring strategy, the competence and experience of the local nursing staff must be considered, as well

as the clinical situation. In most cases at our institution, frequent clinical and Doppler examinations are utilized with confidence.

Salvage

As noted above, the most likely time frame of vascular thrombosis is during the first 12–24 h postoperatively. When monitoring of the replanted digit or extremity reveals a change in blood flow, a decision must be made on a course of action, mainly whether or not a return to the operating room for reexploration and revision is necessary. The details of the particular case must be considered when making this decision, including the mechanism and level of injury, status of the patient, and whether an arterial or venous insufficiency is present based on clinical examination. Many surgeons choose not to return to the operating room for vascular compromise, if they feel the technical aspects of the case cannot be improved upon. That being said, a 75 % salvage rate was accomplished in a series of replanted thumbs upon reexploration [41].

A number of factors can lead to failure of a vascular anastomosis. The most important factor in a microvascular anastomosis is the operator's technical skill. Atraumatic tissue handling, adequate vessel preparation, and precise suture placement can lead to a 100 % patency rate regardless of the anastomosis type or suture selection [42]. However, conditions in the setting of traumatic amputation do not lend themselves to this degree of success. Crush or avulsion injuries have significantly lower success rates than saw-type injuries, which in turn are less successful than sharp injuries, all related to the zone of injury. Failure of blood flow across an anastomosis can be related to technical errors at the anastomosis, vasospasm, or vessel damage from the injury or due to traumatic clamp placement (at, proximal, or distal to the anastomosis).

When postoperative monitoring reveals concern for the viability of the replanted digit or extremity, immediate evaluation and action is warranted. The dressings, which are often saturated, are evaluated for possible constricting points and removed. If a tight closure is present, sutures are strategically removed. If an arterial problem is suspected, the extremity can be placed in a dependent position; similarly, if a venous issue is present, further elevation can aid outflow. Continued warming of the patient's room, pain control, and anxiety control are useful to avoid or reverse vasospasm. An intravenous bolus of heparin (2,500–5,000 units) can be considered in the setting of a presumed arterial thrombus, in which case survival of the digit has been shown to be improved by decreasing coagulation, increasing fibrinolysis, and allowing recanalization early in thrombus formation [8].

Arterial Insufficiency

A return to the operating room is more likely to be necessary (and successful) when an acute loss of arterial inflow is noted. Other interventions, as discussed below, are available to improve venous outflow. An expeditious reexploration to assess and correct the problem will improve the chances of salvage. The anastomoses are assessed for patency or occluding thrombus. If thrombus is found at an anastomosis, a thrombectomy should be performed, along with assessment of the vessel in the region of the anastomosis. Intravenous heparin should be given prior to placing vascular clamps to prevent proximal thrombosis. The prior anastomosis should be resected, at minimum, along with any damaged or abnormal-appearing vessel both proximal and distal. Gapping in the vessel following this resection should be replaced with tension-free vein grafts, following the principles discussed earlier.

Assessing proximal inflow can be difficult. Upon release of the proximal clamp, strong bleeding should be seen immediately. Nonoccluding thrombi or vasospasm can cause areas of sluggish or intermittent flow. Re-anastomosis should not be performed until adequate inflow is noted. Local vasodilators and warming can be utilized to improve bleeding. Assessment of proximal vessel integrity is necessary if inflow does not appear adequate.

Venous Insufficiency

As amputations proceed distally on the upper extremity, the volume of venous outflow decreases. Acute venous congestion in replanted parts proximal to the digits compels a return to the operating room for exploration, thrombectomy, and revision of the anastomosis. In digital replantation, if and when venous congestion is encountered, other methods of venous outflow can be utilized, including heparin scrubs and leech application. In fingertip and zone I amputations, some authors have utilized and described artery-only repair protocols [40, 43]. The protocol implemented in these reports can be used fully or in part in cases of venous congestion postoperatively.

When venous outflow needs to be augmented, typical management includes nail plate removal and the application of leeches (*Hirudo medicinalis*) and/or heparin scrubs. *H. medicinalis* has been utilized medically for over 3,500 years, but their current use is largely limited to cases of venous congestion in plastic surgery and replantation. The sucker of *H. medicinalis* has three jaws with 60–100 pairs of teeth and creates a Y-shaped bite. Relief of venous congestion occurs secondary to the feeding of the leech but also continues after removal of the leech due to the secretion of hirudin, a potent natural anticoagulant. Details of hirudin's activity can be found in the pharmacology section of this chapter. Medical leeches feed at temperatures between 33 and 40 °C and can be stimulated to feed by the application of glucose and saline solution or the presence of blood [44]. Leeches only feed on tissue that is alive and warm.

Leech feeding removes blood from the congested tissue, allowing filling of the tissue with oxygenated blood. The average meal volume is 2.45 mL, and the passive blood loss averages 2.5 mL. When tissue perfusion was evaluated with laser Doppler, a 2-cm^2 area of increased perfusion was noted. Thus, on large tissue flaps or areas, multiple leeches must be utilized [45]. Leeches should be allowed to feed until they fall off of the tissue when a meal is complete. Following removal, a heparin-soaked gauze scrub

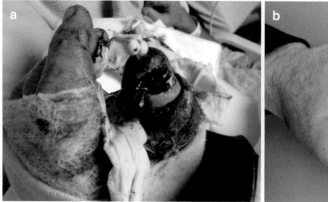

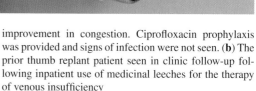

Fig. 8.4 (**a**). On postoperative day 3, this patient underwent dressing change and fabrication of a custom thermoplastic splint. Following this, the replanted thumb became significantly congested acutely. The nail plate was removed at the bedside, and medicinal leeches were applied consistently for approximately 60 h until clinical improvement in congestion. Ciprofloxacin prophylaxis was provided and signs of infection were not seen. (**b**) The prior thumb replant patient seen in clinic follow-up following inpatient use of medicinal leeches for the therapy of venous insufficiency

should be utilized to encourage continued passive bleeding every 15–30 min [44]. Once passive bleeding ceases, a fresh, starved leech should be applied. This continues until neovascularization has occurred and congestion has improved (Figs. 8.4a, b). The success rate of digital replant salvage in a recent review was 43/69 (62.3 %) [46]. The most common complication of leech therapy is infection with *Aeromonas hydrophila*, which lives in the leech digestive tract. These bacteria have an affinity for muscle tissue and can cause serious deep infection with gas formation. Thus, prophylactic antibiotics are strongly recommended for the duration of leech application. Cultures and sensitivities are often available locally or from the provider of medical leeches. The typical antibiotic choice is ciprofloxacin.

Replantation Success

A 2006 meta-analysis reviewed 1,803 digital replantations in 1,299 patients [47]. "Success" rates were evaluated, with "success" based on viability of the replanted part, without regard to functional or long-term outcome. This meta-analysis, therefore, examined the microvascular patency rate in digital replantation. Pertinent findings that can be reasonably generalized to other levels of replantation are reviewed here.

A critical factor in microvascular patency is the type of injury. In the above review, a clean-cut or guillotine injury had the greatest chance of success, with patency in 1,290 of 1,411 digits (91.4 %), compared to crushing injury (128 of 187, 68.4 %) or avulsion (136 of 205, 66.3 %). This clearly relates to the zone of injury of the vasculature, as well as the surrounding tissues.

A social history positive for current smoking was a statistically significant factor for replant failure. In the studies that reported on smoking history, smokers had a 61.1 % chance of replant success (44 of 72 digits) versus nonsmokers who had a 96.7 % success rate (464 of 489).

Females (206 of 221 digits, 93.2 %) had a significantly higher vascular patency rate than males (394 of 460, 85.7 %). The author of the meta-analysis, as well as other authors with similar findings, purported that this difference may be explained by males sustaining trauma of increased severity, including more crush and avulsion-type injuries.

A final indicator for success is a short ischemia time. In the above study, a cutoff of 12 h was used, with digits with a short ischemia time surviving at a greater rate (908 of 975, 93.1 %)

than those with a longer ischemic time (111 of 128, 86.7 %).

Clearly "success" in replantation surgery is not based solely on microvascular patency. A successful replantation is one that becomes functionally useful to the patient, and does not become a hindrance to their productivity. However, without adequate perfusion of the replanted part, the adequacy of repair of the other structures critical for function (bone, tendon, nerve) will never be known. Precise and efficient microsurgery, appropriate anticoagulation, proper postoperative care and monitoring, and expeditious care at the first sign of vascular insufficiency together optimize the chance for long-term functional outcomes in extremity replantation.

References

1. Lie KH, Barker AS, Ashton MW. A classification system for partial and complete DIEP flap necrosis based on a review of 17,096 DIEP flaps in 693 articles including analysis of 152 total flap failures. Plast Reconstr Surg. 2013;132:1401–8.
2. Bourget A, Chang JTC, Wu DBS, Chang CJ, Wei FC. Free flap reconstruction in the head and neck region following radiotherapy: a cohort study identifying negative outcome predictors. Plast Reconstr Surg. 2001;127:1901–8.
3. Yah H, Jackson WD, Songcharoen S, Akdemis O, Li Z, Chen X, Jiang L, Gao W. Vein grafting in fingertip replantations. Microsurgery. 2009;29(4):275–81.
4. Ketchman LD. Pharmacological alteration in the clotting mechanism: use in microvascular surgery. J Hand Surg. 1978;3:407–15.
5. Askari M, Fisher C, Weniger FG, Bidic S, Lee A. Anticoagulation therapy in microsurgery: a review. J Hand Surg. 2006;31(5):836–46.
6. Fu K, Izquierdo R, Hubbard T, Fareed J. Modified crush-avulsion anastomosis model on the rat femoral vein. Microsurgery. 1995;16(8):536–41.
7. Chen LE, Seaber AV, Korompilias AV, Urbaniak JR. Effects of enoxaparin, standard heparin, and streptokinase on the patency of anastomoses in severely crushed arteries. Microsurgery. 1995;16(10):661–5.
8. Noguchi M, Matsusaki H, Yamamoto H. Intravenous bolus infusion of heparin for circulatory insufficiency after finger replantation. J Reconstr Microsurg. 1999;15(4):245–53.
9. Han SK, Lee BI, Kim WK. Topical and systemic anticoagulation in the treatment of absent or compromised venous outflow in replanted fingertips. J Hand Surg. 2000;25(4):659–67.
10. Malm K, Dahlback B, Arnljots B. Low molecular-weight heparin (Dalteparin) effectively prevents thrombosis in a rat model of deep arterial injury. Plast Reconstr Surg. 2003;111:1659–66.
11. Ritter EF, Cronan JC, Rudner AM, Serafin D, Klitzman B. Improved microsurgical anastomotic patency with low molecular weight heparin. J Reconstr Microsurg. 1998;14:331–6.
12. Undas A, Brummel K, Musial J, Mann KG, Szczeklik A. Blood coagulation at the site of microvascular injury: effects of low-dose aspirin. Blood. 2001;98:2423–31.
13. Cooley BC, Gould JS. Experimental models for evaluating antithrombotic therapies in replantation microsurgery. Microsurgery. 1987;8:230–3.
14. Chang WHK, Petry JJ. Platelets, prostaglandins, and patency in microvascular surgery. J Microsurg. 1980; 2:27–35.
15. Nearman HS, Herman ML. Toxic effects of colloids in the intensive care unit. Crit Care Clin. 1991;7:713–23.
16. Disa JJ, Polvora VP, Pusic AL, Singh B, Cordeiro PG. Dextran-related complications in head and neck microsurgery: do the benefits outweigh the risks? A prospective randomized analysis. Plast Reconstr Surg. 2003;112(6):1534–9.
17. Gherardini G, Gurlek A, Cromeens D, Joly GA, Wang BG, Evans GRD. Drug-induced vasodilation: in vitro and in vivo study on the effects of lidocaine and papaverine on rabbit carotid artery. Microsurgery. 1998;18:90–6.
18. Johns RA, DiFazio CA, Longnecker DE. Lidocaine constricts or dilates rat arteriole in a dose-dependent manner. Anesthesiology. 1985;62:141–4.
19. Wadstrom J. Studies on traumatic vasospasm in the central ear artery of the rabbit. Scand J Plast Reconstr Surg Hand Surg Suppl. 1990;21:1–42.
20. Ueda K, Harii K. Comparative study of topical use of vasdilating solutions. Scand J Plast Reconstr Surg Hand Surg. 2003;37:201–7.
21. Casey WJ, Craft RO, Rebecca AM, Smitth AA, Yoon S. Intra-arterial tissue plasminogen activator: an effective adjunct following microsurgical venous thrombosis. Ann Plast Surg. 2007;59:520–5.
22. Greinacher A, Warkentin TE. The direct thrombin inhibitor hirudin. Thromb Haemost. 2008;99: 819–29.
23. Backman C, Nystrom A, Backman C, Bjerle P. Arterial spasticity and cold intolerance in relation to time after digital replantation. J Hand Surg Br Eur. 1993;18:551–5.
24. Betancourt FH, Mah ET, McCabe SJ. Timing of critical thrombosis after replantation surgery of the digits. J Reconstr Microsurg. 1998;14:313–6.
25. Hagau N, Longrois D. Anesthesia for free vascularized tissue transfer. Microsurgery. 2008;29:161–7.
26. Hiltunen P, Palve J, Setala L, Mustonen PK, Berg L, Ruokonen E, Uusaro A. The effects of hypotension and norepinephrine on microvascular flap perfusion. J Reconstr Microsurg. 2011;27:419–26.

27. Harris L, Goldstein D, Hofer S, Gilbert R. Impact of vasopressors on outcomes in head and neck free tissue transfer. Microsurgery. 2012;32:15–9.

28. Chen C, Nguyen MD, Bar-Meir E, Hess P, Lin S, Tobias A, Upton J, Lee B. Effects of vasopressor administration on the outcomes of microsurgical breast reconstruction. Ann Plast Surg. 2010;65:28–31.

29. Kurt E, Ozturk S, Isik S, Zor F. Continuous brachial plexus blockade for digital replantation and toe-to-hand transfers. Ann Plast Surg. 2005;54:24–7.

30. Su HH, Lui PW, Yu CL, Liew CS, Lin CH, Lun YT, Chanh CH, Yang MW. The effects of continuous axillary brachial plexus block with ropivicaine infusion on skin temperature and survival of crushed fingers after microsurgical replantation. Chang Gung Med J. 2005;28:567–74.

31. Phelps DB, Rutherford RB, Boswick JA. Control of vasospasm following trauma and microvascular surgery. J Hand Surg. 1979;4(2):109–17.

32. Chen KT, Mardini S, Chuang DC, Lin CH, Cheng MH, Lin YT, et al. Timing of presentation of the first signs of vascular compromise dictates the salvage outcome of free flap transfers. Plast Reconstr Surg. 2007;120: 187–95.

33. Duffy FJ, Concannon MJ, Gan BS, May JW. Late digital replantation failure: pathophysiology and risk factors. Ann Plast Surg. 1998;40:538–41.

34. Khouri RK, Shaw WW. Monitoring of free flaps with surface temperature recordings: is it reliable? Plast Reconstr Surg. 1992;89:495–9.

35. Reagan DS, Grundberg AB, George MJ. Clinical evaluation and temperature monitoring in predicting viability in replantations. J Reconstr Microsurg. 1994;10:1–6.

36. Stirrat CR, Seaber AV, Urbaniak JR, Bright DS. Temperature monitoring in digital replantation. J Hand Surg. 1978;3:342–7.

37. Kind GM, Buntic RF, Buncke GM, Cooper TM, Siko PP, Buncke Jr HJ. The effect of an implantable doppler probe on the salvage of microvascular tissue transplants. Plast Reconstr Surg. 1998;101:1268–73.

38. Paydar K, et al. Implantable venous doppler monitoring in head and neck free flap reconstruction increases the salvage rate. J Plast Reconstr Surg. 2010;125: 1129–34.

39. Colwell AS, Buntic RF, Brooks D, Wright L, Buncke GM, Buncke HJ. Detection of perfusion disturbances in digit replantation using near infrared spectroscopy and serial quantitative fluoroscopy. J Hand Surg. 2006;31:456–62.

40. Buntic RF, Brooks D. Standardized protocol for artery-only fingertip replantation. J Hand Surg. 2010;35A:1491–6.

41. Sharma S, Lin S, Panozzo A, Tepper R, Friedman D. Thumb replantation: a retrospective review of 103 case. Ann Plast Surg. 2005;55:352–6.

42. Guity A, Young PH, Fischer VW. In search of the "perfect" anastomosis. Microsurgery. 1990;11:5–11.

43. Akyurek M, Safak T, Kecik A. Fingertip replantation at or distal to the nail base: use of the technique of artery-only anastomosis. Ann Plast Surg. 2001;46: 605–12.

44. Green PA, Shafritz AB. Medicinal leech use in microsurgery. J Hand Surg. 2010;35A:1019–21.

45. Conforti ML, Connor NP, Heisy DM, Hartig GK. Evaluation of performance characteristics of the medicinal leech (Hirudo medicinalis) for the treatment of venous congestion. Plast Reconstr Surg. 2002;109:228–35.

46. Whitaker IS, Oboumarzouk O, Rozen WM, Naderi N, Balasubramanian SP, Azzoparki EA, Kon M. The efficacy of medicinal leeches in plastic and reconstructive surgery: a systematic review off 277 reported clinical cases. Microsurgery. 2012;32(3): 240–50.

47. Dec W. A meta-analysis of success rates for digit replantation. Tech Hand Upper Extrem Surg. 2006;10: 124–9.

Toe-to-Hand Transplantation After Failed Replantation

9

Nidal F. ALDeek and Fu-Chan Wei

On the iPhone I tended to draw with my thumb. Whereas the moment I got to the iPad, I found myself using every finger.

David Hockney [1]

Introduction

This concisely describes our time; we are living the digital era, and all of us regardless of our education and work are using our hands, particularly our fingers, thoroughly and completely around the hour.

That said, finger and thumb amputations have a profound impact on the quality of life, the psychosocial functioning, and the ability of our patients to return to work, [2, 3] and when multiple digits are lost, such impact is expected to be debilitating. Therefore, restoring lost integrity and function of the hands is an act of utmost importance, which can be accomplished by two methods. One is similar to raising the dead; it is bringing life back to dead fingers by replantation, a miracle of modern surgery, as W. W. Dzwierzynski likes to call it [4]. The second one, on the other hand, puts the concept of replacing "like with like" in action by utilizing the feet as a donor site for toe transfer to restore function and appearance after digit amputations.

With refinements in microsurgical techniques and accumulation of experience, microsurgical toe transfer is as safe and successful as any free flap, and it is the only procedure that provides functioning digits with sensibility, surpassing results obtained by prosthesis, conventional techniques, and even allotransplantation where lifelong immunosuppressant administration is a major drawback [5, 6]. With toe-to-hand transfer, long-term satisfactory hand function and appearance are achievable [7–12].

Our armamentarium is rich with different forms of toe-to-hand transplantations, ranging from vascularized nail graft to total toe/great-toe transfer to single toe transfer to combined, double, or triple toe transfer and from great toe to fourth or fifth toe transfer. Depending on what is missing and what is available, the surgeon has a wealth of options to give their patients the best alternative to enhance their lives' quality [11–47]. However, for toe-to-hand transfer after failed replantation, in particular, we believe that total or trimmed great-toe, partial great-toe, partial or total lesser-toe, and combined second- and third-toe flaps are the workhorse procedures. Hence, this chapter will focus on the microsurgical transfer of the great, second, and combined second and third toes and their modifications only.

N.F. ALDeek, MSc, MD
Department of Plastic and Reconstructive Surgery,
Chang Gung Memorial Hospital, Taipei, Taiwan
e-mail: nidaldeek@gmail.com

F.-C. Wei, MD (✉)
Department of Plastic Surgery, Chang Gung
Memorial Hospital, Taipei, Taiwan
e-mail: fuchanwei@gmail.com

General Considerations and Patient Selection

The selection criteria for toe-to-hand transfer after failed replantation depend on functional demands. Therefore, failed replantation after single- or multiple-digit amputations in a child, multiple-digit amputations in adult, and thumb amputation at any age are all relatively clear indications for toe-to-hand transfer. Unlike replantation after single-finger amputation [15, 48], toe-to-hand transfer after single-digit amputation is a matter of debate, in which patient's demands and level of amputation are key factors to consider. In relevance to this, it is worth mentioning that a single-finger amputation distal to the proximal interphalangeal (PIP) joint constitutes one of the best indications for toe transfer because of the excellent functional results that can be achieved [12, 29].

Although the indications for toe-to-hand surgery are becoming gradually more clear, this surgical procedure should not become an automated response taken right after replantation failure. Toe transfer involves donor site morbidity and the potential loss of invaluable, limited tissue; therefore, thorough discussion with the patient and their family and full assessment of the patient's age, level of amputation, number of amputated digits and their location, work demands, and motivation level are warranted.

Advanced age is not a contraindication for microsurgical toe transfer; however, nerve regeneration is less and surgical complications are higher in comparison to younger patients [49]. Children, on the other hand, benefit the most from toe-to-hand transfer, similarly to replantation, as gain in function, sensation, and ability to perform daily activities with high psychological satisfaction are achievable [32, 50]. However, given the technical challenges in performing microanastomoses in children younger than 6 months old, definitive reconstructive surgery (i.e., toe transfer) should be postponed until after age 2 [32]. Moreover, in children, the entire toe is transferred without any modifications to protect the epiphyseal plate that is important for toe and finger growth [26].

The number and location of amputated digits deserves to be addressed. The more digits that are lost, the more the functional deficit there will be, and this can be overcome by toe-to-hand transfer as well. In planning for multiple toe transfer, the index and middle fingers are more important for fine manipulation, whereas the ulnar digits (ring and middle) are more necessary for a powerful grasp [51, 52]. When multiple digits are lost, restoration of a stable, strong tripod pinch should be paramount [6, 53]. The scenario of multiple-digit amputation of variable levels presents a formidable challenge to planning toe-to-hand surgery, and it is important to prioritize digits based on patient's work and to harmonize the hand after reconstruction. Confronted with overwhelming multiple-digit loss, for example, when one is left with only metacarpals, the thumb and at least one opposing finger can be reconstructed simultaneously, which has been shown to be both time- and cost-effective [54].

In considering toe-to-hand surgery, donor site morbidity should be fully discussed. Although foot function for most ambulatory activities is not restricted after the resection of one or two toes, it might be limited to some degree for certain sports. Furthermore, when both feet are utilized for transfer, the dominant foot, which is usually the right one, should bear the lesser functional deficit following toe transfer. Within acceptable morbidity, transplantation of the great toe causes the highest functional deficit followed by transfer of the second and third toes simultaneously. The transfer with the least functional deficit is isolated transfer of the second toe [55]. Hence, when toes are utilized from both feet, the great toe on the dominant foot should be spared, if at all possible. Foot cosmesis should not be overlooked as this is important in some cultures and in young patients.

The surgeon attempting replantation is encouraged to consider toe-to-hand transfer as a backup plan, and this has two important implications. First, discussion of this eventual possibility would take place with the patient at the time of the initial consultation for replantation. Second, it means a "tissue preservation" strategy during stump preparation should always be adopted, as the length of bone and neurovascular bundles will determine the type of toe transfer and the extent of donor foot dissection [56, 57].

Timing of Toe-to-Hand Surgery

When Is Toe-to-Hand Transfer Performed After Failed Replantation?

Toe-to-hand transfer can be performed in patients following replantation when failure of the digit to survive looks inevitable or when the amputated part is deemed non-replantable. In both of these settings, which we refer to as *primary transfer*, the potential recipient site wound is fresh.

Occasionally, the patient may decide not to have primary toe-to-hand surgery; the psychological trauma after failed replant of multiple digits may prove too great for the patient to undergo additional surgery, or concern of donor site morbidity might discourage them from proceeding. In this setting, the hand wound is closed using a "tissue preservation strategy" for potential toe-to-hand surgery in the future. When arranged as an elective operation after either a failed replantation or when toe-to-hand surgery is not performed at the time of amputation (e.g., acutely), the operation is called *secondary transfer*.

It is important, however, to mention that primary toe-to-hand transfer may not be suitable in non-replantable finger amputations in children due to low risk-to-benefit ratio, though further studies are needed [50, 58]. Nevertheless, parents should be made aware of such possibility and potential recipient site closure should not compromise future toe-to-hand transfer.

In the literature, few studies compared primary to secondary transfer: When Yim and Wei et al. compared 144 secondary to 31 primary toe-to-hand transplants, survival rate of 96.5 and 96.9 % were reported, respectively. There was no statistical difference between the two groups in terms of intraoperative anastomotic revision, re-exploration, complications, and secondary procedures [45]. Woo et al. had similar results but noted a 30 % reduction in convalescent time and a greater likelihood of patients returning to their original jobs in primary group; interestingly, patient satisfaction was less in primary transfer [59]. Ray et al. demonstrated that primary transfer could reduce cost due to shorter hospital stay;

they also noted faster restoration of hand function and patient's body image [60]. Anecdotally, primary transfer may also be technically easier, because dissection of the neurovascular bundles is not impeded by fibrosis or scar adhesion. Moreover, early transfer may yield better sensory recovery than delayed transfer [61].

Generally, primary toe-to-hand transfer is recommended in well-informed and highly motivated individuals and when wounds are well demarcated and clean [26, 45, 61]. It is also recommended in the setting of multiple-extremity injury when spare parts are available [62]. In our opinion, although some surgeons prefer to delay toe-to-hand transfer until the patient understands the extent of hand injury, the benefits of primary transfer are non-disputable, and we recommend it whenever feasible.

Good preoperative counseling is critical in order for patients to have a realistic set of expectations for results. Although microsurgical toe transfer is a major surgical procedure, patients may fail to appreciate the sophistications of such procedure, especially when the donor foot is painful or has a poor aesthetic appearance [63]. Similarly, the appearance of the toe on the hand is a major concern to the patient, and patients must be counseled that the aesthetic result will not exactly reproduce "normal." In addition, patients must understand that secondary procedures to enhance function may be needed [63–66].

Initial Management and Preparation for Toe-to-Hand Transfer

Replantation and heterotopic replantation, including the use of spare parts, are the gold standard for the management of traumatic amputations [4, 67, 68]. Nevertheless, toe transfer for digit reconstruction must be considered from the time of initial injury either as a backup plan or as a future reconstructive option. This is particularly true in children with a non-replantable digit amputations and adults with multiple-digit amputations or when conditions for replantation are not optimal, such as in extreme contamination, multiple segmental injuries in the amputated part, and severe crushing or avulsion injuries [4, 69, 70]. Bone, tendon, and neurovascular bundle length must be preserved after debridement of all nonviable tissue and provision of adequate soft tissue coverage using "tissue preservation" concept as much as possible [41, 56, 57]. There is no doubt that the length of structures remaining after debridement or definite closure determines the type of toe transplantation and its functional and aesthetic outcome as well as donor foot morbidity.

Tissue Preservation

At the time of initial management, we recommend that excessive bone shortening be avoided and functioning joints or the cartilage surface with the articular capsule be maintained, if possible. In properly selected cases, the transferred toe can be disarticulated, and the joint capsule can be directly repaired with the recipient digit, achieving good functional results, particularly in thumb reconstruction [71, 72]. The temptation to shorten bone at the recipient site in order to facilitate direct vessel repair should be resisted; the pedicle for toe transfer is almost always long enough to reach recipient vessels for direct repair, and, when direct vessel repair is not feasible, vein graft interposition is a reliable procedure to bridge any gap [41, 46, 47]. Bone stumps as short as 5 mm still allow interosseous wire fixation and should be preserved [73].

The same conservative approach applies to tendons, where preservation of length will be important for function and balance. For extensor tendons, the extensor apparatus on the digital stump, the intrinsic insertions on the proximal phalanx, and the extensor hood should all be preserved when possible to maintain the balance between the extrinsic and intrinsic mechanisms. Similarly, flexor tendon length should preserve, if possible, the flexor digitorum superficialis (FDS) insertion. Finally, the integrity of the pulley system, especially the A2 and A4 pulleys, should be kept intact so as to optimize flexor tendon mechanics [56, 57].

As for neurovascular bundles and skin coverage, it is our practice that vessels and nerves are trimmed until healthy lumen and viable fascicles are reached, respectively. As mentioned above, toe transfer has the advantage of providing long vessels and nerves; however, excessive trimming of recipient vessels and nerves should be avoided. This is particularly important for nerve, as the recovery of sensation is faster when neurorrhaphies are performed closer to the transferred toe [49, 74, 75].

Pedicled *local* or *regional* flaps or free tissue transfer for stump closure is discouraged, as they burn potential recipients for toe transfer and increase overall morbidity [41, 57, 76–79].

When faced with skin shortage, our first choice is a pedicled groin flap that provides adequate amount of soft tissue that can protect toe pedicle, create adequate web space, and minimize skin inclusion in a transferred toe, allowing primary closure of the donor site [21, 41].

Surgical Technique

Toe Harvest

We advise that one team prepares the recipient site while the second team harvests the toe. This approach reduces surgery time and saves energy. If a "two-team" approach is not possible, or the availability of recipient structures is in doubt, we recommend that the recipients be prepared first [41, 49].

The toe is harvested through retrograde dissection starting dorsally at the first web space. Many authors report on the anatomic variations of the vascular pedicle at the first web space with different classification systems [80–84]. This creates a sense that the operation is tricky and challenging. Retrograde dissection allows accurate pedicle identification and is invaluable to avoid confusion with vascular anatomy.

We usually first identify the arterial dominance pattern in the distal web space and proceed accordingly with speed and minimum dissection to the foot [85] This technical approach can make a young microsurgeon as efficient in toe surgery as the most senior surgeons [85]. If the first *dorsal* metatarsal artery proves to be the dominant blood supply, dissection continues proximally with ease; however, when the first *plantar* metatarsal artery is the dominant vessel, dissection stops at the midportion of the metatarsal shaft and a vein graft is used to elongate the pedicle, when needed. Tissue dissection, handling, and hemostasis should always be meticulous [86].

Recipient Site Preparation

The recipient site is prepared in a bloodless field with tourniquet control, and the dissection is performed under loupe magnification. We always incise the amputation stump in a cruciate fashion to create four skin flaps for wide exposure and to allow them to interdigitate with the triangular skin flaps of the toe during insetting [63]. If proximal recipient vessels, such as the radial artery in the anatomic snuffbox, are planned, separate incisions are used to identify them, and tunnels connecting the recipient and donor vessels should be loose enough to avoid vascular compression. Periosteal dissection is kept minimal to expose the fixation site in the recipient bone. The bony surface of the stump is leveled to provide good contact and stability. Whenever joint repair is indicated, the joint capsule and ligaments must be carefully dissected while exposing the cartilage surface. The pulley system should be preserved while exposing the flexor tendons, whenever possible. The flexors should be repaired at the mid-palm level to allow smooth excursion. If no flexor tendons are available, the flexor digitorum superficialis tendon from an adjacent finger can be transferred primarily.

The appearance of the nerve fascicles under the microscope determines the site of neurorrhaphy. If the distal nerves have been avulsed, more proximal recipient nerves in the palm, including the palmar cutaneous branch of the median nerve and the dorsal sensory branches of the ulnar nerve, may be selected as proximal recipients. Nerve transfers from the ulnar side of the long or ring finger or sensory branches of the superficial radial nerve on the dorsum of the hand may be used, as well.

When the vascular anastomosis can be performed at the level of the proper digital artery, the artery on the ulnar side is selected more often than the proper digital artery on the radial side because of its larger diameter. In the setting of extensive crush injury, common digital arteries in the palm are less prone to spasm and may be preferred, provided the arterial arch in the hand was not involved in the initial injury. The radial artery in the anatomic snuffbox or the princeps pollicis artery can also be used when the damage extends to the palm, but a vein graft may be needed. One healthy vein on the dorsum of the hand can serve as a recipient vein. Usually, one artery and one vein are adequate for revascularization of the transferred toe.

Toe Flap Inset

Skeletal Fixation
In toe-to-hand transfer, intraosseous wires, Kirschner wires, plates, and intramedullary fixation have been described for bone fixation [73, 87–90]. We prefer intraosseous wires technique (see Chap. Chap. 2). This technique allows rapid fixation with minimal dissection and provides adequate stability for early movement. As mentioned earlier, it can also be applied to bone segments as short as 5 mm [73].

For composite joint repair, the volar plate and collateral ligaments of the toe are attached to the corresponding structures on the finger with nonabsorbable sutures [71, 72]. The volar plate has to be repaired with proper tension to prevent postoperative hyperextension of the joint.

Tendon Repair
The extensor tendon is repaired next. The extensor longus tendon of the toe is joined to the extensor in the finger using a Pulvertaft weave technique (see Chap. 2) with the proximal interphalangeal joint and metacarpophalangeal joints in full extension to avoid flexion contracture. After that, the long flexor tendon of the toe is sutured to the proximal flexor digitorum profundus (FDP) tendon stump of the amputated digit

using modified Kessler's method. In distal finger amputations, if the insertion of the flexor digitorum superficialis is intact, the long flexor tendon of the toe can be repaired to the distal end of the FDP, if present, or sutured to the distal portion of the FDS insertion. For proximal finger amputations, only the FDP is repaired, usually in zone 3, to prevent entrapment in zone 2. The tension between the flexor and extensor tendons should be adjusted so that the finger forms a natural cascade with the other digits. Claw deformity, due to the relative higher power of flexor musculature, has the potential to be relatively common in toe-to-hand surgery. In our experience, the best way to prevent this complication is tight extensor tendon repair and night splint application with the finger in full extension for at least 1 year [12, 41, 47, 63].

Nerve Repair

The nerves are coapted in an end-to-end fashion with 10-0 nylon under as little tension as possible. Repair priority is given to the proper digital nerve in order to restore pulp sensation. If enough recipient nerves are available, the deep and superficial peroneal nerves can be repaired, as well as potentially adding dorsal sensation to the digit. When only one recipient digital nerve is available proximally, the two proper digital toe nerves can be sutured together to this nerve or to a common digital nerve more proximally.

Skin Closure

At this point, the skin can be tailored and temporarily closed before vascular anastomosis to minimize swelling expected after reperfusion. We always interdigitate the recipient skin flaps with the donor skin flaps to create smooth contour, and we trim thick skin flaps to avoid a bulbous appearance [66].

Vascular Anastomosis and Wound Closure

The arterial anastomosis is done before venous anastomosis to confirm adequate back flow and to rule out compression of the vascular pedicle of the transferred toe. Typically one dorsal vein will be repaired. The remaining wounds in the finger are closed without tension. When closure appears tight, it is advisable to release some stitches and to use a skin graft to temporarily cover raw surfaces.

Donor Site Closure

The donor site is closed primarily using one layer of 3-0 nylon. Drains are not used and skin grafts should be avoided.

Toe Transfer Variations

Total or Trimmed Transplantation of the Great Toe (Figs. 9.1a–f and 9.2a–g)

Total or trimmed great-toe transfer to replace a thumb is indicated when the amputation level is at the proximal phalanx or metacarpal bone. It aims to reconstruct a new thumb with good range of motion and broad pulp surface for more powerful pinch. The trimmed transplantation of the great toe [14, 43, 63] is indicated when there is an unacceptable size difference between the thumb on the normal contralateral side and the great toe, especially when a mobile IP joint is desired. In the trimmed great-toe technique, both skin and skeleton including proximal and distal phalanges as well as interphalangeal joint are reduced to increase resemblance to the thumb. The nail bed is not trimmed to avoid nail deformity. For amputations distal to IP joints, functional deficit is usually less [91, 92] and some patients may not prefer any reconstruction [93]. However, partial great-toe transfer or modified wraparound flap can achieve good satisfactory results [26]. Degloving injuries with intact skeleton can be managed with wraparound techniques either from the great or second toe [94, 95]. In both variants, the donor proximal phalanx is osteotomized, preserving at least 1 cm of the base of the proximal phalanx, which maintains foot span for a better appearance and to preserve push-off function of the donor foot [47].

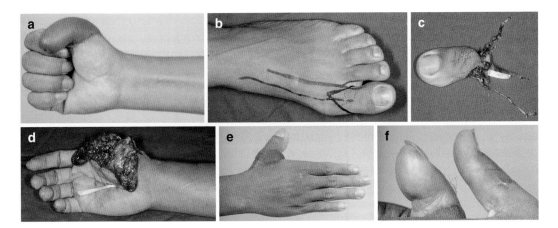

Fig. 9.1 (**a–f**) Total great-toe transfer to an unreplantable thumb amputation at proximal phalanx. (**a**) Coverage reconstruction of the amputation stump of the thumb with a pedicle groin flap before a total great-toe transfer. (**b**) Design of a total great-toe transfer at the donor left foot. (**c**) Harvested great toe. (**d**) Preparation of the recipient site. Note the use of transferred flexor digitorum profundus (FDP) of the ring finger for flexor function of the new thumb. (**e**, **f**) Appearance 3 months after toe-to-thumb reconstruction

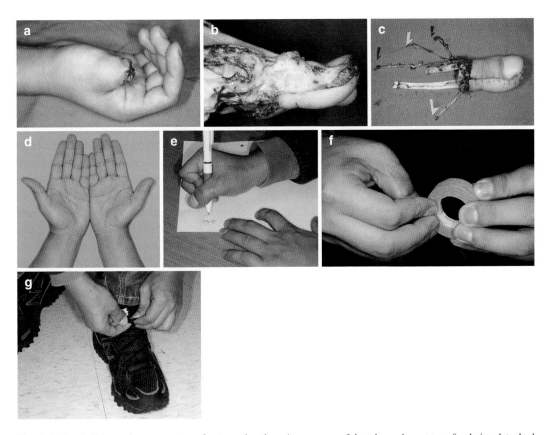

Fig. 9.2 (**a–g**) Trimmed great-toe transfer to a thumb after failed replantation. (**a**) Thumb stump appearance after failed replantation. (**b**) Both proximal, distal phalange and interphalangeal joint trimmed smaller. (**c**) Appearance of the trimmed great toe after being detached from its donor site. (**d–g**) Appearance and function of the new thumb 7 years after reconstruction

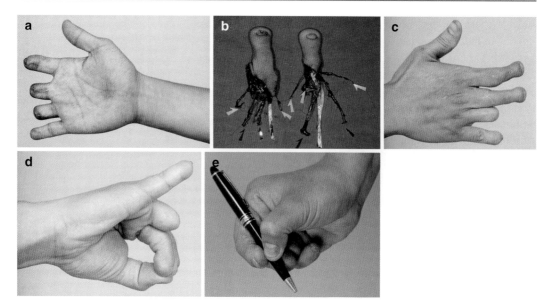

Fig. 9.3 (**a–e**) Two total second-toe transfers to right index and middle finger. (**a**) Right index, middle, and ring finger amputated at proximal interphalangeal joint, proximal phalanx, and proximal phalanx respectively. (**b**) Two second toes from both feet harvested. (**c–e**) Appearance and function of transferred toes (new fingers) 3 years after reconstruction

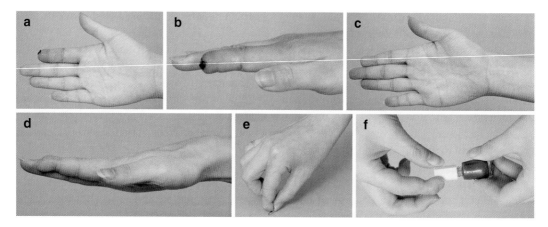

Fig. 9.4 (**a–f**) Partial second-toe transfer to an unreplantable distal index finger. (**a**, **b**) Appearance of amputation stump. (**c**, **d**) Appearance of reconstructed index finger 4 years after partial second-toe transfer. (**e**, **f**) Function of the reconstructed index finger 2 years after partial second-toe transfer

Total or Partial Transplantation of the Second Toe (Figs. 9.3a–e and 9.4a–f)

The second-toe transfer is another reliable procedure after failed replantation; it can be transferred for reconstruction of either the thumb or fingers. Thumb amputation proximal to (CMC) joint may, in particular, benefit from lesser-toe transfer that provides valuable bone length up to proximal metatarsus, which contrasts with the proximal phalanx harvest level in great-toe transfer. Partial transplantation of the second toe is used for finger amputations distal to the insertion of the superficial flexor tendon, whereas total transplantation is used for the reconstruction of more proximal finger amputations [12, 52, 74, 84, 87, 96–102].

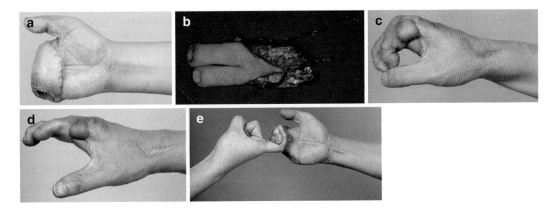

Fig. 9.5 (**a–e**) Type I metacarpal hand reconstructed with a combined second- and third-toe transfer. (**a**) Type I metacarpal hand initially treated with a pedicled groin flap for coverage. (**b**) Harvested combined second and third toe. (**c–e**) Appearance and function 2 years after combined second- and third-toe transfer reconstruction

Combined Transplantation of the Second and Third Toes
(Fig. 9.5a–e)

Combined second- and third-toe transfer is indicated for reconstruction of two adjacent fingers after traumatic amputation proximal to the digital webs. Advantages of combined second and third tow transfer over bilateral transplantation of both second toes are multiple. First, only a single set of recipient vessels is required; second, less operative time is required; third, potential morbidity in the donor site is limited to one foot [103].

The level of digit amputation is used to determine the osteotomy level, and we recommend that the second and third plantar arteries be preserved to be used for a second arterial anastomosis when arterial perfusion to third toe is in doubt [104].

Postoperative Care

Directly after surgery, aspirin (325 mg/day) is administered for 2 weeks to reduce the risk of platelet aggregation. Dextran is not routinely used due to risk of systemic complications, particularly pulmonary edema in elderly patients (see Chap. 8). Heparin is only given when there is intraoperative vascular compromise, as it may cause a hematoma or other bleeding problems. We occasionally use brachial plexus blockade, which has been shown to prevent vessel spasm and to provide early pain relief in related patients [105].

No splints are used; rather, the proximal portion of the palm and wrist is gently wrapped with the fingers uncovered for continuous observation. The hand and forearm are kept slightly elevated atop a smooth support to reduce edema formation. The dressing is kept simple and light; bulky dressings are not recommended because blood clots may be retained around the wounds, and when the dressing is removed, disruption of the clots may risk induction of vasospasm. Lastly, bulky dressings make it impossible to start early postoperative rehabilitation.

In Chang Gung Memorial Hospital, every free flap patient, such as great- and second-toe transfers, is hospitalized for an average of 5 days in specially designed microsurgery intensive care unit, where trained nurses closely monitor the transplanted toe and the patient's general condition. The toe is monitored hourly by the nursing staff, and when there is any change from the base line, the attending surgeon is notified.

Toe flap monitoring is done clinically by skin color, turgor, and capillary refill observation every hour by experienced nurse. When in doubt, the pulp of the toe can be pricked with 25-gauge needle. Also, we objectively monitor the toe by measurement of the surface temperature in the toe in comparison to the adjacent normal finger and opposite hand. Also, the Doppler ultrasound and laser Doppler are used for evaluation and assessment [106]. Of these monitoring techniques, the laser Doppler has the highest sensitivity and specificity compared to digital thermometry and ultrasonic Doppler [107].

The donor foot is gently covered with nitrofurazone (Furacin)-impregnated gauze over the wound and a light fluff dressing. No splints are used on the donor foot. Two days later the foot is uncovered, and no further dressings are used.

Rehabilitation

Motor Rehabilitation

The rehabilitation program developed in our unit consists of five stages starting on the first postoperative day [108]:

1. Protective stage (days 1–3). During this stage, interaction between the patient and the hand therapist is established.
2. Early mobilization stage (day 4 to week 4). Rehabilitation is directed at preventing excessive swelling and joint stiffness. We start with 15-degree gentle passive range of motion exercises. In the second week, the joint distal to the bony union site is moved through a full range of motion while keeping the wrist in neutral position. In the third and fourth weeks, the proximal joints are moved more aggressively, with full range of motion avoided so as not to interfere with bone healing. A protective splint is provided between exercises.
3. Active motion stage (weeks 5–6). Gentle active exercise is started, and the splint is changed to a dynamic one, if necessary. During the sixth week, blocking flexion and extension exercises are initiated.
4. Activities of daily living training stage (weeks 7–8). According to patient capabilities, different manual jobs that simulate daily manual activities are assigned.
5. Prevocational training stage (week 8 and beyond). This training aims to further improve muscle strength and hand dexterity and coordination.

Sensory Rehabilitation

Sensory recovery is important for functional recovery [49, 108] and is primarily accomplished by reeducation, which is directed at helping the patient interpret the altered sensory impulses reaching the brain from peripheral nerves [108, 109].

The program of sensory reeducation is divided into early and delayed stages. In the early stage, reeducation focuses on facilitating the perception of touch submodalities with correct localization and continues according to a sequence of sensory recovery reported by Dellon [109]. Late-phase sensory reeducation focuses on size and shape discrimination and object identification. In a study of sensory recovery after toe-to-hand transplantation, the senior author and his colleagues found a good relationship between Meissner corpuscle number and two-point discrimination.

Donor Site Rehabilitation

For the first 2 weeks following toe harvest, the patient should remain non-weight-bearing on the donor foot. The patient is allowed to walk a few steps on the heel of the donor foot after the second week. It must be emphasized that any contact with the anterior plantar weight-bearing surface should be avoided during this recovery period. The sutures in the donor foot should not be removed earlier than 3 weeks following the operation. After 4 weeks, the patient is allowed to walk with a normal gait.

Outcome

Yam and Wei et al. reported on 96.8 % survival rate in 31 primary transfers vs. 96.5 % in 144 secondary transplantations [56]. There was no statistical difference between the two groups in terms of survival, intraoperative anastomotic revision, re-exploration, future secondary procedure, infection, and complications [56]. Rosson and

Buncke compared outcomes between thumb replantation and great-toe transplantation, when the thumb proved non-replantable, for isolated amputations of the thumb and reported higher success rate in transplantation group (93 % vs. 85 %) [54]. Woo et al. and Ray et al. reported in multiple series on immediate partial great-toe transfer with a 100 % success rate [26, 59, 60]. Together, all these reports lay a strong foundation for the safety and reliability of primary toe-transplantation surgery for the management of fresh digit amputations.

Another measure of outcome is objective measurement of hand function. Long-term follow-up of successful immediate partial great-toe transfer showed that mean static two-point discrimination was 8.2 ± 1.2 mm, key pinch was 66 % of the intact contralateral side, and grip power was 57 ± 17.4 % (range, 30–85 %) of the contralateral hand [26]. Huang et al. showed that the mean static two-point discrimination in partial great-toe transfer and second-toe transfer groups was 7.8 ± 1.3 mm and 7.6 ± 1.2 mm, respectively. The grip strength was 78 ± 6.3 % the normal contralateral hand in partial hallux transfer vs. 68 ± 9.7 % in second-toe transfer group [110]. Rosson and Buncke's [54] study mentioned previously noted that the IP joint motion was greater in hallux transplantation group compared with replantation after crush/avulsion injury but was the same between both after sharp cut amputations. Total MCP motion and grip and pinch strength were essentially the same between the two groups.

Data demonstrating that the transplanted toe has better sensation than both the donor toe and the replanted thumb [49, 100] suggests that the great-toe transplantation maybe functionally better than thumb replantation in crush/avulsion injury and as good as thumb replant in sharp cut amputation [54].

The best measurement of outcome is the use and function of the hand. With regard to this, there is only one well-designed study over long-term follow-up (range 3–13 years) [55]. In this study, Wei and Cheng showed that toe transfer patients had statistically significantly better overall hand function, work performance, aesthetics, and satisfaction. Functional testing demonstrated that strength and dexterity of the toe transfer hands were comparable to the opposite normal hands.

Complications

The most dreadful complication is free toe transfer failure; however, primary toe transplantation has a very high survival rate (range 93–100) [26, 45, 54, 59, 60, 110]. Failed toe transfer tends to happen in more frequently in transferred great toes compared with second-toe transplantation and in crush/avulsion compared to sharp injury [45, 54]. Notably, timing of transfer does not play any adverse effect on transplant survival [45]. There is no statistical difference in re-exploration rate between primary and secondary toe transfer. Risks of arterial or venous compromise can be minimized by maintaining meticulous hemostasis during the surgery, tension-free closure, and wide subcutaneous tunnels for the vessels. When perfusion is in doubt during the primary procedure, second artery should be utilized as a life boat [26, 45, 59, 60, 105, 110]. Vasospasm may complicate toe transfers just as it may threaten replanted digits; risk reduction for this and management are discussed elsewhere in this book (Chap. 8).

Conclusion

Toe transfer for restoration of finger or thumb function has a well-established role in settings where replantation is either impossible or has previously failed. Outcomes from both functional and aesthetic standpoints are good and compare favorably to primary replants. The mechanics of performing toe-to-hand transfer are essentially the same as those involved in replantation surgery and should come naturally to the experienced hand surgeon. The potential need for a toe transfer should guide management of the recipient hand during the initial surgery at the time of injury so that no reconstructive bridges are burned at the primary treatment. The techniques described above combined with a motivated patient may convert an otherwise "assist" hand to one with functional grasp and pinch.

References

1. www.brainyquote.com/quotes/authors/d/david_hockney_4.html.
2. Waljee JF, Chung KC. Toe-to-hand transfer: evolving indications and relevant outcomes. J Hand Surg Am. 2013;38(7):1431–4.
3. Matsuzaki H, Narisawa H, Miwa H, Toishi S. Predicting functional recovery and return to work after mutilating hand injuries: usefulness of Campbell's Hand Injury Severity Score. J Hand Surg Am. 2009;34(5):880–5.
4. Dzwierzynski WW. Replantation and revascularization. In: Neligan PC, Chang J, editors. Plastic surgery. 3rd ed. Philadelphia: Elsevier Saunders Publishing; 2013.
5. Wei FC, Carver N, Lee YS, et al. Sensory recovery and Meissner corpuscle number after toe-to-hand transplantation. Plast Reconstr Surg. 2000;105:2405–11.
6. Wei FC, El-Gammal TA, Lin CH, et al. Metacarpal hand: classification and guidelines for microsurgical reconstruction with toe transfers. Plast Reconstr Surg. 1997;99:122–8.
7. Kotkansalo T, Vilkki S, Elo P. Long-term results of finger reconstruction with microvascular toe transfers after trauma. J Plast Reconstr Aesthet Surg. 2011;64(10):1291–9.
8. Kotkansalo T, Vilkki SK, Elo P. The functional results of post-traumatic metacarpal hand reconstruction with microvascular toe transfers. J Hand Surg Eur Vol. 2009;34(6):730–42.
9. Gülgönen A, Gudemez E. Toe-to-hand transfers: more than 20 years follow-up of five post-traumatic cases. J Hand Surg Br. 2006;31(1):2–8.
10. Chung KC, Kotsis SV. Outcomes of multiple microvascular toe transfers for reconstruction in 2 patients with digitless hands: 2- and 4-year follow-up case reports. J Hand Surg Am. 2002;27(4):652–8.
11. Chen HC, Tang YB, Wei FC, Noordhoff SM. Finger reconstruction with triple toe transfer from the same foot for a patient with a special job and previous foot trauma. Ann Plast Surg. 1991;27:272–7.
12. El-Gammal TA, Wei FC. Microvascular reconstruction of the distal digits by partial toe transfer. Clin Plast Surg. 1997;24:49–55.
13. Koshima I, Soeda S, Dakase T, Yamasaki M. Free vascularized nail grafts. J Hand Surg Am. 1998;13:29–32.
14. Logan A, Elliot D, Foucher G. Free toe pulp transfer to restore traumatic digital pulp loss. Br J Plast Surg. 1985;38:497–500.

15. O'Brien BM, Brennen MB, MacLeod AM. Simultaneous double toe transfer for severely disabled hands. Hand. 1978;10:232–40.
16. Rose EH, Buncke HJ. Simultaneous transfer of the right and left second toes for reconstruction of amputated index and middle fingers in the same hand: case report. J Hand Surg Am. 1980;5:590–3.
17. Tan BK, Wei FC, Lutz BS, Lin CH. Strategies in multiple toe transplantation for bilateral type II metacarpal hand reconstruction. Hand Clin. 1999;15:607–12.
18. Tan BK, Wei FC, Chang KJ, Lutz BS. Combined third and fourth toe transplantation. Hand Clin. 1999;15:589–96.
19. Tsai TM. Second and third toe transplantation to a transmetacarpal amputated hand. Ann Acad Med Singapore. 1979;8:413–8.
20. Wei FC, Coskunfirat K, Lin CH, Lin YT. Isolated third toe transfer: indications, technique, and reliability. Plast Reconstr Surg. 2005;115:1314–21.
21. Wei FC, Jain V, Chen SHT. Toe-to-hand transplantation. Hand Clin. 2003;19:165–75.
22. Wei FC, Lutz BS, Cheng SL, Chuang DCC. Reconstruction of bilateral metacarpal hands with multiple toe transplantations. Plast Reconstr Surg. 1999;104:1698–704.
23. Wei FC, Mardini S. Reevaluation of the technique of toe-to-hand transfer for traumatic digital amputations in children and adolescents. Plast Reconstr Surg. 2003;112:1870–4.
24. Wei FC, Strauch RJ, Chen HC, Chuang CC. Reconstruction of four damaged or destroyed ipsilateral fingers with free toe-to-hand transplantations. Plast Reconstr Surg. 1994;93:608–14.
25. Wei FC, Yim KK. Single third-toe transfer in hand reconstruction. J Hand Surg Am. 1995;20:388–94.
26. Woo SH, Lee GJ, Kim KC, et al. Immediate partial great toe transfer for the reconstruction of composite defects of the distal thumb. Plast Reconstr Surg. 2006;117:1906–15.
27. American Replantation Mission to China. Replantation surgery in China. Plast Reconstr Surg. 1973;52:476–89.
28. Cobbett JR. Free digital transfer: report of a case of transfer of a great toe to replace an amputated thumb. J Bone Joint Surg Br. 1969;51:677–9.
29. del Piñal F. The indications for toe transfer after "minor" finger injuries. J Hand Surg Br. 2004;29:120–9.
30. El-Gammal TA, Wei FC. Microvascular toe transfer in children. Part B: the traumatic deficit. In: Scheker KS, editor. Growing hand. London: Harcourt; 1999. p. 1000–8.
31. Foucher G, Medina J, Navarro R, Nagel D. Toe transfer in congenital hand malformations. J Reconstr Microsurg. 2001;17:1–7.
32. Jones NF, Hansen SL, Bates SJ. Toe-to-hand transfers for congenital anomalies of the hand. Hand Clin. 2007;23:129–36.
33. May JW. Microvascular great toe to hand transfer for reconstruction of the amputated thumb. In: McCarthy

JG, editor. Plastic surgery. Philadelphia: WB Saunders; 1990. p. 5154–8.

34. O'Brien BM, Black MJ, Morrison WA, et al. Microvascular great toe transfer for congenital absence of the thumb. Hand. 1978;10:113–24.

35. O'Brien BM, MacLeod AM, Sykes PJ, Donahoe S. Hallux-to-hand transfer. Hand. 1975;7:128–33.

36. Ohmori K, Harii K. Transplantation of a toe to an amputated finger. Hand. 1975;7:134–8.

37. Tamai S, Hori Y, Tatsumi Y, Okuda H. Hallux-to-thumb transfer with microsurgical technique: a case report in a 45-year-old woman. J Hand Surg Am. 1977;2:152–5.

38. Wei FC. Thumb reconstruction. In: Weiss APC, Berger RA, editors. Hand surgery. Philadelphia: Lippincott Williams & Wilkins; 2003.

39. Wei FC, Chen HC, Chuang CC, Noordhoff SM. Simultaneous multiple toe transfers in hand reconstruction. Plast Reconstr Surg. 1988;81:366–77.

40. Wei FC, Chen HC, Chuang DCC, Noordhoff MS. Reconstruction of the thumb with a trimmed great toe transfer technique. Plast Reconstr Surg. 1988;52:506–13.

41. Wei FC, El-Gammal TA. Toe-to-hand transfer: current concepts, techniques and research. Clin Plast Surg. 1996;23:103–16.

42. Wei FC, Jain V. Discussion on the chapter of "revascularisation and replantation and toe to hand transfer" by Harry J. Buncke, Gregory M. Buncke, Gabriel M. Kind, and Rudolf F. Buntic. In: Goldwyn RM, Cohen MN, editors. The unfavorable result in plastic surgery: avoidance & treatment. 3rd ed. Philadelphia: Lippincott, Williams & Wilkins; 2001. p. 800–4.

43. Wei FC, Jain V. Discussion on the chapter of "thumb reconstruction" by Rosa L. Dell'Oca and Vincent R. Hentz. In: Goldwyn RM, Cohen MN, editors. The unfavorable result in plastic surgery: avoidance & treatment. 3rd ed. Philadelphia: Lippincott, Williams & Wilkins; 2001. p. 825–9.

44. Yang D, Yudog G. Thumb reconstruction utilizing second toe transplantation by microvascular anastomosis—report of 78 cases. Chin Med J. 1979;92:295–301.

45. Yim KK, Wei FC, Lin CH. A comparison between primary and secondary toe-to-hand transplantation. Plast Reconstr Surg. 2004;114:107–12.

46. Henry SL, Wei FC. Thumb reconstruction with toe transfer. J Hand Microsurg. 2010;2(2):72–8.

47. Wei FC, Henry SL. Toe-to-hand transplantation. In: Wolfe SW, editor. Green's operative hand surgery. 6th ed. New York: Elsevier Churchill Livingstone publishing; 2011.

48. White WL. Why I, hate the index finger. Orthop Rev. 1980;6:23.

49. Dellon AL. Sensory recovery in replanted digits and transplanted toes: a review. J Reconstr Microsurg. 1986;2:123–9.

50. Kaplan JD, Jones NF. Outcome measures of microsurgical toe transfers for reconstruction of congenital and traumatic hand anomalies. J Pediatr Orthop. 2014;34(3):362–8.

51. Wei FC, Coessens B, Ganos D. Multiple microsurgical toe-to-hand transfer in the reconstruction of the severely mutilated hand: a series of fifty-nine cases. Ann Chir Main Memb Super. 1992;16:177–87.

52. Wei FC, Colony LH. Microsurgical restoration of distal digital function. Clin Plast Surg. 1989;16:443–55.

53. Wei FC, Colony LH. Microsurgical reconstruction of opposable digits in mutilating hand injuries. Clin Plast Surg. 1989;16:491–504.

54. Rosson GD, Buncke GM, Buncke HJ. Great toe transplant versus thumb replant for isolated thumb amputation: critical analysis of functional outcome. Microsurgery. 2008;28:598–605.

55. Chung K, Wei FC. An outcome study of thumb reconstruction using microvascular toe transfer. J Hand Surg Am. 2000;25:651–8.

56. McKee NH. Amputation stump management and function preservation. In: McCarthy JG, editor. Plastic surgery. Philadelphia: WB Saunders; 1990. p. 4329–43.

57. Wei FC. Tissue preservation in hand injury—the first step to toe-to-hand transplantation. Plast Reconstr Surg. 1998;102:2497–501.

58. Yildirim S, Calikapan GT, Akoz T. Reconstructive microsurgery in pediatric population-a series of 25 patients. Microsurgery. 2008;28(2):99–107.

59. Woo SH, Kim JS, Seul JH. Immediate toe-to-hand transfer in acute hand injuries: overall results, compared with results for elective cases. Plast Reconstr Surg. 2004;113:882–92.

60. Ray EC, Sherman R, Stevanovic M. Immediate reconstruction of a nonreplantable thumb amputation by great toe transfer. Plast Reconstr Surg. 2009;123(1):259–67.

61. Chu NS, Wei FC. Recovery of sensation and somatosensory evoked potentials following toe-to-digit transplantation in man. Muscle Nerve. 1995;18:859–66.

62. Chang J, Jones NF. Simultaneous toe-to-hand transfer and lower extremity amputations for severe upper and lower limb defects: the use of spare parts. J Hand Surg Br. 2002;27(3):219–23.

63. Wei FC, Chen HC, Chuang DC, et al. Aesthetic refinements in toe-to-hand transfer surgery. Plast Reconstr Surg. 1996;98:485–90.

64. Woo SH, Lee GJ, Kim KC, et al. Cosmetic reconstruction of distal finger absence with partial second toe transfer. J Plast Reconstr Aesth Surg. 2006;59:317–24.

65. Wallace CG, Wei FC. Further aesthetic refinement for great toe transfers. J Plast Reconstr Aesthet Surg. 2010;63(1):e109–10.

66. Yim KK, Wei FC. Secondary procedures to improve function after toe-to-hand transfers. Br J Plast Surg. 1995;48:487–91.

67. Chen CT, Wei FC, Chen HC, et al. Distal phalanx replantation. Microsurgery. 1994;15:77–82.

68. Foucher G, Norris RW. Distal and very distal digital replantation. Br J Plast Surg. 1992;45:199–203.

69. Tamai S. Twenty years' experience of limb replantation: review of 293 upper extremity replants. J Hand Surg Am. 1982;7:549–56.

70. Urbaniak JR. Replantation. In: Green DP, editor. Operative hand surgery. 3rd ed. New York: Churchill Livingstone; 1993. p. 1085–102.

71. Wilson CS, Buncke HJ, Alpert BS, Gordon L. Composite metacarpophalangeal joint reconstruction in great toe-to-hand free tissue transfers. J Hand Surg Am. 1984;9:645–8.

72. Strauch RJ, Wei FC, Chen SHT. Composite finger metacarpophalangeal joint reconstruction in combined second and third free toe-to-hand transfers. J Hand Surg Am. 1993;18:972–7.

73. Yim KK, Wei FC. Intraosseous wiring in toe-to-hand transplantation. Ann Plast Surg. 1995;35:66–9.

74. Kato H, Ogino T, Minami A, Usui M. Restoration of sensibility in fingers repaired with free sensory flaps from the toe. J Hand Surg Am. 1989;14:49–54.

75. Chu NS, Wei FC. Peripheral recovery and central response following toe-to-finger transplantation. Suppl Clin Neurophysiol. 2006;59:317–20.

76. Foucher G. Discussion in: resurfacing of thumb-pulp loss with a heterodigital neurovascular island flap using a nerve disconnection/reconnection technique. J Reconstr Microsurg. 1997;13:122–3.

77. Kessler I. Cross transposition of short amputation stumps for reconstruction of the thumb. J Hand Surg Br. 1985;10:76–8.

78. Orticochea M. Reconstruction of the thumb using two flaps from the same hand. Br J Plast Surg. 1971;14:345–50.

79. del Piñal F, García-Bernal FJ, Delgado J, et al. Overcoming soft-tissue deficiency in toe-to-hand transfer using a dorsalis pedis fasciosubcutaneous toe free flap: surgical technique. J Hand Surg Am. 2005;30:111–9.

80. Gilbert A. Vascular anatomy of the first web space of the foot. In: Landi A, editor. Reconstruction of the thumb. London: Chapman & Hall; 1989. p. 205.

81. Gordon L. Toe-to-thumb transplantation. In: Green DP, editor. Operative hand surgery. New York: Churchill Livingstone; 1993. p. 1253–82.

82. Leung PC, Wong WL. The vessels of the first metatarsal web space: an operative and radiographic study. J Bone Joint Surg Am. 1983;65:235–8.

83. Gu XD, Zhang GM, Chen DS, Cheng XM, Xu JG, Wang H. Vascular anatomic variations in second toe transfers. J Hand Surg. 2000;25A:277–81.

84. Santamaria E, Chen HTS, Wei FC. Second toe/free joint transfer. In: Russell RC, Zamboni W, editors. Manual of free flaps. St Louis: CV Mosby; 2001.

85. Wei FC, Silverman TS, Hsu WM. Retrograde dissection of the vascular pedicle in toe harvest. Plast Reconstr Surg. 1995;96:1211–4.

86. Wei FC, Demirkan F, Chen HC, Chuang DC, Chen SH, Lin CH, Cheng SL, Cheng MH, Lin YT. The outcome of failed free flaps in head and neck and extremity reconstruction: what is next in the reconstructive ladder? Plast Reconstr Surg. 2001;108(5):1154–60; discussion 1161–2.

87. Foucher G, Moss AL. Microvascular second toe to finger transfer: a statistical analysis of 55 transfers. Br J Plast Surg. 1991;44:87–90.

88. Leung PC. Use of an intramedullary bone peg in digital replantation, revascularization and toe-transfers. J Hand Surg Am. 1981;6:281–4.

89. Urbaniak JR. Wrap-around procedure for thumb reconstruction. Hand Clin. 1985;1:259–69.

90. Valauri FA, Buncke HJ. Thumb and finger reconstruction by toe-to hand transfer. Hand Clin. 1992;8:551–74.

91. Morrison WA. Thumb reconstruction: a review and philosophy of management. J Hand Surg Br. 1992; 17:383.

92. Goldner RD. One hundred eleven thumb amputations: replantation vs revision. Microsurgery. 1990; 11:243–50.

93. Matev IB. The bone-lengthening method in hand reconstruction: twenty years' experience. J Hand Surg Am. 1989;14:376.

94. Morrison WA, O'Brien BM, MacLeod AM. Thumb reconstruction with a free neurovascular wrap-around flap from the big toe. J Hand Surg Am. 1980;5:575–83.

95. Wei FC, Chen HC, Chuang DCC, et al. Second toe wrap-around flap. Plast Reconstr Surg. 1991;88: 837–43.

96. Buncke HJ. Thumb and finger reconstruction by microvascular second toe and joint autotransplantation. In: McCarthy JG, editor. Plastic surgery. Philadelphia: WB Saunders; 1990. p. 4409–29.

97. Buncke HJ. Digital reconstruction by second-toe transplantation. In: Buncke HJ, editor. Microsurgery: transplantation, replantation: an atlas text. Philadelphia: Lea & Febiger; 1991. p. 61–101.

98. Gilbert A. Discussion in: the second toe flap. In: Serafin D, editor. Atlas of microsurgical composite tissue transplantation. Philadelphia: WB Saunders; 1996. p. 616–8.

99. Koshima I, Eoh H, Moriguchi T, Soeda S. Sixty cases of partial or total toe transfer for repair of finger losses. Plast Reconstr Surg. 1993;92:1331–8.

100. Leung PC. Thumb reconstruction using second-toe transfer. Hand Clin. 1985;1:285–95.

101. Wei FC, Chen HC, Chuang CC, Chen SH. Microsurgical thumb reconstruction with toe transfer: selection of various techniques. Plast Reconstr Surg. 1994;93:345–51.

102. Wei FC, Epstein MD, Chen HC, et al. Microsurgical reconstruction of distal digits following mutilating hand injuries: results in 121 patients. Br J Plast Surg. 1993;46:181–6.

103. Wei FC, Colony LH, Chen HC, et al. Combined second and third toe transfer. Plast Reconstr Surg. 1989;84:651–61.

104. Cheng MH, Wei FC, Santamaria E, et al. Single versus double arterial anastomoses in combined second- and third-toe transplantation. Plast Reconstr Surg. 1998;102:2408–12.

105. Kurt E, Ozturk S, Isik S, et al. Continuous brachial plexus blockade for digital replantations and toe-to-hand transfers. Ann Plast Surg. 2005;54:24–7.

106. Bakri K, Moran SL. Monitoring for upper extremity free flaps and replantations. J Hand Surg. 2008;33A: 1905–8.

107. Hovius SER, van Adrichem LNA, Mulder HD, et al. Comparison of laser Doppler flowmetry and thermometry in the postoperative monitoring of replantations. J Hand Surg. 1995;20A:88–93.

108. Wei FC, Ma HS. Delayed sensory reeducation after toe-to-hand transfer. Microsurgery. 1995;16:583–5.

109. Dellon AL. Sensory re-education after fingertip injury and reconstruction. In: Foucher G, editor. Fingertip and nailbed injuries. New York: Churchill Livingstone; 1991. p. 27–39.

110. Huang D, Wang HG, Wu WZ, Zhang HR, Lin H. Functional and aesthetic results of immediate reconstruction of traumatic thumb defects by toe-to-thumb transplantation. Int Orthop. 2011;35(4):543–7.

Heterotopic Digital Replantation

10

Cheng-Hung Lin and Fu-Chan Wei

Introduction

Reconstruction of the mutilated hand is one of the most difficult challenges for hand surgeons [1]. Replantation of amputated digits is without doubt the best option to restore function, especially when multiple digits are involved [2]. Refinements in microsurgical technique and effective postoperative monitoring have seen the survival rate of digital replantation approach 90 % [3–5]. However, the challenge is not only to restore circulation to a digit but also to create a functional hand. To this end, restoration of an opposable thumb and at least two fingers to work against, each pain-free and sensate with mobile and stable joints, is the key priority when treating a mutilated hand [6, 7].

Orthotopic digital replantation (ODR) restores amputated digits in their original anatomical position. This is the most straightforward and established procedure following digital amputation. However, for cases where amputated parts or their recipient stumps are unsalvageable or unavailable, ODR cannot be performed. In such circumstances, heterotopic digital replantation (HDR), tempo-rary ectopic implantation, or toe-to-hand transfer should be considered [8–12]. HDR would seem the most practical and reliable method to reconstruct the mutilated hand in the acute setting. HDR is defined as replacing an amputated digit in a position other than its original anatomical site. The greatest advantage of HDR over ODR is the functional, rather than anatomical, approach to reconstruction. Another advantage is limiting donor site morbidity to the zone of trauma. Despite these advantages, the optimal replantation strategy in terms of where to position the amputated digits remains a topic for debate [13–15].

In this article, the clinical results of our reconstructions are presented and used as a basis for a guideline for the management of mutilating hand injuries with HDR.

Indications/Guidelines for HDR

One of the main reconstructive goals following multiple digit amputation is recreating a tripod pinch. For HDR in the mutilated hand, this presents three main considerations: (i) thumb reconstruction, (ii) at least two fingers to oppose against the thumb, and (iii) management of any associated hand injury.

The first consideration is to the thumb because it contributes 40–50 % of hand function [3]. Reconstruction should aim to restore length and sensation. Moreover, if there is an associated injury to thenar muscles, which may compromise the function of the thumb, the author advocates

C.-H. Lin, MD (✉)
Department of Plastic and Reconstructive Surgery, Chang Gung Memorial Hospital, Taipei, Taiwan
e-mail: lukechlin@gmail.com

F.-C. Wei, MD
Department of Plastic Surgery, Chang Gung Memorial Hospital, Taipei, Taiwan
e-mail: fuchanwei@gmail.com

A.N. Salyapongse et al. (eds.), *Extremity Replantation: A Comprehensive Clinical Guide*,
DOI 10.1007/978-1-4899-7516-4_10, © Springer Science+Business Media New York 2015

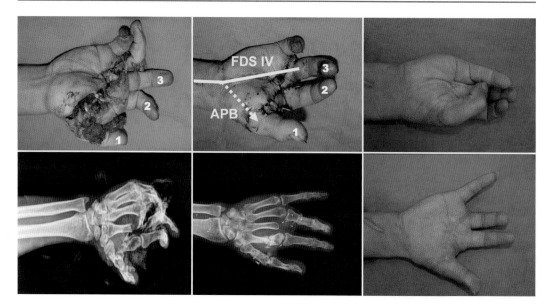

Fig. 10.1 Immediate opponensplasty with flexor digitorum superficialis from the amputated finger. *Left*: crush injury of right hand, resulted in incomplete amputation of right thumb, index, long, and ring fingers with severance of the thenar muscle, destruction of right third metacarpophalangeal joint, and long-segmented comminuted bone fracture of right ring finger. *Middle*: heterotopic replantation of amputated long finger to right ring finger stump was performed for optimal restoration of the skeleton. Immediate Bunnell opponensplasty was also carried out for improving thumb function. *Right*: opposition 7/10 on Kapandji's scale was achieved at 1 year after surgery

that an immediate opponensplasty, using the redundant flexor digitorum superficialis of the amputated finger that was replanted onto the thumb, greatly improves thumb function with no additional donor site morbidity (Fig. 10.1).

The second consideration is to provide at least two opposable fingers. Amputation of the fingers can be classified as a metacarpal hand (loss of all digits), loss of radial (index ± middle ± ring) or ulnar (little ± ring ± middle) digits, loss of alternate fingers (index and ring; middle and little), or other combinations, such as loss of central (middle and/or ring) digits or loss of both radial and ulnar digits. A metacarpal hand requires restoration of at least two functional digits [6]. Wei et al. found grip strength to be greater when replanting digits to the ulnar stumps of the hand. In contrast, if the patient requires better dexterity for more delicate work, digits are best reconstructed on the radial side of the hand. A compromise position is to reconstruct middle and ring fingers. This provides some degree of power grip, an adequate first web space, as well as precision grip [6, 16].

Replantation of multiple radial or ulnar digit amputations should start from adjacent to an uninjured finger to avoid a mid-hand gap. This principle also governs reconstruction of amputations of alternate digits, where reestablishing three contiguous fingers is the priority. If this is not possible, ray amputation of the intervening amputated digit should be considered [17]. Management of other rare amputation combinations should prioritize reconstruction of the central rays in the first instance (middle and ring fingers). This is reflected in the higher percentage of middle (77.3 %) and ring finger (78.9 %) reconstructions undertaken than for index (40 %) and little finger (21.4 %) in our series (unpublished). In summary, the vast majority of multiple amputations can be managed by reconstructing digits in the following order: middle, ring or index, index or ring, followed by the little finger (Fig. 10.2).

The third consideration is management of any associated hand injury. When the amputated digit is judged unsuitable for replantation, it should be borne in mind that the remnant can be used for "spare parts" to reconstruct other injuries within the hand. Useful components may include skin, soft tissue, nail bed, nerve, vessel, bone, joint, and tendon [17, 18]. It may even be possible to design a small free flap or vascularized joint transfer to improve function (Fig. 10.3).

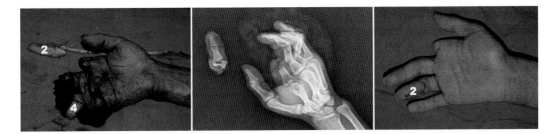

Fig. 10.2 Heterotopic digital replantation for avoiding a mid-hand gap. *Left, middle*: crush avulsion injury of right hand with avulsion amputation of index finger and segmental amputation of ring finger. *Right*: transplantation of amputated index finger to the ring finger stump for better coordination of the fingers and esthetic result

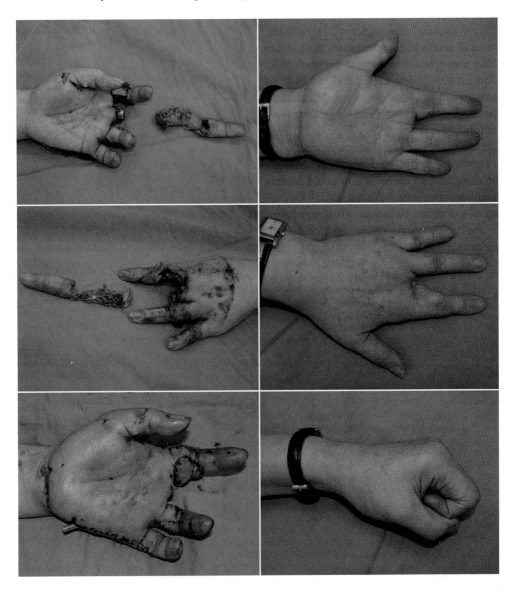

Fig. 10.3 Spare parts surgery: transfer parts of the tissue from the less functional amputated part or stump. *Left*: crush injury of left hand, resulted in long-segmented comminuted bone fracture of amputated long finger, and soft tissue defect at the ulnar index finger. Amputation of left long finger to the metacarpophalangeal joint and free fillet flap from amputated long finger for reconstruction of left index finger was performed. *Right*: good functional and esthetic outcomes at 9 months after surgery

When all possible functional requirements are met, an attempt should be made to restore the normal length sequence of the digits. This can improve the overall cosmetic appearance of the hand that many patients appreciate.

Conclusion

Following mutilating hand injuries where multiple digits are amputated, HDR has many advantages over ODR when trying to achieve the best possible functional reconstruction. The "best" amputated parts are reserved for thumb reconstruction and two opposable adjacent fingers which, together, can achieve tripod pinch. Most other injuries which would otherwise compromise hand function could be corrected simultaneously with the concept of "spare parts." As with all ventures in reconstruction of the mutilated hand, the operative plan must take into account the mechanism of injury, patient's occupation, functional demands, expectations and motivation, age and comorbidities, associated injuries, and psychological status [19]. The ultimate functional outcomes will be influenced by the success of patient education, rehabilitation, and any secondary reconstructive surgery performed [14].

References

1. Weinzweig J, Weinzweig N. The "tic-tac-toe" classification system for mutilated injuries of the hand. Plast Reconstr Surg. 1997;100:1200–11.
2. del Piñal F. Severe mutilated injuries to the hand: guidelines for organizing the chaos. J Plast Reconstr Aesthet Surg. 2007;60:816–27.
3. Waikakul S, Sakkarnkosol S, Vanadurongwan V, et al. Results of 1018 digital replantations in 552 patients. Injury. 2000;31:33–40.
4. Buncke HJ, Buncke GM, Lineaweaver WC, et al. The contributions of microvascular surgery to emergency hand surgery. World J Surg. 1991;15:418–28.
5. Chiu HY. Indications and contraindications of digital replantation. J Formos Med Assoc. 1992;91:S214–21.
6. Wei FC, el-Gammal TA, Lin CH, et al. Metacarpal hand: classification and guidelines for microsurgical reconstruction with toe transfers. Plast Reconstr Surg. 1997;99:122–8.
7. Wilhelmi BJ, Lee WP, Pagenstert GI, May Jr JW. Replantation in the mutilated hand. Hand Clin. 2003;19:89–120.
8. An PC, Kuo YR, Lin TS, et al. Heterotopic digit replantation in mutilated hand injury. Ann Plast Surg. 2003;50:113–8.
9. Brooks D, Buntic R, Buncke HJ. Use of a venous flap from an amputated part for salvage of an upper extremity injury. Ann Plast Surg. 2002;48:189–92.
10. Druecke D, Homann HH, Kutscha-Lissberg F, et al. Crossover extremity transfers. Limb salvage in amputations with segmental defects. Chirurg. 2007;78:954–8.
11. Lin CH, Hu TL, Lin CH. Split second- and third-toe transplantation in mutilating-hand-injury reconstruction. Ann Plast Surg. 2008;60:267–71.
12. Wei FC, el-Gammal TA. Toe-to-hand transfer. Current concepts, techniques, and research. Clin Plast Surg. 1996;23:103–16.
13. Chiu HY, Lu SY, Lin TW, et al. Transpositional digital replantation. J Trauma. 1985;25:440–3.
14. Lin CH, Wei FC, Chen HC. Microsurgical transfer of avulsed index finger to degloved thumb – a case report. J Surg Assoc ROC. 1993;26:223–7.
15. Soucacos PN, Beris AE, Malizos KN, et al. Transpositional microsurgery in multiple digital amputations. Microsurgery. 1994;15:469–73.
16. Wei FC, Colony LH. Microsurgical reconstruction of opposable digits in mutilating hand injuries. Clin Plast Surg. 1989;16:491–504.
17. Brown RE, Wu TY. Use of "spare parts" in mutilated upper extremity injuries. Hand Clin. 2003;19:73–87.
18. Russell RC, Neumeister MW, Ostric SA, et al. Extremity reconstruction using nonreplantable tissue ("spare parts"). Clin Plast Surg. 2007;34:211–22.
19. Gerostathopoulos N, Efstathopoulos D, Misitzis D, Bouchlis G, Anagnostou S, Daoutis NK. Mid-palm replantation. Long-term results. Acta Orthop Scand Suppl. 1995;264:9–11.

Replantation in the Child and Adolescent

Joshua M. Abzug, Scott H. Kozin, and Dan A. Zlotolow

Introduction

Fortunately, traumatic amputations in the pediatric population are relatively rare events. However, when they do occur, they are emotionally devastating injuries for the child, the child's family, and the health-care team caring for the child. While the majority of aspects regarding replantation in children are analogous to replantation in adults, several important and distinct differences exist. This chapter will highlight these differences, while permitting the reader to obtain the detailed discussions of each component from the other chapters in this book.

Mechanism and Etiology

The true incidence of pediatric traumatic amputations remains unknown; however, white males, with an average age of 10 years, are the most commonly injured pediatric population [1, 2]. Amputations that occur at the elbow, midpalm, or digital levels are the most common locations that are seen in the

pediatric population [2]. The most common mechanisms of injury, especially around the hand and digits, are cutting/piercing mechanisms that may occur with a saw or axe [1, 3]. Alternatively, bicycle chain injuries and door slams are commonly seen in distal digital injuries, causing either crushing injuries or avulsions [3] (Fig. 11.1a–d). Rare mechanisms can also occur due to young children placing their fingers in things that older children and adults would not (Figs. 11.2 and 11.3). More proximal injuries are commonly the result of motor vehicle collisions, train accidents where the limb is hit by the moving train causing the amputation, or power tool injuries [3].

Another unusual mechanism of injury seen in the pediatric population is trauma caused by home exercise equipment. Injuries sustained due to treadmills typically result in abrasions, burns, or minor lacerations [4]; however, injuries sustained by exercycles/stationary bicycles can lead to traumatic amputations [5] (Fig. 11.4). Benson et al. reviewed 32 traumatic digital injuries, in 19 children, that occurred as the result of injuries sustained secondary to exercycles/stationary bicycles. Thirteen digits were injured by the wheel spokes, including 3 amputations, and 19 digits were injured by the chain or sprocket, including 16 amputations. Due to the recognition of home exercise equipment as a mechanism of injury involved in pediatric amputation, the authors recommended that manufacturers design shielding for the wheel spokes and enclose the entire chain axis and gear interface. Additionally, children between the ages

J.M. Abzug, MD (✉)
Department of Orthopaedics, University of Maryland
Medical System, Timonium, MD, USA
e-mail: jabzug@umoa.umm.edu

S.H. Kozin, MD • D.A. Zlotolow, MD
Department of Orthopaedic Surgery, Shriners
Hospital for Children, Philadelphia, PA, USA
e-mail: skozin@shrinenet.org; dzlotolow@yahoo.com

A.N. Salyapongse et al. (eds.), *Extremity Replantation: A Comprehensive Clinical Guide*,
DOI 10.1007/978-1-4899-7516-4_11, © Springer Science+Business Media New York 2015

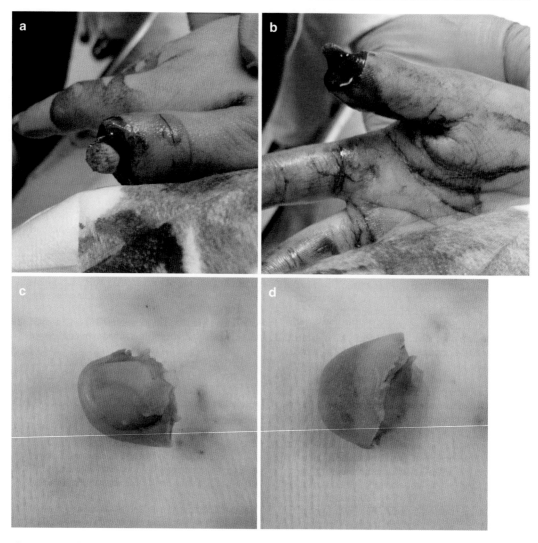

Fig. 11.1 (**a–d**) Avulsion-type amputation in a 7-year-old child that occurred due to a door slam. (**a**) Dorsal view of the thumb with exposed distal phalanx. (**b**) Volar view with the exposed distal phalanx. (**c**) Dorsal view of the amputated part. (**d**) Volar view of the amputated part. Note the bruising of the pulp indicating a crushing component of the injury (Published with kind permission of Joshua Abzug. © Joshua Abzug 2014. All Rights Reserved)

of 18 months and 5 years should not be permitted near the home exercise equipment [5].

Anatomic and Physiologic Differences

Children are not just little adults. There are differences related to their anatomy and physiology that are important to consider, especially in traumatic situations, such as an amputation. With regard to the bony anatomy, preservation of the physis is critical when performing any replantation, to permit continued growth. Additionally, during early childhood, the bones of the amputated part may still be primarily cartilaginous, making radiographic interpretation difficult. Lastly, with regard to the bony anatomy of children, the periosteum is thick and has

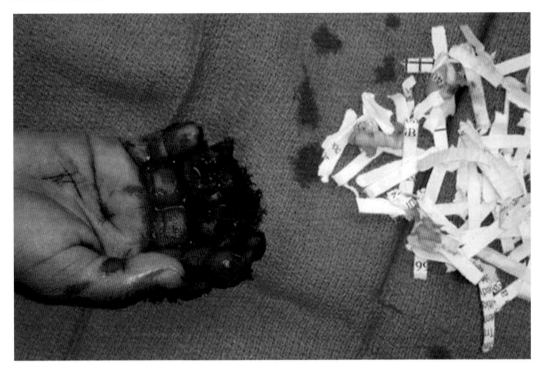

Fig. 11.2 Multiple digit crush amputation caused by a young child placing his or her fingers in a paper shredder (Published with kind permission of Joshua Ratner, MD. © Joshua Ratner 2014. All Rights Reserved)

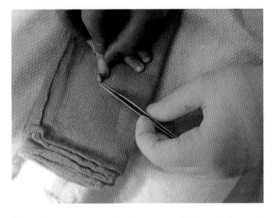

Fig. 11.3 Near amputation that occurred due to a 15 month-old child placing his finger in the cage of a domestic parrot (Published with kind permission of Joshua Abzug. © Joshua Abzug 2014. All Rights Reserved)

a rich vascular supply, permitting for rapid bone healing.

The soft tissue structures also heal more rapidly with less scarring in children compared to

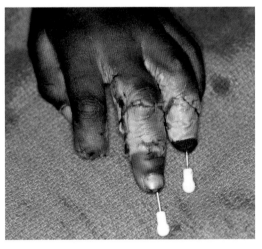

Fig. 11.4 Successful replantation of the long and ring fingers following an exercycle injury. Note the revision amputation required on the index finger due to the severity of injury caused by the wheel spokes (Published with kind permission of Shriners Hospital for Children, Philadelphia, PA. © Shriners Hospital for Children (Philadelphia, PA) 2014. All Rights Reserved)

adults. Most importantly, this permits faster and better recovery of nerve regeneration following repair. Furthermore, the shorter distance required for neural input following repair allows for improved muscle and sensory recovery. On the contrary, vasospasm occurs more easily in children and may be more severe than in adults. Therefore, early recognition and treatment of this is necessary [6]. However, overall, children have more favorable outcomes following replantation than adults [3, 7–9].

Initial Evaluation

The evaluation of a child who sustains an amputation begins at the scene of the accident with the first responders. As life comes before limb, the child as a whole needs to be evaluated including assessment of the airway, breathing, and circulation, prior to any evaluation of the amputated area. Therefore, standard advanced trauma life support (ATLS) and pediatric advanced life support (PALS) protocols should be initiated as soon as personnel arrive on the scene. Once the ABCs have been performed, evaluation and early treatment of the amputated part can begin.

Initially, direct pressure should be applied to any areas of bleeding, to minimize blood loss and prevent the child from going into hypovolemic shock. If the bleeding is uncontrollable and the child is hemodynamically unstable, a tourniquet should be applied to maintain adequate perfusion to the rest of the child. It is important that the time be noted when the tourniquet was applied, as this is a useful information for the replantation team and can alter decision-making processes based on the child's overall condition. A clamp/hemostat should not be applied directly on the end of a vessel to control bleeding, as this may severely damage the vessel and prevent the opportunity for replantation.

Once the child is stabilized, attention should be turned to the amputated part. Prehospital personnel should be trained in the appropriate handling of amputated parts, which begins by placing the part in a moist sterile gauze (Fig. 11.5) and then inside a waterproof bag. Subsequently, the

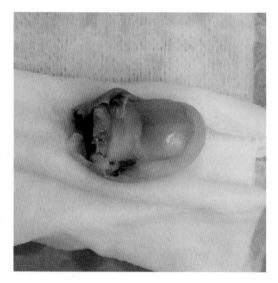

Fig. 11.5 Amputated part wrapped in moist sterile gauze. The part should then be placed in a waterproof bag and then on ice (Published with kind permission of Joshua Abzug. © Joshua Abzug 2014. All Rights Reserved)

bag is placed in a bucket of ice. The part should never be placed directly on the ice, as this will cause frostbite and/or freezing of the tissues, again preventing the opportunity for replantation. It is also important to note that the part should never be placed on dry ice.

Following stabilization and packaging of the patient and amputated part, rapid transport to a center capable of performing replantation in children is critical. Upon arrival in the emergency department, a formal assessment of the patient and amputated part will be made by the replantation team to determine the feasibility of replantation. Therefore, we feel that prior to this determination, it is important that the patient and their family not be told that the part will definitely undergo a replantation attempt. Thus, the replantation team needs to be notified early in the prehospital evaluation to permit adequate time for the appropriate personnel and resources to be available when the child arrives in the emergency department.

The replantation team will perform a thorough evaluation of the proximal stump and amputated part in the operating room. Therefore, the dressings applied to the proximal stump in the prehospital environment that are maintaining hemostasis should not be removed by additional prehospital personnel, emergency department providers, or the trauma team. Furthermore, the part should remain wrapped in the moist gauze inside the waterproof bag on ice, as excessive handling of the part may lead to more damage or the part being misplaced. The unnecessary performance of these tasks may delay the replantation team and/or disrupt the hemostasis that has already occurred. A photograph taken at the scene of initial evaluation with a digital camera may be helpful to show providers the injury and thus prevent the temptation of the aforementioned processes.

While the patient is in the emergency department being evaluated by the replantation team, a simultaneous resuscitation following ATLS and PALS protocols should be occurring. This includes the establishment of two large-bore intravenous catheters, infusion of warm Lactated Ringer's solution, and warming of the patient. Blood or crystalloid transfusions should be performed liberally as blood loss at the scene of the accident is usually underestimated. More than 40 % of children who undergo a replantation require postoperative blood transfusions [10, 11]. Antibiotic prophylaxis with a first-generation cephalosporin should also be given in the emergency department. If the scene of the accident was on a farm or involved soil, penicillin should be added. The child should also receive tetanus prophylaxis.

Surgical Indications

The vast majority of microsurgeons feel that any amputated part in a child should undergo an attempt at replantation as future function and psychosocial adaptation may be improved, analogous to congenital hand anomaly correction [10]. This is due to the excellent healing potential present in the pediatric population, which permits the ability to regain motion easier and have enhanced nerve regeneration. However, Chung and colleagues recently showed that replantation only occurs in approximately 40 % of pediatric finger amputations [1]. Additionally, the authors noted that Caucasian patients and those with private health insurance more commonly undergo replantation, even after controlling for confounding factors, compared to blacks, Hispanics, or children without health insurance [1].

The specific mechanism of injury that caused the amputation may determine whether or not replantation should be attempted. Older children who sustain amputations due to guillotine mechanisms are the best candidates for replantation and have the best outcomes [3]. Crushing and avulsion amputations, typically occurring in children around 5 years of age, have less predictable outcomes [3]. Any amputation that results in a hemodynamically unstable patient should not be considered for replantation as a prolonged procedure may lead to the patient becoming critically ill or even dying.

While single-digit replantation is typically contraindicated in adults, replantation should be attempted in a child with a clean guillotine-type amputation, as functional sensation and motion are typically restored. Even very distal replantation (distal to the distal interphalangeal joint) has been shown to be technically feasible with either composite grafting or artery repair alone [11–13]. Composite grafting works best in younger children, typically less than 3 years of age, and more distal amputations. Microsurgical anastomosis yields better results than composite grafting, even when arterial repair alone is performed, and therefore should be undertaken when technically feasible [12, 13]. Thumb, multiple digit, mid-palm, and proximal amputations should all undergo replantation if at all technically feasible. However, it is imperative to ensure that the child is not too sick, the ischemia time is not prolonged, there are not significant injuries at multiple levels, and the brachial plexus has not been avulsed, especially in proximal amputations.

Operative Technique

The technical aspects of replantation in children are analogous to adults with a few caveats. When shortening the bone, the physis should be preserved if at all possible to permit continued growth of the part. Additionally, fixation across the physis should be limited to smooth wires/pins if possible as this will limit the potential for physeal arrest or bar formation. Plates can be utilized in the diaphysis of long bones in more proximal injuries.

Another potential caveat in children is that amputations sustained at the distal interphalangeal joint or distal to this point can undergo composite grafting [11]. This technique should be limited to younger patients, typically those 3 years old or less and those with more distal amputations. The suture placed should be absorbable to avoid causing unnecessary pain and discomfort for the child during suture removal. Despite reported success with this technique, microsurgical anastomosis, even if only the artery was repaired, yields better results and is preferred when technically possible [12, 13]. Shi and colleagues performed 12 replantations in children at or distal to the nail base and only had one that failed [13].

The postoperative management of a child who has undergone replantation is mainly analogous to that of adults with a few minor differences (Fig. 11.6). We admit children to the pediatric intensive care unit for 5 days while they receive a

low-dose heparin drip. During this time, sedation with narcotics and/or anxiolytics may be necessary to minimize pain, fear, and/or anxiety. This is important to do as activation of the sympathetic nervous system may induce vasospasm [14].

Outcomes

The success of replantation in children is reported to be higher than that for adults, with rates as high as 97 % and 151° of active finger motion [15, 16]. Additionally, thumb motion has been shown to be 130°, two-point discrimination was normal in 88 % of children, and grip strength was equal to the contralateral limb in 79 % of patients [16]. These results can be attributed to faster soft tissue healing, less scar formation, improved nerve regeneration, easier joint mobilization, and enhanced tendon gliding.

The factors that are most likely to yield a successful outcome in pediatric replantation include age under 34 months, guillotine-like amputations, body weight greater than 11 kg, repair of more than one vein, bone shortening, intraosseous fixation, and vein grafting of arteries and veins. No correlation has been shown to occur when assessing survival of the replantation compared to the total ischemia time or digit position [11].

Proximal replantation results are not as favorable compared to digital replantation, with success rates of 77 % reported for complete amputations and 80 % for revascularization procedures. Furthermore, on average, additional 2.8 procedures were needed to attempt to improve function. These suboptimal results are likely due to myonecrosis causing sepsis [14].

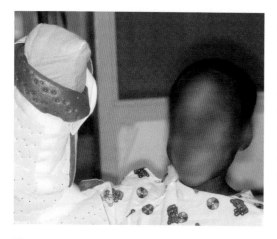

Fig. 11.6 Example of the bulky postoperative dressing utilized for the child who underwent successful replantation of the long and ring fingers following an exercycle injury. Note the elevation of the limb to aid in venous return (Published with kind permission of Shriners Hospital for Children, Philadelphia, PA. © Shriners Hospital for Children (Philadelphia, PA) 2014. All Rights Reserved)

Conclusion

Amputations in children are rare injuries, but when they occur, they are emotionally devastating events for the child, the family, and the health-care providers. Successful replantation can occur; however, the child's life must always take precedence before proceeding. Indications are broader than those in adults and the outcomes are improved. This is due to the improved healing potential of children with less scar formation and their increased ability to regenerate nerves.

References

1. Squitieri L, Reichert H, Kim HM, Steggerda J, Chung KC. Patterns of surgical care and health disparities of treating pediatric finger amputation injuries in the United States. J Am Coll Surg. 2011;213:475–85.
2. Galway HR, Hubbarb S, Mowbray M. Traumatic amputations in children. In: Kostvik JP, editor. Amputation surgery and rehabilitation – the Toronto experience. Edinburgh: Churchill Livingstone; 1981.
3. Jaeger SH, Tsai TM, Kleinert HE. Upper extremity replantation in children. Orthop Clin North Am. 1981;12:897–907.
4. Carman C, Chang B. Treadmill injuries to the upper extremity in pediatric patients. Ann Plast Surg. 2011; 46:15–9.
5. Benson LS, Waters PM, Meier SW, Visotsky JL, Williams CS. Pediatric hand injuries due to home exercycles. J Ped Orthop. 2000;20:34–9.
6. Duteille F, Lim A, Dautel G. Free flap coverage of upper and lower limb tissue defects in children: a series of 22 patients. Ann Plast Surg. 2003;50:344–9.
7. Van Beek AL, Wavak PW, Zook EG. Microvascular surgery in young children. Plast Reconstr Surg. 1979; 63:457–62.
8. O'Brien BM, Franklin JD, Morrison WA, et al. Replantation and revascularization surgery in children. Hand. 1980;12:12.
9. Berger A, Meissl G, Walzer L. Techniques and results in replantation surgery in children. Int J Microsurg. 1981;3:9.
10. Boyer MI, Mih AD. Microvascular surgery in the reconstruction of congenital hand anomalies. Hand Clin. 1998;14:135–42.
11. Baker GL, Kleinert JM. Digit replantation in infants and young children: determinants of survival. Plast Reconstr Surg. 1994;94:139–45.
12. Heisten JB, Cook PA. Factors affecting composite graft survival in digital tip amputations. Ann Plast Surg. 2003;50:299–303.
13. Shi D, Qi J, Li D, Zhu L, Jin W, Cai D. Fingertip replantation at or beyond the nail base in children. Microsurgery. 2010;30:380–5.
14. Beris AE, Soucacos PN, Malizos KN, et al. Major limb replantation in children. Microsurgery. 1994;15: 474–8.
15. Wang S, Young K, Wei J. Replantation of severed limbs – clinical analysis of 91 cases. J Hand Surg Am. 1981;6:311–8.
16. Cheng GL, Pan DD, Zhang NP, Fang GR. Digital replantation in children: a long-term follow-up study. J Hand Surg Am. 1998;23(4):635–46.

Lower Limb Replantation

12

Pedro C. Cavadas and Alessandro Thione

Introduction

Lower extremity traumatic amputations are not infrequent injuries in developed countries, affecting a relatively young population group and commonly associated with motor-vehicle accidents. Optimal treatment of these injuries has not been established, although the literature tends to support primary revision amputation and prosthesis [1–3]. This apparently straightforward approach has distinct complications, including stump neuromas, irritation and ulceration of the skin, substantial long-term costs, and derangement of the patient's body self-image [4].

Replantation of lower extremity amputations is not a widely accepted procedure, even some decades after the first reported case [5]. Most of the literature discourages replantation, arguing high complication rates, protracted treatment times, high economic costs, and marginally functional results [6, 7]. Most reports on lower limb replantation are either anecdotal successful case reports [5, 8–13] or short case series with mixed results [14–16]. The series reported by the authors in 2009 and the cases performed since then demonstrate that consistently good results

can be obtained, following some modifications in the approach to these injuries [17].

Above the knee replantation has been very infrequently reported [18]. These unfortunate injuries should be approached cautiously and differently from infrapopliteal amputations due to the volume of energy absorbed and injury sustained, the limited available information about outcomes, and the definite risk of fatal complications. The authors do not have experience in transfemoral replantation, and therefore this discussion will be limited to infrapopliteal amputations. Theoretically, a clean distal or middle-third femoral amputation with at least half of the quadriceps preserved and innervated in the stump, without associated life-threatening injuries, could benefit from replantation in the right environment. This clinical scenario is nevertheless very infrequent and should be considered cautiously.

The single most important characteristic of a native leg, compared to a below-knee prosthesis, is plantar sensation [19–21]. It is a sensate sole that can make a replanted foot better than a prosthesis. In this regard, lower limb replantation can be considered as a replantation of a functional sole of the foot. Restoring a properly aligned, stable skeleton with excellent skin coverage is the other integral part of the procedure to obtain a limb that is better than a prosthesis. From this basic situation, the more ankle and foot active motion achieved, the more favorable this outcome will be for the patient.

P.C. Cavadas, MD, PhD (✉)
A. Thione, MD, PhD
Department of Reconstructive Surgery,
Clinica Cavadas, Hospital de Manises, Valencia, Spain
e-mail: pcavadas@telefonica.net; althione@gmail.com

A.N. Salyapongse et al. (eds.), *Extremity Replantation: A Comprehensive Clinical Guide*,
DOI 10.1007/978-1-4899-7516-4_12, © Springer Science+Business Media New York 2015

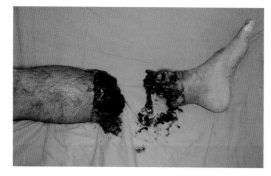

Fig. 12.1 A relatively sharp injury. After proper debridement and bone shortening, direct wound closure could be achieved with minimal wound necrosis. A flap was not needed

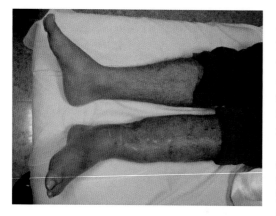

Fig. 12.2 A case of Fig. 12.1 after bone lengthening; the final result was good. This is a very unusual situation in the authors' practice

Timeframe is another key element in treating these injuries. The goal should be to have all treatment finished by 1 year. Shorter times may not be realistic, and longer times can be prohibitively burdensome to the patients.

Complications in lower limb replantation are the rule, rather than the exception. Only rarely, in sharp injuries, do wounds not develop edge necrosis (Figs. 12.1 and 12.2). Expectant approaches after the initial replantation have led to unacceptable rates of failure and poor function [17]. Prevention and treatment of these almost ubiquitous complications should be considered crucial elements of the replantation procedure. Lower limb replantation, in sharp contrast to upper limb injuries, should be considered a

staged procedure, the emergency replantation being but the first stage. Soft-tissue management with secondary debridement and early free flap coverage and bone lengthening are, respectively, the second and third stages that have to be carefully planned and timely executed. This aggressive approach, when performed by trained and highly involved teams, yields consistently good results [17].

Indications

The risk-benefit ratio is very delicately balanced in lower limb replantation, and indications should be carefully evaluated [19–22]. Because the staged process is labor-intensive and requires highly committed teams for consistent results, the first consideration should include the ability and willingness of the team to assume such cases. Otherwise, referral to the proper team, if time and general condition of the patient allow, is appropriate.

Given the complexity of the whole process, and the high risk of complications, absolute indications cannot be unequivocally established. A balanced interplay between the type of injury, the general condition of the patient, and the technical capacity and involvement of the surgical team is critical for deciding a particular indication. Complex replantations, as in the case of the lower limb, should not be "attempted." Instead, a clear plan of reconstruction possibilities, likely complications, and the solution for them should be formulated at the outset, and then, if the chances for success are considered high, replantation should proceed. Absolute contraindications are infrequent and include anatomic destruction of the sole of the foot, massive crushing of the extremity, concurrent destruction of the knee joint in a young patient, sacral root avulsion, and extended ischemia time (over 8–10 h). Ischemia times in the 6–8 h range can be managed with temporary arterial catheter perfusion [23]. While there exists a whole collection of injury severity scores for lower limb trauma, with cutoff numbers for salvage, their usefulness for the experienced surgeon is very limited.

Age, per se, is not a contraindication, but previous ambulatory state is important. A physically fit patient in his or her seventies could benefit from replantation. A previously nonambulatory patient has no indication for replantation regardless of the age. Pediatric injuries have a wider indication for replantation [4, 19–21]. The combination of advanced age, severe peripheral occlusive arterial disease, and/or severe comorbidities contraindicates replantation. A patient's desire is difficult to assess in the emergency situation. The association of severe, potentially lethal injuries is a general contraindication (life before limb). Surgically treatable conditions can be corrected, and a low-impact temporary ectopic replantation can be considered as a temporizing measure (see below).

Injury-related factors are also important in decision-making. Massive bone loss, either primary or resulting from adequate debridement, is a contraindication. Complication rates of bone lengthening of the tibia abruptly increase when more than 15 cm are elongated [24]. Unilateral defects over 18–20 cm contraindicate replantation, even if a good tibial nerve repair can be done. Significant tibial nerve injury precluding satisfactory repair even after aggressive bone shortening also contraindicates replantation. If the tibial nerve can be directly coapted, the sole is relatively intact, the skeletal defect is manageable, and the anticipated soft-tissue problems are deemed solvable, the replanted limb can be more functional than a prosthesis.

Knee joint preservation is crucial in lower limb infrapopliteal amputations. Unless the joint is massively disrupted, every effort should be made to keep at least a below-knee level of amputation if formal replantation is not indicated. Salvage replantation in the form of replanting portions of the otherwise discardable foot may improve the function of the residual limb. As stated above, the authors have no experience in transfemoral replantation, but under optimal circumstances, it would be reasonable to convert the AK into a BK level through replantation of the knee and proximal third of the tibia, especially in bilateral cases. Theoretically, this approach would be relatively straightforward, with short

recovery time before prosthetic fitting (bone healing only). Femoral bone shortening could easily be compensated with the prosthesis, obviating the need of bone lengthening.

Crushing of the stump, contamination, and double-level proximal vascular injuries are not per se contraindications and can be managed with adequate debridement or a temporary ectopic replantation.

Heel, calcaneal, and sole amputations should be replanted, since the reported results are superior to any available reconstruction [25, 26]. Toe replantation, especially the great toe, has been described, although with marginal benefit for the patient [27].

Surgical Technique

Although the general surgical steps in lower limb replantation are similar to upper limb replantation, the philosophy is somewhat different. Complications are very frequent, and their treatment is an integral part of the replantation process. Lower limb replantation should be viewed as a three-stage surgical procedure, the urgent replantation being but the first stage. Soft-tissue coverage and bone lengthening are the other two stages.

Stage One: Replantation

Generally, this will be more straightforward than most upper limb cases, although general replantation guidelines apply, with some modifications. Using temporary arterial catheter perfusion and artery-last sequence of repairs allows for optimization of ischemia times [23]. Because of the higher risk of soft-tissue necrosis and the relatively lower functional impact of extensive muscle loss compared to the upper limb, debridement should be very aggressive. Bone shortening should also be very liberal to allow for direct wound closure (if possible) and, most importantly, a high-quality tibial or plantar nerve repair. Bone fixation is performed with K-wires in amputations distal to the ankle joint

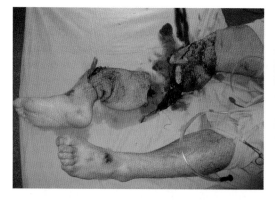

Fig. 12.3 A crushing injury, with double-level tibial injury. The sole of the foot was intact. Tibial nerve was repairable. Replantation was performed, anticipating severe skin necrosis

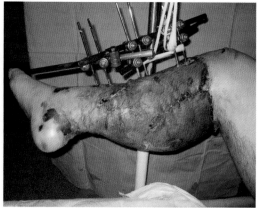

Fig. 12.4 A case of Fig. 12.3: Extensive circumferential skin necrosis without deep infection at 4th postoperative day

and with modular external fixation in transtibial amputations for expediency. Perfect anatomic reduction or completely stable constructs are not necessary in above-ankle replantations, since this fixation is temporary. Vessel repair should include as many arteries and deep veins as possible if the amputation is distal to the popliteal trifurcation. The risk of skin necrosis is high, and superficial veins should not be relied upon as the main outflow of the limb. Regarding muscles, at least the tibialis anterior muscle and the triceps surae muscle should be repaired. Other muscles can be repaired only under optimal (and unusual) conditions. Wounds are loosely closed if possible; otherwise, the vascular and neural structures are temporarily covered with skin grafts until definitive closure is performed a few days later [28]. Fasciotomies are rarely necessary and only performed if ischemia time exceeds 6–7 h (Fig. 12.3).

Stage Two: Definitive Wound Coverage

Because skin-edge necrosis is the rule rather than the exception, early flap coverage will almost always be the second stage of the replantation procedure and should be performed within a few days after the replant. Occasionally, the wounds can be covered with skin grafts (Figs. 12.1 and 12.2), but more frequently a free flap is required

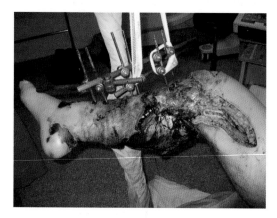

Fig. 12.5 A case of Figs. 12.3 and 12.4: After debridement and construction of a vascular loop to the first portion of the popliteal artery, a free latissimus dorsi flap was used for coverage

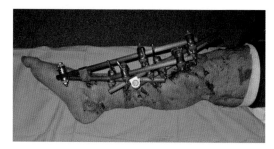

Fig. 12.6 Healed wounds with 9 cm bone shortening

(Figs. 12.4, 12.5, and 12.6). If vascular repairs are not directly underneath the necrotic skin, 1 week is allowed for demarcation. The recipient vessels are usually proximal to the amputation

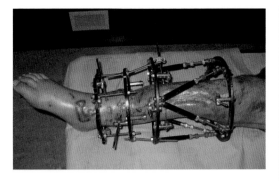

Fig. 12.7 The tubular external fixator was exchanged for a ring fixator for bone lengthening

level, and end-to-side or double end-to-end "T" constructs are mandatory. Distal vessels within the replanted leg can be used as recipients for flap coverage of associated double-level defects. Workhorse flaps as latissimus dorsi, gracilis, or ALT flaps are recommended to avoid unnecessary complexity. Early delayed definitive coverage is preferable to emergency free flaps in most cases.

Stage Three: Skeletal Lengthening

In amputations distal to the ankle, bone shortening is inconsequential and does not need further correction. In transtibial amputations, bone shortening has to be corrected through callus distraction (distraction osteogenesis), especially in unilateral cases (Figs. 12.6, 12.16, and 12.21). It is preferable to place the osteotomy for distraction at the proximal metaphysis rather than the fracture site [29, 30]. Bone lengthening should be performed soon after the wounds are healed, usually by the 3rd month, to reduce overall treatment times. Monorail half-pin frames are easier to manage than ring fixators and are preferable in most cases (Figs. 12.7, 12.8, 12.9, and 12.17). A normal lengthening of 1 mm/day is used, and early exchange of the external fixator for a locked, intramedullary nail is advisable to allow weight bearing and further shorten treatment times (Fig. 12.10, 12.11, and 12.12). The proximal metaphyseal osteotomy for distraction could theoretically be performed initially,

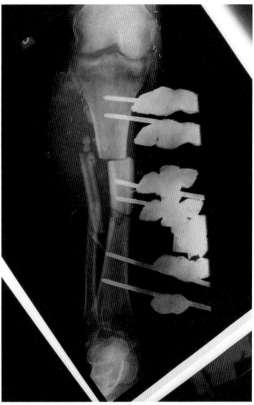

Fig. 12.8 The short proximal fragment after metaphyseal osteotomy required a ring fixator

during replantation surgery, and the monorail fixator placed primarily to shorten the overall treatment time further. The authors do not use this option for two reasons: firstly, placing the monorail fixator accurately adds complexity and time to the initial procedure, and secondly and most important, in the unlikely case of replant failure, the tibial stump would be compromised unnecessarily.

Replantation in Unfavorable Situations

If the injured limb is considered amenable to replantation, but the local or general condition of the patient precludes an immediate replantation, there are three useful techniques, namely, ectopic, heterotopic, and salvage replantation, that help overcome these transient difficulties.

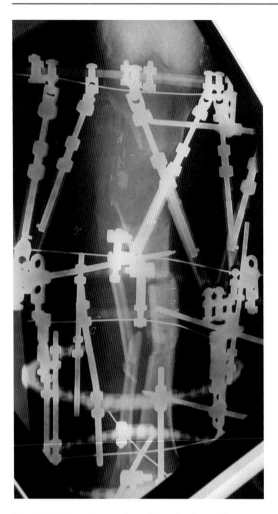

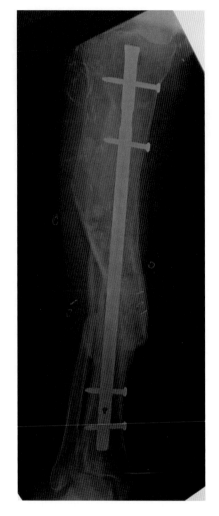

Fig. 12.9 Ring fixator allowed lengthening of 9 cm and distal fracture healing

Fig. 12.10 Stable skeleton after exchange of the ring fixator for a reamed locked nail at postoperative month 15

Temporary Ectopic Replantation

This is a low-impact, straightforward technique that allows maintenance of perfusion in the amputated part while the local or general condition of the patient improves enough to permit orthotopic transfer [31, 32]. Severe crushing, contamination or double-level injuries of the stump, and hemodynamic instability or treatable potentially lethal associated injuries are the main indications (Figs. 12.13, 12.14, 12.15, 12.16, 12.17, and 12.18). The recipient vessels for the ectopic replantation can be the contralateral femoral artery and saphenous vein or the distal posterior tibial vessels (Figs. 12.19 and 12.23). The latter have the distinct advantage of allowing simultaneous elevation of a perforator flap with

the vascular pedicle upon orthotopic transfer, the possibility of repairing two venae comitantes, and possibly the greater saphenous vein too, and the length of the vascular pedicle if the whole posterior vascular bundle is harvested upon transfer [33] (Figs. 12.20, 12.21, 12.22). The main drawback of using the posterior tibialis vessels as recipients is that, should a free fibular flap be necessary later on for the treatment of complications during bone lengthening in the replanted limb, the contralateral "healthy" leg would be left with only the anterior tibial artery, unless the peroneal artery is simultaneously reconstructed with a vein graft, in this unlikely but possible scenario. The ectopically replanted part should be fixed

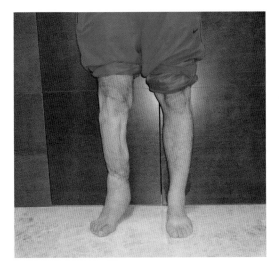

Fig. 12.11 Postoperative situation at 24 months. Plantar sensation was protective

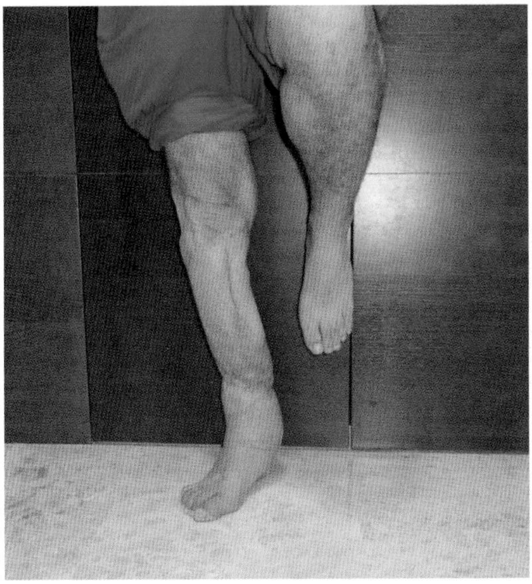

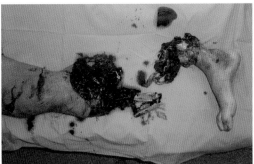

Fig. 12.13 In severe injuries with proximal double-level lesions, if the sole is intact, the tibial nerve is repairable, and the skeletal defect manageable, replantation can be performed as a staged ectopic replantation

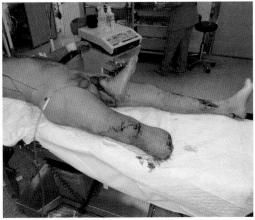

Fig. 12.14 Ectopic replantation to the contralateral femoral artery and saphenous vein. The proximal injuries were treated meanwhile. At postoperative day 6 orthotopic transfer was planned. Note the concomitant latissimus dorsi free flap for anticipated soft-tissue shortage

Fig. 12.12 Postoperative situation at 24 months. The patient could walk without aid

with a modular external fixator to the contralateral femur or tibia to secure a stable fixation. Once the local condition of the stump improves through sequential debridement and wound care, or the general status of the patient is stabilized, the replanted leg can be transferred to the stump. This typically happens about 1 week after the accident. Longer times make dissection of the scarred vessels and identification of structures more difficult. The ectopic time also allows for

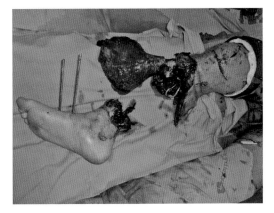

Fig. 12.15 The free flap was connected to the anterior tibial vessels and the replant to the posterior tibial vessels

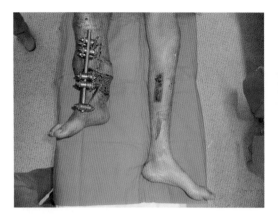

Fig. 12.16 Healed wounds with 11 cm shortening, before lengthening

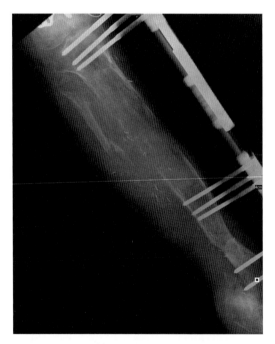

Fig. 12.17 Rx view: A half-pin monorail fixator was used for lengthening of the tibia

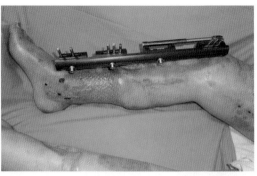

Fig. 12.18 Clinical view: a half-pin monorail fixator was used for lengthening of the tibia

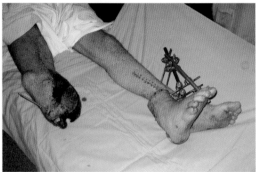

Fig. 12.19 The contralateral posterior tibial vessels are preferable if available as recipients for ectopic replantation

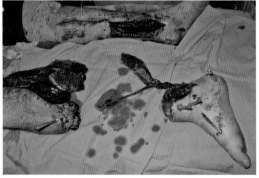

Fig. 12.20 A posterior tibial perforator flap can be elevated with the posterior tibial vessels to address soft-tissue defects of moderate size without additional morbidity

the skin-edge necrosis to develop, and definitive debridement can be performed with the orthotopic transfer (Fig. 12.23). Soft-tissue shortage should be anticipated when orthotopic transfer is performed, and simultaneous free or regional flaps are usually necessary. Ectopic replantation, although initially a low-impact, straightforward technique, adds considerable complexity to the overall replantation procedure and should be considered cautiously.

Heterotopic or "Crossover" Replantation

In bilateral cases, replanting the "best foot to the (contralateral) best stump" has been described as *heterotopic or "crossover" replantation* [31, 34–37]. Cosmesis is poor, with the hallux at the

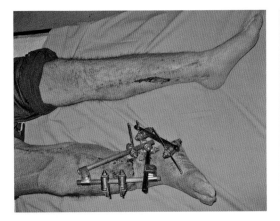

Fig. 12.21 Healed wounds before bone lengthening

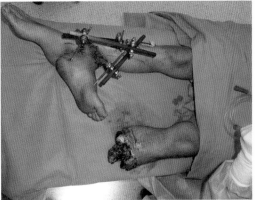

Fig. 12.23 The ectopic transfer allows the skin-edge necrosis to develop outside the replantation wound. Skin is trimmed upon orthotopic transfer thus reducing wound problems

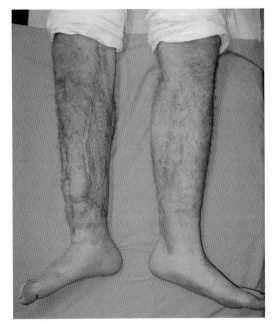

Fig. 12.22 Final result at 4 years. The patient has independent deambulation without aids

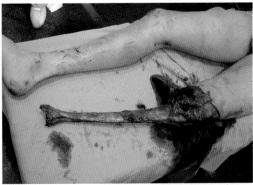

Fig. 12.24 A lower leg avulsion with femur fracture and knee ligamentous injury. The destruction of tissues contraindicated formal replantation

lateral side of the foot, but the functional result justifies this technique in well-motivated patients.

Salvage Replantation

In cases of severe limb destruction contraindicating formal replantation, with loss of skin coverage of the knee, and surgically treatable knee injuries, every attempt should be made to preserve knee function and a below-knee amputation level. The soft-tissue envelope of the amputated foot can be replanted as a free fillet flap for stump coverage [38]. The flap typically includes the dorsum and sole of the foot, and the tibial nerve is usually coapted to provide sensation. The innervated sole of the foot has excellent weight-bearing and shear-resisting characteristics for stump coverage (Fig. 12.24, 12.25, and 12.26a, b). In cases of a very short proximal tibial remnant, the calcaneus bone can be included in the fillet flap to lengthen the stump (Figs. 12.27, 12.28, 12.29, and 12.30a, b). In some cases, when the knee joint is massively dislocated and the vascularity of the proximal tibia is uncertain, the joint cannot be preserved.

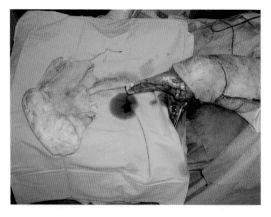

Fig. 12.25 The tibia was trimmed and the BK-level stump was covered with a foot fillet flap

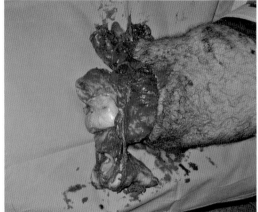

Fig. 12.27 A high transtibial amputation with knee dislocation and femoral fracture. The tibial remnant was short. The amount of injury in the leg contraindicated formal replantation

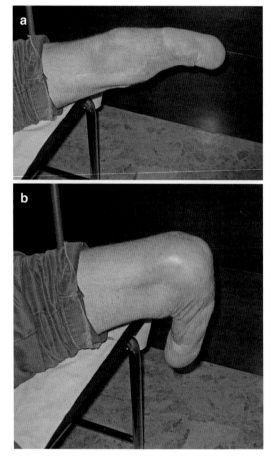

Fig. 12.26 (**a**, **b**) Functional result at 9 years with uneventful prosthetic fitting

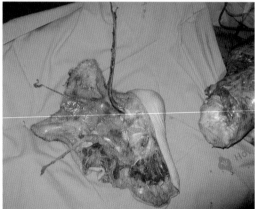

Fig. 12.28 A foot fillet flap including the calcaneus was replanted to lengthen the BK stump and facilitate prosthetic fitting

The same applies to massive bone loss of the joint. In these two scenarios, the replantation of the distal third of the leg, ankle, and foot, axially rotated 180°, allows for reconstruction of the knee with the ankle. This technique is based on the time-honored Borggreve-Van Nes rotationplasty used in orthopedic oncology [39, 40]. The tibia is plated to the femur, the quadriceps is sutured to the calcaneal tendon, the hamstrings are repaired to the tibialis anterior and peroneus brevis tendons, the tibialis nerve is coapted, and vascular repairs are performed (Figs. 12.31 and 12.32a, b). The combined tibiotalar and subtalar motion allows almost 90° of "knee" flexion-extension. The toes are generally removed to reduce the visual impact.

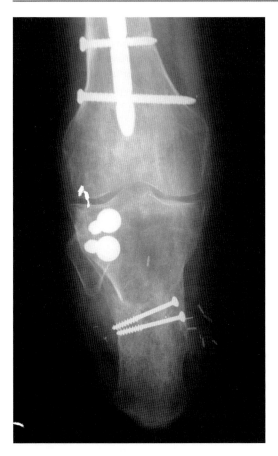

Fig. 12.29   X-ray of the healed tibia and calcaneus

Below-knee prostheses in these patients usually include an articulated femoral brace to improve lateral stability of the reconstructed knee.

Perioperative Considerations

Lower limb amputations occur in high-energy accidents. Serious associated injuries are frequent and should be ruled out before considering replantation. Basic rules of trauma care and resuscitation apply to these patients. Hemodynamic stability is a prerequisite. Constant communication with the anesthesiology team is essential throughout the procedure. Blood pressure should be stable with judicious use of volume replacement and blood transfusion. Lung injury secondary to massive transfusion or volume overload should be avoided. Liberal use of the tourniquet, rapid surgical technique, and artery-last sequence of repairs help reduce the always substantial blood loss involved in these procedures. Anticoagulants have not demonstrated effectiveness beyond the surgeon's subjective comfort, and there is no solid reason to use them, apart from standard pulmonary thromboembolism prophylaxis.

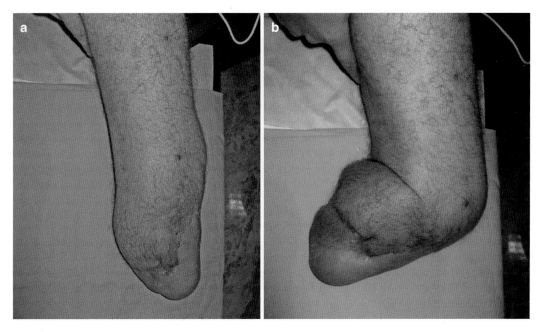

Fig. 12.30   (**a**, **b**) Functional result al 6 years with successful prosthesis fitting

Medical postoperative care of these patients is not different from upper limb replantation patients. Dangling, which is usually delayed because of the almost constant early free flap performed, starts on the 10th day post free flap. Rehabilitation protocols are dictated by the skeletal injury. Passive and active knee movement is started on the first post-op week if vascular grafts do not cross the joint level. Otherwise, a further week is allowed before starting knee movement. Passive ankle dorsiflexion is started depending on the quality of muscle-tendon repairs. The goal is to achieve 90° (neutral ankle) during the first few weeks and maintain it with a custom-made ankle-foot orthosis. Weight bearing is gradually started during the bone lengthening, if a ring Ilizarov system is used, and after intramedullary nail placement, if a monorail system is used for lengthening. Full weight bearing is allowed after X-ray evidence of healing.

Complications and Results

As stated earlier, some complications are so frequent that they can be considered part of the normal course of the injury. Soft-tissue necrosis occurs in more than 90 % of the cases and should be debrided and covered early to avoid infection and replant failure or late consequences such as unstable scars or nonunions [24]. In the series published by the authors, there was an 83 % incidence of significant soft-tissue necrosis, with a 17 % incidence of deep infections [17]. These high rates of wound complications could be attributed to the frequency of crushing-avulsion mechanism of injury and the low threshold for replantation. Debridement at the initial replantation surgery and in the first few postoperative days plays a key role in preventing wound

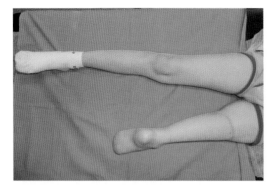

Fig. 12.31 A 10-year-old boy with a mid-shaft femoral amputation and loss of the knee in the amputated part. The lower leg was replanted as a microvascular rotationplasty. The compound femur-tibia construct was made longer than the contralateral femur to compensate for growth difference

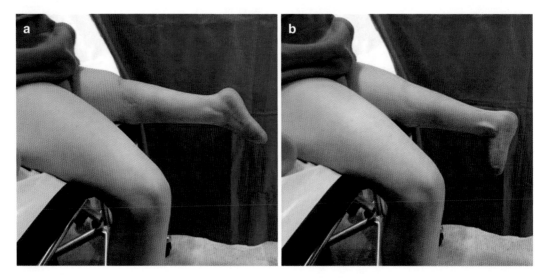

Fig. 12.32 (**a**, **b**) Flexion and extension of the "knee" at 2 years. The patient uses a BK prosthesis with hinged femoral brace

complications. Deep infection at the replantation wound should be aggressively treated surgically since it is a major cause of thrombosis and failure. Systemic complications may occur and are not different from other major surgical procedures. The cumulative risk of the various surgical stages of limb replantation is significant and should be carefully weighed by the surgeon and the patient continuously.

Bone shortening is a consequence of treatment, rather than a complication, and its management is an integral part of the procedure. Malunion or nonunion during the lengthening process is not different from non-replantation cases, and their management does not differ significantly. Nonetheless, the secondary surgical procedures in a replanted limb have the added difficulty of distorted anatomy, extensive scarring, and the presence of critical vascular and neural repairs.

With proper planning and execution, frequently cited complications such as persistent pain, malalignment of the foot, chronic bone infection, or plantar ulcers are infrequently seen. Secondary amputation is the reported treatment of these conditions. It represents a failure in the management of these injuries, either a poor judgment to perform the replantation or an inability to deal with complications. With adequate training and involvement, this outcome is virtually nonexistent.

The results of the authors' series of 20 complete replantations compare favorably to previously reported series. The functional grading of Chen was used for outcome measurement (Table 12.1) [19, 41]. Kutz et al. [16] report on 9

lower limb infrapopliteal replantations, with a 33 % success rate. Hierner et al. [14, 42] report a 63 % success rate, with 93 % of Chen's grade I and II results. Battiston et al., in a series of 14 replantations below the knee in 12 patients, report a 100 % initial success, although a secondary amputation was performed in 36 % of the cases due to severe complications. Of the remaining nine limbs, 78 % achieved a Chen grade I or II [15, 43]. In the authors' series, the success rate was 100 %, with 92 % of cases being grades I and II (good or excellent) according to the criteria of Chen [17]. Sensory recovery of the sole has not been systematically studied in replanted feet. In the authors' series, the monofilament test was 2.0 g for the anterior sole and 4.0 g for the posterior sole (with great variability), which is comparable to the results of published series of tibial nerve repair [44, 45], and well above the accepted threshold of 5.0 g for plantar breakdown in diabetic patients [46, 47].

Even with a highly proactive treatment strategy, the treatment times are long. The mean of 11 months at the authors' series compares favorably with the published series, and it may represent a reasonable timeframe. It is essential to discuss this topic thoroughly with the patients and their families before embarking in a long and costly treatment. There is no published study comparing outcomes and costs of lower leg replantation versus revision amputation and prosthesis. In a recent review, no difference in outcome was found between these two treatment options in type IIIb and IIIc open tibial fractures [21], although amputation tends to be a more expensive treatment in the long term [1, 2].

Table 12.1 Chen criteria of replanted lower limb

Grade I: Return to previous work; normal gait walk; almost normal sensory recovery at the sole; almost normal range of movement (ROM) of knee and ankle joints

Grade II: Return to light work; walk with slight limp; good sensory recovery of the sole; ROM over 40 % of normal

Grade III: Useful in daily life; use of higher heel; poor sensibility at the sole without trophic ulcers

Grade IV: Use of crutches; no sensory recovery at the sole; trophic ulcers

Used with permission from Chen [41]

Conclusion

Lower limb replantation is a more complex treatment than its upper limb counterpart. The urgent surgical reattachment is relatively simple, but the postoperative management is considerably more complex. Surgeon's involvement and experience are critical for consistent results. Complications are the rule and their management constitutes an integral part of the procedure itself. Expectant approaches lead to unacceptable failure rates and account for the bad reputation of lower limb replantation. A highly committed surgical team conversant with modern orthopedic, plastic, and microvascular reconstructive surgical techniques working in a very proactive way is crucial to obtain consistent good results and restore the patients to their active life with the least medical, psychological, and economic impact.

References

1. Bondurant FJ, Colter HB, Buckle R, Miller-Crotchett P, Browner BD. The medical and economic impact of severely injured lower extremities. J Trauma. 1988;28:1270.
2. Helfert DL, Howy T, Sanders R, Johansen K. Limb salvage versus amputation. Clin Orthop Relat Res. 1990;256:80.
3. Hansen Jr ST. Overview of the severely traumatized lower limb reconstruction versus amputation. Clin Orthop Relat Res. 1989;243:17.
4. Gayle LB, Lineaweaver WC, Buncke GM, Oliva A, Alpert BS, Billys JB, Buncke HJ. Lower extremity replantation. Clin Plast Surg. 1991;18:437.
5. Usui M, Minami M, Ishii S. Successful replantation of an amputated leg in a child. Plast Reconstr Surg. 1979;63:613.
6. Clarke P, Mollan RAB. The criteria for amputation in severe lower limb injury. Injury. 1994;25:139.
7. Robertson PA. Prediction of amputation after severe lower limb trauma. J Bone Joint Surg (Br). 1991;73:816.
8. Yaffe B, Borenstein A, Seidman D, Amit Y. Successful replantation of both legs in a child—5 year follow-up: case report. J Trauma. 1991;31:264.
9. Bajec J, Srakar F. Complete bilateral amputations of both legs in a 2-year-old child with a 10 year follow-up. Injury. 1994;25.
10. Buckley JR, Dunkley P. Successful replantation of both feet. J Bone Joint Surg (Br). 1988;70:667.
11. Vilkki SK. Replantation of a leg in an adult with 6-years' follow-up. Acta Orthop Scand. 1986;57:447.
12. Kusunoki M, Toyoshima Y, Okajima M. Successful replantation of a leg. A 7-year follow-up. Injury. 1984;16:118.
13. Krylov VS, Milanov NO, Peradze TY, Borovikov AM, Shilov BL. Lower leg replantation in children: railroad amputation. J Reconstr Microsurg. 1987;3:321.
14. Hierner R, Betz A, Pohlemann T, Berger A. Long-term results after lower leg replantation—does the result justify the risks and efforts? Eur J Trauma. 2005;4:389.
15. Battiston B, Tos P, Pontini I, Ferrero S. Lower limb replantations: indications and a new scoring system. Microsurgery. 2002;22:187.
16. Kutz JE, Jupiter JB, Tsai TM. Lower limb replantation a report of nine cases. Foot Ankle. 1983;3:197.
17. Cavadas PC, Landín L, Ibáñez J, Roger I, Nthumba P. Infrapopliteal lower extremity replantation. Plast Reconstr Surg. 2009;124(2):532.
18. Patradul A, Ngarmukos C, Parkpian V. Major limb replantation: a Thai experience. Ann Acad Med Singap. 1995;24(4 Suppl):82.
19. Chen Z-W, Yang HL. Lower limb replantation. In: Urbaniak JR, editor. Microsurgery for major limb reconstruction. St. Louis: The C.B. Mosby Comp; 1987. p. 67. Chapter 11.
20. Yur–Ren Kuo, Sagalongos O, Chiang YC. Replantation of the lower extremity. In: Lee LQ Pu, Levine JP, Fu-Chan Wei, editors. QMP Publishing, St. Louis Missouri. Reconstructive surgery of the lower extremity, chapter 72. p. 1217. Edited by QMP 2013.
21. Saddawi-Konefka D, Kim HM, Chung KC. A systematic review of outcomes and complications of reconstruction and amputation for type IIIB and IIIC fractures of the tibia. Plast Reconstr Surg. 2008;122:1796.
22. Hidalgo DA, Shaw WW. Lower limb replantation. In: Shaw WW, Hidalgo DA, editors. Microsurgery in trauma. Mount Kisco: Futura Publishing; 1987. p. 95–104. Chapter 7.
23. Cavadas PC, Landin L, Ibañez J. Temporary catheter perfusion and artery-last sequence of repair in macroreplantations. J Plast Reconstr Aesthet Surg. 2009; 62(10):1321.
24. Hierner R, Berger AK, Frederix PR. Lower leg replantation. Decision-making, treatment, and long-term results. Microsurgery. 2007;27:398.
25. Libermanis O. Replantation of the heel pad. Plast Reconstr Surg. 1993;92:537.
26. Chiang YC, Wei FC, Chen LM. Heel replantation and subsequent analysis of gait. Plast Reconstr Surg. 1993;91:729.
27. Lin CH, Lin CH, Sassu P, Hsu CC, Lin YT, Wei FC. Replantation of the great toe: review of 20 cases. Plast Reconstr Surg. 2008;122:806.
28. Thione A, Cavadas PC, Landin L, Ibañez J. Microvascular pedicle coverage with split thickness skin graft: indications and surgical tips. Indian J Plast Surg. 2011;44(3):528.
29. Betz AM, Stock W, Hierner R, Baumgart R. Primary shortening with secondary limb lengthening in severe injuries of the lower leg: a six year experience. Microsurgery. 1993;14:446.
30. Datiashvili RO, Oganesian OV, Chichkin VG, et al. Rehabilitation of patients after lower limb replantations by the bone distraction method. J Trauma. 1993;35.
31. Kayikçioğlu A, Ağaoğlu G, Nasir S, Keçik A. Crossover replantation and fillet flap coverage of the stump after ectopic implantation: a case of bilateral leg amputation. Plast Reconstr Surg. 2000;106:868.

32. Wang JN, Wang SY, Wang ZJ, Liu D, Zhao GQ, Zhang F. Temporary ectopic implantation for salvage of amputated lower extremities: case reports. Microsurgery. 2005;25:385.

33. Cavadas PC, Landin L, Thione A. Secondary ectopic transfer for replantation salvage after severe wound infection. Microsurgery. 2011;31(4):288.

34. Betz A, Stock W, Hierner R, Schweiberer L. Crossover replantation after bilateral traumatic lower leg amputation—a case report with a six year follow-up. J Reconstr Microsurg. 1996;12:247.

35. Girot J, Marin-Braun F, Merle M, Xenard J. Crossover replantation in case of bilateral amputation of the legs. Rev Chir Orthop. 1987;74:259.

36. Daigeler A, Fansa H, Schneider W. Orthotopic and heterotopic lower leg reimplantation. Evaluation of seven cases. J Bone Joint Surg. 2003;85(4):554–8.

37. Cinar C, Arslan H, Ogur S, Pilanci O, Yucel A, Cetinkale O. Crossover replantation of the foot after bilateral traumatic lower extremity amputation. Ann Plast Surg. 2007;58:667.

38. Jupiter JB, Tsai TM, Kleinert HE. Salvage replantation of lower limb amputations. Plast Reconstr Surg. 1982;69:1.

39. Gupta SK, Alassaf N, Harrop AR, Kiefer GN. Principles of rotationplasty. J Am Acad Orthop Surg. 2012;20(10):657–67.

40. Druecke D, Homann HH, Kutscha-Lissberg F, Schinkel C, Steinau HU. Crossover extremity transfers. Limb salvage in amputations with segmental defects. Chirurg. 2007;78(10):954–8.

41. Chen Z-W, Qian YQ, Yu ZJ. Extremity replantation. J World Surg. 1978;2:513.

42. Cavadas PC. Salvage of replanted upper extremities with major soft-tissue complications. J Plast Reconstr Aesthet Surg. 2007;60:769.

43. Hierner R, Bets AM, Comtet JJ, Berger AC. Decision making and results in subtotal and total leg amputations: reconstruction versus amputation. Microsurgery. 1995;16:830.

44. Kim DH, Murovic JA, Tiel R, Kline DG. Management and outcomes in 353 surgically treated sciatic nerve lesions. J Neurosurg. 2004;101:8.

45. Ruch DS, Smith AM. Articulating external fixation to overcome nerve gaps in lower extremity trauma. J Orthop Trauma. 2003;17:290.

46. Jeng C, Michelson J, Mizel M. Sensory thresholds of normal human feet. Foot Ankle Int. 2000;21:501.

47. Nather A, Neo SH, Chionh SB, Liew SC, Sim EY, Chew JLJ. Assessment of sensory neuropathy in diabetic patients without diabetic foot problems. Diabetes Complicat. 2008;22:126.

Management of Complications After Replantation

13

Guang Yang and Kevin C. Chung

Introduction

Successful replantation is composed of a sequence of multiple procedures, and what might be considered a single, seemingly slight problem may set off a chain reaction resulting in total loss of the replantation or long-term dysfunction. Therefore, careful attention must be paid to each step from the beginning to the end of the procedure. Neglecting critical steps, taking shortcuts during the seemingly "easy" components of the operation, or failing to recognize problems as they arise can all result in failure. And failure, while disheartening for the surgeon, most importantly impacts the well-being of the patient over the individual's lifespan.

Early Complications

Preparation and Prevention

Replantation is a long and exhausting procedure for the surgical team, and the need to return acutely to the operating theater is physically taxing for all

G. Yang, MD
Department of Hand Surgery,
China-Japan Union Hospital of Jilin University,
Changchung, Peoples Republic of China
e-mail: y_guang@jlu.edu.cn

K.C. Chung, MD, MS (✉)
Section of Plastic Surgery, University of Michigan
Health System, Ann Arbor, MI, USA
e-mail: kecchung@med.umich.edu

involved. Avoidance of early complications will minimize the probability of such a return as well as maximize the chance of a successful replantation. The early complications that will most commonly present include venous congestion, arterial thrombosis, bleeding, and, while slightly more subacute, infection.

The successful replantation procedure begins with aggressive and adequate debridement in order to accomplish two principal aims. The first is to rid the amputated segment of contaminated and nonviable tissue that can lead to infection. This is important, as infection is one factor that may predispose the replant to vascular occlusion during postoperative days 3–10. Identification of contamination is relatively straightforward; however, nonviable skin or subcutaneous tissue may not be evident until after the distal segment reperfuses. Since most replants will involve some degree of bone shortening, contamination at the raw, cancellous surface will often be addressed as part of the bone stabilization. Removal of crushed, possibly contaminated bone facilitates performance of a tension-free microvascular repair. This is critical, since anastomoses performed under tension will result in shearing forces at the suture line, tearing of the vascular wall, bleeding, vasospasm, vascular congestion, and ultimately thrombosis (Fig. 13.1). Conservative shortening will not have great effect as long as the shortening is limited to about 1.5 cm in the digits. An addition of 1–2 mm of vessel length provides more leeway to improve

A.N. Salyapongse et al. (eds.), *Extremity Replantation: A Comprehensive Clinical Guide*,
DOI 10.1007/978-1-4899-7516-4_13, © Springer Science+Business Media New York 2015

anastomosis quality. When possible, tensionless anastomoses obtained by bony shortening are simpler and require one fewer anastomosis than using vein grafts or "harvest veins." During the debridement of bone, the bone surfaces should be rendered smooth and contoured so that the matching surface areas of the proximal and distal segments are maximized. Good bone contact will improve rigid fixation and minimize the late complication of bone nonunion.

The second aim of debridement is the identification of vessels and nerves. Prevention of early vascular complications begins with careful identification and preparation of the vessels. In cases of digital replantation, it is relatively easy to find the proper palmar digital nerves and arteries that run along the sides of each finger (Fig. 13.2). The digital nerves are usually identi-

fied first, because they do not retract very far. Next, the nerves are tagged with 6-0 Prolene sutures. When gentle tension is placed on the digital nerve, the retracted artery at the dorsolateral aspect of the nerve will emerge. The arteries are also dissected free and tagged with 6-0 Prolene for easy retrieval. A bilateral mid-axial incision is helpful to identify the volar neurovascular bundle and dorsal venous plexus [1]. Often it is difficult to identify the dorsal veins in the amputated part before restoring the arterial blood supply. Our preferred method is to incise the dermal layer of the skin about 1–3 mm distal to the edge of the wound on the dorsum while taking care not to cut too deeply as this might damage the minute veins located between the skin and extensor tendon. The veins are then identified in the incision (Fig. 13.3a, b). Careful debridement and exposure of the vessels so they are not under tension also allows rotation of the vessels during the anastomosis and vessel eversion with no luminal exposure of the adventitia.

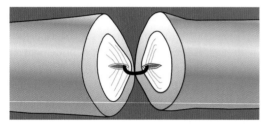

Fig. 13.1 Shearing force of the suture under tension will lead to tearing of the vascular wall

Bone

While early complications related to management of the bone are rare, anticipation of outcomes such as nonunion and malunion should

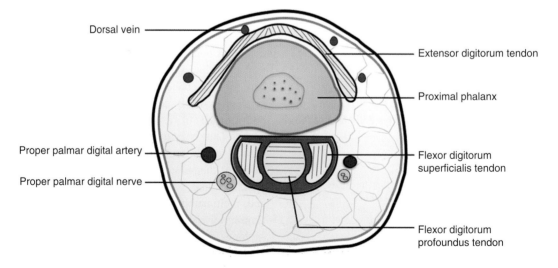

Fig. 13.2 Cross-section anatomy of the proximal phalange of the middle finger. The proper palmar digital nerves and arteries run along the sides of the finger, and the dorsal veins are located between the skin and the extensor digitorum tendon

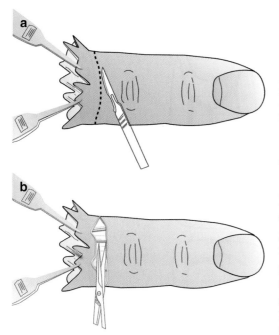

Fig. 13.3 The method to identify the dorsal veins. (**a**) Incise the dermis of the skin about 1–3 mm distal to the edge of wound on the dorsum. (**b**) Then, look for the veins in the incision

direct decision making in an attempt to avoid secondary procedures. One of two possible scenarios will occur, either the amputation involved or destroyed part of a joint or the damage is primarily extra-articular. In cases of joint damage or loss, primary arthrodesis may be indicated. Techniques for achieving rigid fixation in either of these settings are well described in the chapters devoted to replantation at each level of the extremity. The replant surgeon should emphasize that, if possible, any joints that must be immobilized by fixation techniques should be stabilized in the "functional position." In the case of the metacarpophalangeal joint, this would be roughly 60° of flexion, whereas the proximal and distal interphalangeal joints should rest at 0°. To some degree, joint stiffness following replantation is inevitable; anticipating this complication may allow placement of stiffness in the best possible position to facilitate later therapy and rehabilitation.

Although most fixation methods are designed to achieve fracture control in multiple planes,

occasionally, the fracture may dictate use of only a single K-wire. In this setting, periosteal repair is useful to prevent finger rotation. Furthermore, the risk of tendon adhesion may be reduced by periosteum covering the fracture site [2]. Prevention of malrotation may obviate the need for a corrective osteotomy at a later date.

Tendon

Extensor and flexor tendons are repaired in this order. Because the strength of finger flexion is greater than extension, the extensor tendon repair must be reliable to avoid rupturing when the patient performs motion exercises postoperatively. By first repairing the extensor tendon, the surgeon can confirm that no gapping occurs following the limited application of stress applied by the secondarily repaired flexor tendon. Additionally, identification and careful repair of the lateral bands of the extensor tendon and intrinsic tendons at the level of the proximal phalanx should be attempted to avoid a severe flexion deformity of the distal interphalangeal joint. Details regarding optimizing specific tendon repairs are addressed in Chap. 2 of this book.

Vascular

Prevention of vascular complications began with debridement and vessel preparation as noted above. The next step relies on optimizing the quality of the microvascular repair. At least some debate remains as to the optimal method for performing these repairs. One controversy centers on whether the arteries or veins should be repaired first during digital replantation. In more proximal amputations, which contain muscle, restoration of inflow takes precedence, and the point is moot. Some replantation surgeons champion repairing digital arteries before the veins [3, 4], which carries with it the obvious advantage of greater ease in identifying veins in the amputated part after restoring arterial blood supply. Furthermore, repairing the veins first appears to place the "cart before the horse," assuming arterial inflow will be adequate, an assumption that may not hold true, especially in the case of avulsion/amputation. In that setting, repair of the veins may be seen as a "waste of time" [3]. The other side of the debate supports the repair of veins prior to arteries. These authors argue that it is easier to perform anastomosis on the veins before restoring arterial inflow when the surgical field is not stained with blood [5]. In our experience, venous anastomosis in the diffuse bloody field can be avoided by using an arm or finger tourniquet. Perhaps the strongest argument in favor of repairing the digital veins first is that it comprises the most difficult part of the replantation. Performing this portion first, with full vigor at the beginning of the operation, allows the surgeon to devote the attention and detail that this repair requires and avoids relegating venous anastomosis to the end of the operation when one is tired and tends to take shortcuts by not repairing as many veins as possible.

An additional question that often arises is how many veins and arteries should be repaired. In our experience, if possible, both arteries should be repaired to maximize perfusion thus reducing the risk of loss secondary to arterial thrombosis. If both arteries are impossible to repair, the dominant digital artery (the one with lager diameter in bilateral arteries) should be repaired. Ideally, two veins are repaired per artery repaired as robust venous drainage is helpful to relieve edema after replantation and is essential to obtain good digital sensibility. While it is relatively impossible to find more than four veins with diameters over 0.5 mm to anastomose in most replanted fingers [6], the diameter of the veins increases as the number of veins decreases. On the occasion of being unable to match the veins at the appropriate position of the amputated finger and the proximal finger secondary to bony shortening, the veins can be mobilized for anastomosis by dividing and ligating their branches (Fig. 13.4a, b).

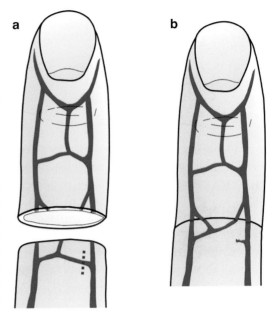

Fig. 13.4 The method of mobilization of the veins. (**a**) The veins at the appropriate position of the amputated finger and the proximal finger did not match. (**b**) The veins were moved for anastomosis by dividing and ligating their branch

avoiding neuroma and achieving some degree of distal sensibility. In a review in 1990, Glickman found that overall mean static two-point discrimination was 11 mm in the thumb and 12 mm in fingers following digital replantation [7]. According to recent systematic reviews, the mean 2-point discrimination was on average 10 mm in the replanted fingers after avulsion injuries and 7 mm in replanted fingers after distal digital amputation [8, 9]. Nerve defects that cannot be repaired in a tensionless manner can be repaired by nerve grafts or with interposition nerve conduits immediately during the replant procedure or later on. One well-know late complication, finger pulp atrophy, is directly related to low quality of nerve repair. Therefore, precise nerve repair under the microscope is a critical component of the replantation effort.

Nerve

Primary nerve repair is usually not difficult if the bones are adequately shortened for replantation. Prevention of complications here includes

Common Early Complications

Bleeding

Bleeding is one of the common complications after replantation. Leung reported that 9 of 20 patients suffered from marked oozing of blood from the hand dressing [10]. Adequate hemostasis should therefore be achieved during the operation to minimize postoperative bleeding that consequently may compress the underlying anastomosis. Although one might theorize that external bleeding offers a source of venous outflow (analogous to leech therapy), quite the opposite is true. Bleeding may represent poor outflow through the repaired veins. Decreased blood flow in the anastomosed veins increases the risk of thrombosis. External bleeding that saturates the dressing should raise consideration of return to the operating theater. Obvious bleeding at the wound edges should be stopped by suturing or with bipolar cautery, and suturing should be performed carefully to avoid injury of the vessels.

Vascular Compromise

Even though the blood flow is patent at the operating table, vascular complications including vasospasm, arterial thrombosis, and venous congestion may occur postoperatively, causing failure of the replantation. To avoid vasospasm, patients should be maintained in a comfortable and warm room in the hospital for at least 5 days after replantation. There are four "NOs" in the perioperative period: "No pain, No cold, No smoking, and No full bladder." Each of these interventions is made in order to avoid or prevent vasospasm. If vasospasm occurs, identification of factors that make patients uncomfortable (e.g., inadequate pain control) should be addressed prior to instituting more aggressive medical or surgical interventions. Additional chemotherapeutic methods of maintaining vascular patency are addressed in Chap. 8.

Color, pulp turgor, capillary refill, and skin temperature are the indicators to identify arterial or venous crisis not only in the injured finger but also in the replanted finger (Fig. 13.5 and Table 13.1). Needle prick of the finger pulp using an 18-gauge needle to observe the bleeding is a reliable method to identify vascular crisis of the replanted finger. Absence of bleeding suggests arterial insufficiency; dark blood from the pinprick site suggests venous insufficiency.

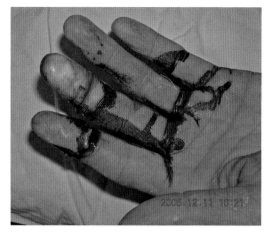

Fig. 13.5 The appearance of arterial and venous crisis in injured fingers. The patient suffered from a crush injury in the index finger and middle finger with open wounds. The index finger was in venous crisis, because the dorsal veins were damaged and volar arteries were intact. On the contrary, the middle finger was in arterial crisis, because the volar arteries were ruptured

Table 13.1 Indicators of vascular crisis after digital replantation

	Normal	Arterial crisis	Venous crisis
Color	Rosy	Pale	Purple
Skin temperature	>32 °C	Low	Low
Pulp turgor	Moderate	Flaccid	Engorged, blister
Capillary refill	1–2 s	Slow or no	Fast
Bleeding	Red arterial blood	No blood	Purple venous blood

Once arterial thrombosis is confirmed, the only solution is to return to the operating room within 4–6 h for re-exploration, reanastomosis, or venous grafting. Venous congestion is not uncommon and usually happens during the first 12–24 postoperative hours. Nevertheless, it is often unrecognized immediately until 2 or 3 days postoperatively heralded by venous backflow from the skin edges. While return to the operating room for redo venous anastomosis can be performed, prevention, as noted above, seems to be the most effective method when the replantation is attempted proximal to the distal interphalangeal joint. Should poor venous outflow occur, leech therapy is an excellent solution to augment venous outflow and increase vascular patency (refer to Chap. 8 for the mechanism of action of hirudin, in maintaining vascular patency). While not all hospitals have this resource, when available, leeches should be used as the first line of defense for venous insufficiency. If arterial and venous congestion occurs greater than 5 days after replantation, the chance of reanastomosis will be fruitless as late thrombosis events are usually caused by infection.

Late Complications

Although the survival rate of replanted extremities is high, the function of extremity replantations is most satisfactory in replantation distal to the proximal interphalangeal joint. This should not be surprising, given that complications such as stiffness and tendon adhesions will have much lower impact on hand function distal to the PIPJ. The late complications that affect the recovery of hand function include nonunion and malunion of the bone, stiffness of the finger, rotation deformity, sensory impairment, and cold intolerance. Some of these complications can be managed by secondary surgery. According to a review in 2002, the overall incidence of secondary surgery after replantation ranged from 2.9 to 93.2 % [11]. Timing and order of surgery after replantation comply with the principles of late hand function reconstruction. In most cases, this will be dictated by the patient's functional progress through hand therapy, as addressed in Chap. 15. A secondary procedure after replantation should not be considered until survival of the replanted finger can be guaranteed. Secondary surgery can be extremely difficult, particularly for volar exposure because of potential injury to the artery and the nerves that are encased in scar tissue. Therefore, any secondary surgical procedure must be weighed carefully.

The complications listed above seldom occur alone, so the surgeon must develop a plan of management to achieve the maximal restoration of function. Although different patients have different problems to deal with, the sequence of reconstructive management follows a generalized order outlined in Table 13.2.

Table 13.2 Order of reconstructive managements after replantation

	Tissues	Managements
1	Skin	Skin graft, flap
2	Bone	Arthrodesis, osteotomy, bone graft
3	Nerve	Nerve graft
4	Tendon	Tenolysis, tendon graft

Nonunion and Malunion of the Bone

Nonunion and malunion of the bone after replantation, regardless of the cause, need to be carefully addressed, as not doing so not only has effects on the replanted digit but also impacts functional recovery of the adjacent fingers. In cases of nonunion, bone graft or fusion is used for reconstruction, and for rotation or angulation, osteotomy is used. A longitudinal dorsal incision over the nonunion or malunion site is performed in most cases. The extensor tendon is split sharply in the middle to expose the phalanx. The length of the bone graft should be appropriate to prevent stretching of the neurovascular bundle and devascularization of the finger. Arthrodesis is a favorable choice especially when severe tendon problems, such as tendon defects and extensive tendon adhesion, coexist in the same finger. We prefer to use plates and screws as stable fixation rather than K-wires in secondary surgery (Fig. 13.6a–i). More details related to secondary surgery are addressed in Chap. 14.

Stiff Finger

Stiffness of the finger after replantation is often due to tendon adhesion or rupture. Static progressive and dynamic splints are effective to improve passive range of motion, but improvement of active motion of the finger is difficult to achieve. This is secondary to a myriad of effects at the operative site including scar and adhesions involving the skin, bone, flexor and extensor tendons, and tendon sheath. Tenolysis is the most common procedure after digital replantation [11, 12]. Flexor tenolysis is often performed with a palmar approach using the Z-shaped incision for maximal exposure rather than the mid-lateral approach. Some authors have reported good outcomes of

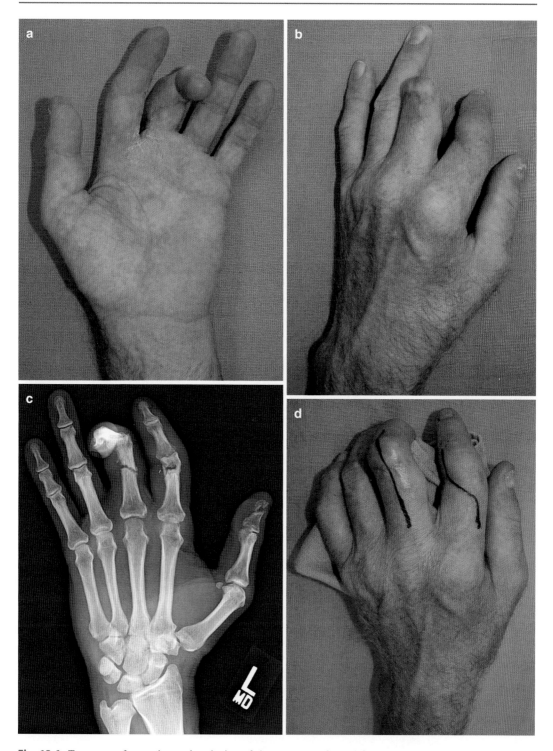

Fig. 13.6 Treatment of nonunion and malunion of the bone after replantation using plate and screw. (**a**, **b**) The deformities of the index and middle finger occurred after replantation. (**c**) The preoperative X-ray showed nonunion and malunion at the proximal phalanx of the index finger and the middle finger. (**d**) Longitudinal dorsal incisions were performed for osteotomy in the index finger and arthrodesis in the middle finger. (**e**, **f**) The plates and screws were used to fix the bones after osteotomy and arthrodesis. (**g–i**) Appearance and function of the fingers a month after deformity correction and internal fixation

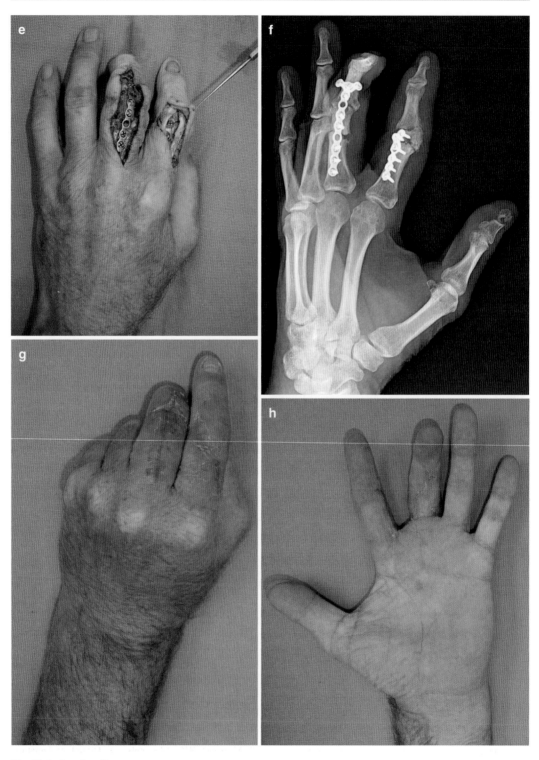

Fig. 13.6 (continued)

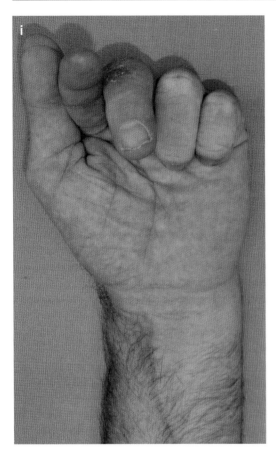

Fig. 13.6 (continued)

flexor tenolysis after replantation of fingers [12–14]. It is difficult to perform tenolysis in replanted fingers compared to an isolated tendon injury. The surgeon must be very careful to preserve the palmar neurovascular bundle during tenolysis. Arterial injury may not cause the finger to die, but insufficient blood supply may cause ischemic problems to the replanted digit.

Cold Intolerance

Cold intolerance that occurs in some replantation patients is related to the original injury rather than insufficient blood supply to the replanted digit [15]. The symptoms and signs of cold intolerance include pain, numbness, tingling, and color changes. The incidence of cold intolerance after replantation is inconsistently reported in the litera-

ture. Dabernig et al. reported that 86.7 % of patients after replantation complained of cold sensitivity [16]. In 2013, Adani reported that 5 of 29 (17.2 %) patients with successful replantation of ring avulsions complained of cold intolerance [17]. Cold intolerance also has a higher incidence in children. Cheng et al. reported that cold intolerance was slight or moderate in 40 % of children with digit replantation [18]. Fingertip injuries have a lower incidence of cold intolerance. In a study by Venkatraman, the authors found that none of their 24 patients reported cold intolerance, even though the digital nerves were not repaired [19]. According to Backman's observations, symptoms will not disappear but may relieve during 2 years after replantation [20]. Because the exact mechanism is unknown, there are currently no effective methods to treat this complication.

Summary

Replantation spans the entire spectrum of injuries often encountered by the hand surgeon and, as a result, brings with it the potential for all of the complications associated with each individual system. Dealing successfully with these complications requires addressing each mentally at the outset, performing the replantation with an eye towards prevention, and then monitoring the patient carefully to allow early identification and intervention postoperatively. In the case of late complications, management follows established treatment for each individual component of the original repair. The complexity derives from balancing and often incorporating the secondary treatments into a single operation.

References

1. Chung KC, Alderman AK. Replantation of the upper extremity: indications and outcomes. J Am Soc Surg Hand. 2002;2:78–94.
2. Morrison WA, McCombe D. Digital replantation. Hand Clin. 2007;23:1–12.
3. Goldner RD, Urbaniak JR, editors. Green's operative hand surgery. Philadelphia: Elsevier/Churchill Livingstone; 2011. p. 355–89.

4. Beris AE, Lykissas MG, Korompilias AV, et al. Digit and hand replantation. Arch Orthop Trauma Surg. 2010;130:1141–7.

5. Chang J, Jones N. Twelve simple maneuvers to optimize digital replantation and revascularization. Tech Hand Up Extrem Surg. 2004;8:161–6.

6. Sukop A, Nanka O, Dusková M. Clinical anatomy of the dorsal venous network in fingers with regard to replantation. Clin Anat. 2007;20:77–81.

7. Glickman LT, Mackinnon SE. Sensory recovery following digital replantation. Microsurgery. 1990;11:236–42.

8. Davis Sears E, Chung KC. Replantation of finger avulsion injuries: a systematic review of survival and functional outcomes. J Hand Surg Am. 2011;36(4):686–94.

9. Sebastin SJ, Chung KC. A systematic review of the outcomes of replantation of distal digital amputation. Plast Reconstr Surg. 2011;128:723–37.

10. Leung PC. An analysis of complications in digital replantations. Hand. 1980;12:25–32.

11. Wang H. Secondary surgery after digit replantation: its incidence and sequence. Microsurgery. 2002;22:57–61.

12. Yu JC, Shieh SJ, Lee JW, et al. Secondary procedures following digital replantation and revascularisation. Br J Plast Surg. 2003;56:125–8.

13. Matsuzaki H, Kouda H, Maniwa K. Secondary surgeries after digital replantations: a case series. Hand Surg. 2012;17:351–7.

14. Jupiter JB, Pess GM, Bour CJ. Results of flexor tendon tenolysis after replantation in the hand. J Hand Surg Am. 1989;14:35–44.

15. Lithell M, Backman C, Nyström A. Cold intolerance is not more common or disabling after digital replantation than after other treatment of compound digital injuries. Ann Plast Surg. 1998;40:256–9.

16. Dabernig J, Hart AM, Schwabegger AH, et al. Evaluation outcome of replanted digits using the DASH score: review of 38 patients. Int J Surg. 2006;4:30–6.

17. Adani R, Pataia E, Tarallo L, et al. Results of replantation of 33 ring avulsion amputations. J Hand Surg Am. 2013;38:947–56.

18. Cheng GL, Pan DD, Zhang NP, et al. Digital replantation in children: a long-term follow-up study. J Hand Surg Am. 1998;23:635–46.

19. Venkatramani H, Sabapathy SR. Fingertip replantation: technical considerations and outcome analysis of 24 consecutive fingertip replantations. Indian J Plast Surg. 2011;44:237–45.

20. Backman C, Nyström A, Backman C, et al. Arterial spasticity and cold intolerance in relation to time after digital replantation. J Hand Surg Br. 1993;18:551–5.

Secondary Procedures in Replantation

14

S. Raja Sabapathy, Jenny Tzujane Chen,
and Ahmed M. Afifi

Introduction

Since the first replant performed over 50 years ago, the desired outcome of replantation has shifted from the survival of the repaired part to full functional restoration. In order to achieve this goal, the surgeon must adhere to the fundamental surgical principles of replantation that have been detailed in other chapters in this book, including appropriate debridement, stable skeletal fixation, precise nerve and tendon repair, and early soft tissue coverage followed by timely therapy [1]. However, there are many cases where primary repair of all structures, or an "ideal" repair, cannot be done at the time of the primary replant, due to the general condition of the patient, the nature of the injury, doubts about survivability of the replant, surgeon fatigue, etc. In these cases,

secondary procedures are valuable in improving the functional outcome. The experience gained from these secondary procedures has encouraged surgeons to push the boundaries and expand the indications for replantation (Fig. 14.1a–n). Unfortunately, little has been published about secondary procedures after replantation, and surgeons need to rely on anecdotal evidence, expert opinion, and personal experience.

The incidence of secondary procedures in replantation varies between 2.95 and 93.2 %. These secondary procedures are more common with proximal injuries, multiple digit amputations, and more severe injuries [2]. Yaffe et al. in their series of 22 successful arm and forearm replantations found that each replantation required around three additional secondary operations. Fufa et al. in their series of 121 successful replantations found that 59 % of their digits required at least one secondary procedure, with an average of 1.7 procedures per replantation. In their series, the most common secondary procedure was actually revision amputation, followed distantly by tenolysis and contracture release [3]. Just as the indications for replantation in children are much wider, surgeons should have a lower threshold for performing secondary procedures in younger patients. The possible need for secondary procedures must be made known to the patient at the time of the primary procedure itself [4].

We are entering an era of many advances in the treatment of upper extremity and hand amputations, including elaborate patient-controlled prostheses,

S.R. Sabapathy, MD, MCh, DNB, FRCS, MAMS (✉)
Department of Plastic Surgery, Hand and
Reconstructive Microsurgery, and Burns,
Ganga Hospital, Coimbatore, India
e-mail: rajahand@vsnl.com

J.T. Chen, MD
Division of Plastic Surgery, University of Wisconsin
Hospital and Clinics, Madison, WI, USA
e-mail: tchen@uwhealth.org

A.M. Afifi, MD
Division of Plastic Surgery, University of Wisconsin
Hospital and Clinics, Madison, WI, USA
e-mail: afifi@surgery.wisc.edu

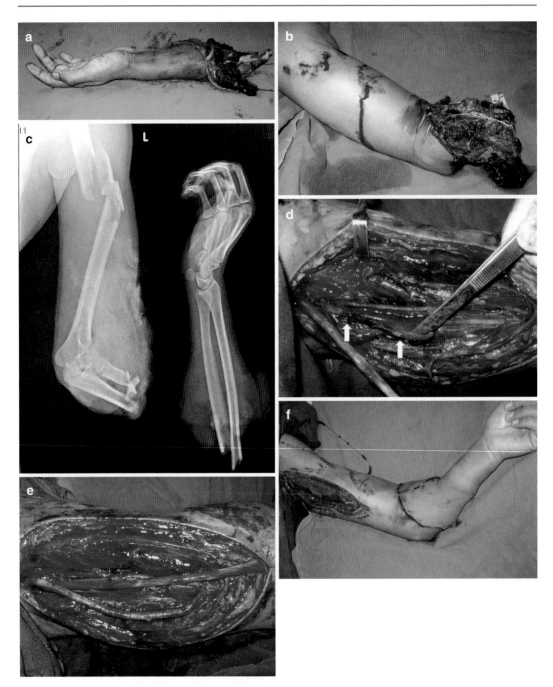

Fig. 14.1 (**a**, **b**) Avulsion amputation of the left fore-arm. (**c**) Radiograph showing the level of amputation and the proximal fracture in the humerus. (**d**) Rupture of the brachial artery (between *arrows*) at the site of fracture. (**e**) Brachial artery reconstructed with a vein graft after fixation of the humerus and the replant completed (**f**). (**g**) Preparation for secondary reconstruction of elbow flexors; the line of the brachial artery marked using the Doppler before raising the skin flaps. (**h**, **i**) Bipolar transfer of pectoralis major for elbow flexion. (**j**, **k**) Reinnervation of thenar muscles due to nerve recovery occurred at 12 months. (**l**) After recovery of thenar muscles and adductor of the thumb (4/5), finger flexors were reconstructed by free functioning gracilis muscle transfer with artery attached to end to side to the brachial artery and nerve to a fascicle of the median nerve. (**m**, **n**) Patient has Chen grade 2 recovery with good elbow flexion and finger flexion capable of good hook grip and gross holding power

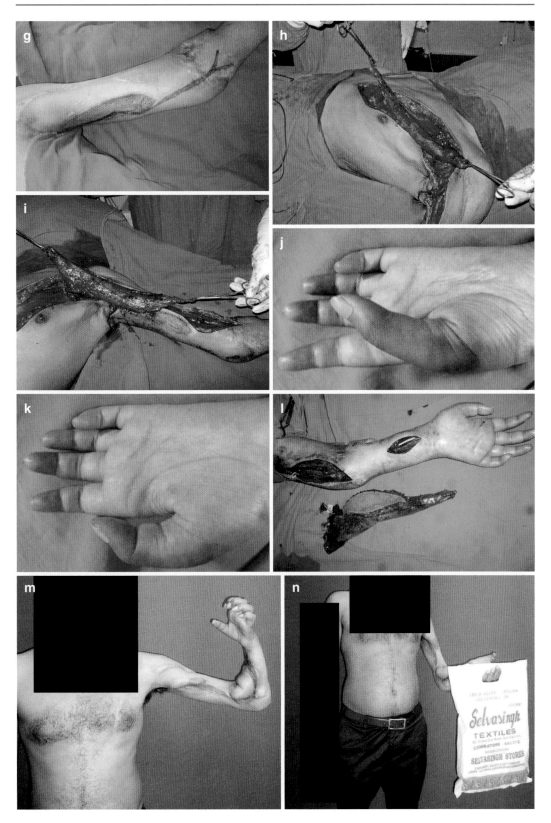

Fig. 14.1 (continued)

and hand transplantation [5]. However, upper limb prosthesis technology has not advanced as much as that of the lower limb, and reconstructed upper extremities continue to score higher functional outcomes than the best available prosthesis on the long term. The alternative of hand transplantation is yet to become a routine procedure. Hence, proficiency with replantation and the required secondary procedures remains critical.

Classification of Secondary Procedures

Most authors divide secondary procedures into early and late according to the timing of the procedure relative to the time of injury. Yu et al. found that early procedures (within 2 months following replantation) were mainly for soft tissue coverage (92 %), while late procedures (after 2 months) were mainly for tendon reconstruction (67 %) [6]. Sabapathy et al. preferred to classify secondary procedures based on the type of procedure performed, rather than its timing, as similar procedures may be done at different time points [7]:

Group 1: *Procedures to restore continuity of structures that were not repaired during the primary procedure*. This mainly involves bridging gaps in soft tissues, nerves, and tendons. This is usually done early but could be performed later such as when a skin grafted area is replaced by a flap to gain access for bony or tendon procedures.

Group 2: *Procedures to promote healing or enhance function of structures repaired during the original procedure*. The most common procedures in this group are tenolysis of repaired tendons and bony procedures for the correction of malunion and nonunion.

Group 3: *Procedures not part of the normal steps of replantation but which are done secondarily to enhance function and cosmesis*. This usually involves altering the normal anatomy of the replanted part and includes selective arthrodesis of joints, bone lengthening, tendon transfers, and free functioning muscle transfers.

General Considerations

Maintaining Good Records of the Primary Procedure

Detailed documentation is critical during the primary replantation as it will facilitate the planning of secondary procedures. This should include a detailed note of the structures repaired as well as the type and the location of repair. Equal emphasis must be given to recording the structures that have *not* been repaired, the reasons thereof, and the location of the proximal and the distal ends if known. These data must be documented and not be trusted to memory. While the proximal end of the nerve could be located based on the Tinel's sign, it is not possible to preoperatively localize the distal nerve end while planning a secondary neurorrhaphy. Inclusion of photographs in the medical record is another possible option that further helps in planning the incisions for secondary exploration and facilitating the dissection. In particular, the course of the repaired vessels and nerves needs to be documented. The repaired vessels may not be in their anatomical location, particularly if vein grafts are used. Many replants are dependent on the repaired blood vessels for a long time or even permanently, and it is important to avoid vessel injury during the secondary procedure. Griffin et al. described a report of late arterial occlusion 9 years after replantation of a thumb, requiring the excision of a segment of the thrombosed arterial vein graft to restore blood flow [8]. A Doppler study may be done to mark the course of the vessel prior to the secondary surgery. A good operative note becomes even more valuable if the secondary surgery is done at another center.

Timing of Secondary Procedures

Adequate soft tissue coverage is critical in hand replantation and is the most common type of early secondary procedure [6]. If the site of vessel repair is exposed, it must be covered with a flap as part of the primary procedure. Delay in such instances can be disastrous. In situations where the vessels are not exposed, timing depends upon the nature of the defect. If the raw area could accept a skin graft, it can be done within 72 h. Recently, VAC dressings have been applied to the raw areas at the end of replantation. Zhou et al. compared the progress of 18 wounds after replantation treated with regular dressing change to 26 wounds treated by VAC therapy. The intervals between wound treatment and secondary wound coverage procedure were 12.0 ± 1.7 days in the dressing change group and 6.1 ± 0.7 days in the VAC group. Flaps were applied for wound coverage in 50 % of wounds in the dressing change group and in 19.2 % of wounds in the VAC group ($P<0.05$) (the remaining wounds were covered by a skin graft). The results showed that VAC therapy could promote the growth of granulation tissue of the wound, decrease the need of flap for wound coverage, and did not change the survival of replantation [9]. There are obvious concerns with the negative pressure jeopardizing flow in the repaired vessels and the difficulty in applying the VAC and securing a seal around the wound. The authors do not have personal experience in using VAC after replantation and continue to rely on early soft tissue coverage appropriate to the wound condition.

Among the secondary procedures in replantation, achieving bone union is a priority. We cannot operate on other structures unless bone union has occurred or is progressing satisfactorily. If bone grafts are needed, they are usually done between 8 and 12 weeks. We usually do not combine bone grafting procedures with tendon and nerve graft procedures for two reasons. First, adhesions may be more common if performed together. Second, tendon graft rehabilitation protocols are easier to adhere to if they are performed in isolation.

The timing for secondary repair of tendons and nerves follows the same principles as any other complex injury management. The status of the soft tissue at the proposed surgery site is the most important factor in determining the timing of the secondary surgery, and the skin and the suture line must be soft and supple prior to secondary procedures. To reduce the induration which accompanies any surgical procedure,

anti-edema procedures like hand elevation, massage of the suture lines, and regular use of compression garments are instituted early on in the postoperative period [10]. Normally, the wound becomes supple by about 2 months from replantation, and that is when secondary procedures become feasible.

Group 1 Procedures: Surgery for Bridging Gaps in Tissues that Were Not Repaired During the Original Procedure

Bridging Gaps in Skin and Soft Tissues

Skin and soft tissue cover after replantation is done either early (at the end of the primary procedure or within a few days of the surgery) or late (to cover a tendon or bone reconstruction or for esthetic reasons). Skin grafting of the raw areas at the edge of replantation is the most common procedure performed [2]. If critical structures like nerves or vessels are exposed, we do not advocate skin grafts over them even as a temporary procedure. If performed, the skin graft must be replaced with a flap before the skin graft is adherent to the underlying structures. An adherent graft is very difficult to shave off the deeper structures should a flap be needed at a subsequent stage. Local flaps such as random transposition or rotation flaps can be used, but they are limited in their size and reach. The posterior interosseous artery flap is a useful flap to cover the wrist and the dorsum of the hand after replant. It is not dependent upon any major vessel and can be safely used in wrist- and transmetacarpal-level amputations (Fig. 14.2a–g). For circumferential defects, proximal defects, and volar defects, a free flap is often necessary. The recipient vessel is chosen well proximal to the level of the replant, and most often an end-to-side anastomosis is done. In the forearm, if one vessel is used for replantation, the other vessel can be used for the free flap. The gracilis muscle flap is our free flap of choice. Unlike a skin flap, it does not require accurate planning of the size and shape, can fill deeper

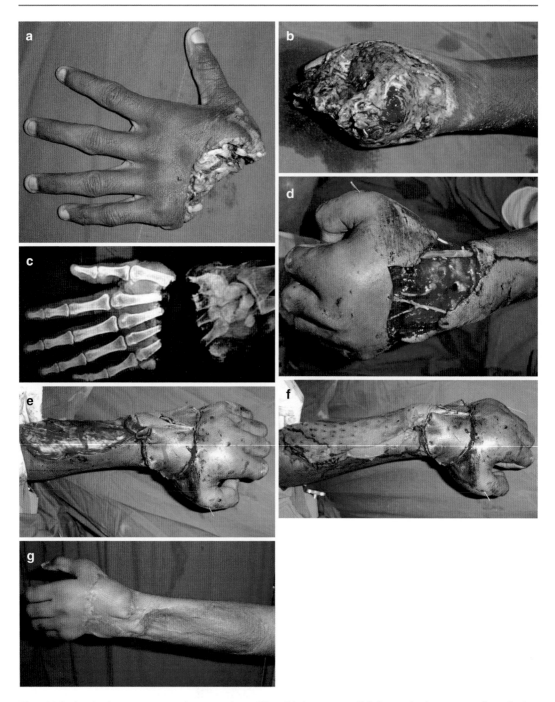

Fig. 14.2 (**a–c**) A transmetacarpal amputation. (**d**) Replantation required vein grafts to veins, and due to soft tissue loss, they were exposed at the end of the procedure. (**e**) A reverse pedicled posterior interosseous flap raised to cover the vital structures. (**f**) Donor area skin grafted without narrowing to avoid tension. (**g**) After healing of the wound

cavities, drapes well, and can cover a wide area. Finally, pedicled abdominal flaps still have a role in these difficult cases, and we have used abdominal flaps to cover the raw area after replant. A common indication is a raw area on the dorsum of the hand without exposed vessels. Our distant pedicled flap of choice is the hypogastric flap, based on the superficial inferior epigastric vessels.

The vessel is constant, and large flaps can be raised while keeping the base as small as 4 cm, centered on the line of the femoral artery. This flap is preferable to a standard groin flap, since the replanted hand can be well supported on the abdomen (Fig. 14.3a–h).

There is no objective evidence in the literature about the effect of tourniquet use shortly after replantation on vessel patency. In the absence of definite evidence, we have used the tourniquet during procedures for flap coverage within 48–72 h after the primary procedure without complications. A bolus dose of heparin (50 units/kg body weight of the patient) is given 5 min before the inflation of the tourniquet. The tourniquet can also be used during the initial replantation surgery while raising the flaps from the same limb. We allow an interval of 20 min after reperfusion of the

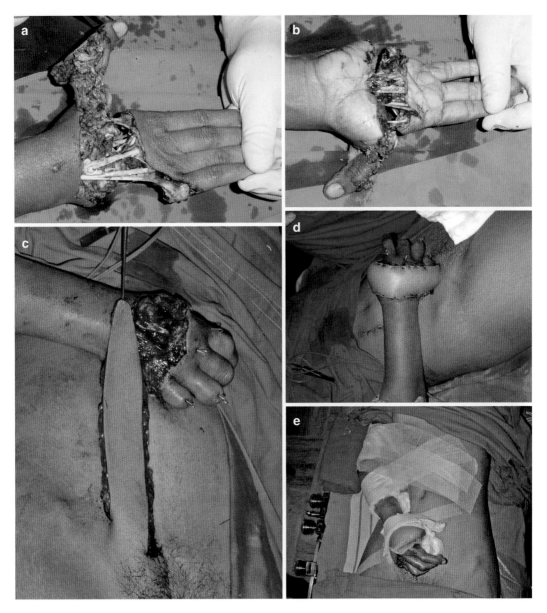

Fig. 14.3 (**a, b**) A transmetacarpal near total amputation with non-salvageable thumb. (**c, d**) The raw area on the dorsum is covered by the axial pattern flap based on the superficial inferior epigastric artery. (**e**) The type of restraint used in the immediate postoperative period. (**f–h**) The final result with a well settled flap

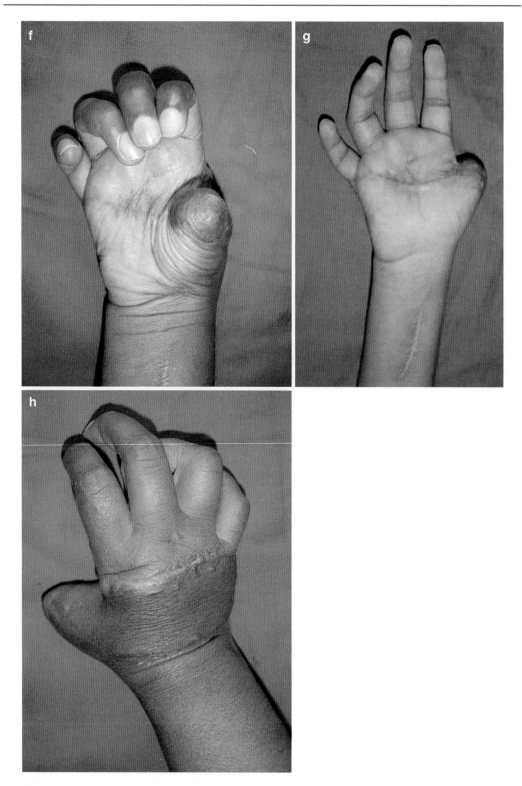

Fig. 14.3 (continued)

limb following microvascular repair before reinflating the tourniquet for raising the flaps.

Delayed soft tissue coverage may be needed to facilitate secondary procedures on the bone or tendons. At that time, the general principles practiced while providing soft tissue coverage in any complex injury are followed, with additional precautions taken not to injure the repaired vessels. One of the most common indications for flap coverage of the hand in the delayed situation is a first web contracture. We commonly use the pedicled groin flap or the posterior interosseous artery flap in these situations; these flaps share the benefit of not requiring any proximal dissection to identify recipient vessels.

Bridging Gaps in the Tendons

These procedures will vary depending on the level of the replant.

Arm

In avulsion amputations of the arm, the biceps and brachialis muscles often avulse proximally and hang on the distal tendon. The muscle in such instances does not get revascularized after replantation and likely is removed with the debridement. In other cases, the musculocutaneous nerve may be avulsed. In either case, elbow flexion needs to be restored. In contrast, the triceps muscle rarely needs reconstruction, because proximal innervation of the triceps typically allows preservation of function following repair. In the very rare instance that both biceps and triceps are lost, preference is given to the reconstruction of the flexors of the elbow.

The most common procedure performed for elbow function is the transfer of the latissimus dorsi or the pectoralis major muscles. Both transfers can result in a good outcome. These muscles have also been transferred at the time of replantation both to restore flexion and to provide soft tissue cover for the blood vessels and nerves [11]. In upper third arm replantations or when vein grafts for vessel reconstruction have been used near the axilla, routing of the latissimus dorsi muscle may be difficult. In these cases, a pectoralis major muscle transfer is a reasonable option. It has the advantage of obviating the need for position change for flap harvest, albeit the expense of an unsightly scar in front of the chest. In lower arm replants, we prefer the latissimus dorsi transfer, which seems to generate more powerful flexion of the elbow than the pectoralis major. The line of the brachial artery is marked with the Doppler before marking the skin incision, and the vessels are protected while insetting the flaps. Bipolar technique of transfer of these muscles yields better results, by allowing for a direct line of pull [12]. The detached insertion of the latissimus dorsi or the pectoralis major is attached to the coracoid process and the other end is woven into the biceps tendon. A few centimeters of rectus sheath is harvested along with the pectoralis muscle to provide a more secure attachment to the biceps tendon. If the humerus has been shortened considerably during replantation, there may be a slack in the muscle. The upper attachment of the muscle in such circumstances is moved more proximally onto the clavicle. Establishing correct tension of the muscle while insetting the transfer is important. To accomplish this, we focus on reestablishing resting tension that was present prior to muscle harvest. After dissecting the entire muscle and before detaching the origin and insertion, marks are placed at 4 cm apart on the muscle with the arm abducted to 90°. The distance between the marks must be measured with the shoulder fully adducted and abducted. During transfer, the tension is adjusted such that the distance between marks during flexion and extension of the elbow nearly matches that observed during shoulder adduction/abduction prior to harvest. Elbow is immobilised in 100° flexion for 4 weeks, and then a detachable splint is used to maintain the position for a further period of 4 weeks when gradual loading and strengthening exercises are started.

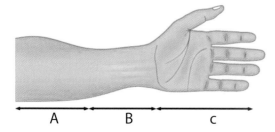

Fig. 14.4 Classification of complex flexor tendon injury. *Zone A*: From flexor muscle origin to musculotendinous junction. *Zone B*: From the musculotendinous junction to the proximal margin of the carpal tunnel. *Zone C*: Flexor tendons in the hand

Forearm

Proximal third forearm-level replantations need more secondary surgery than distal forearm replants or lower third arm-level replants [13]. In traction or crush amputations, there may be segmental loss of muscle secondary to either injury or debridement. If the loss involves the motor nerves to the muscles or the neuromuscular junction, then all function is lost. Chuang et al. retrospectively studied 27 patients who had replantation after crush or traction avulsion amputation and recommended immediate free tissue transfer for soft tissue coverage and delayed free functional muscle transfer for the patients whose injuries resulted in denervation. Delayed free functional muscle transfer is performed after the patient's condition has stabilized, and the limb is no longer swollen, which can be as early as 3–6 months after replantation. In two-stage reconstruction of both flexor and extensor motor units, the extensor reconstruction should precede the flexor reconstruction by 4–6 months [13].

Sabapathy and Elliot have classified the long flexor loss in complex injuries into three zones for the purpose of reconstruction (Fig. 14.4) [14]. Direct reconstruction of flexor loss in zone A may not be possible and free functioning muscle transfers are recommended. The procedure is usually performed 3 months after replantation. The gracilis musculocutaneous flap is our preferred free flap. The skin island not only serves for flap monitoring in the immediate postoperative period but

also allows for a tension-free skin closure. Most replantations at this level are not able to accommodate the volume of the free muscle flap, and the skin island obviates the need for skin graft and permits easy skin closure.

The free flap can receive its blood and nerve supply from the forearm or the arm, depending on the extent of the injury. The anterior interosseous nerve or the motor branches from the median nerve to the flexor muscles have been recommended as the donor nerve, with the radial or ulnar artery supplying the blood flow. In our experience, we have found it difficult to identify a good motor nerve in the scarred forearm, particularly after proximal third replants. We often anastomose the free flap end to side to the brachial artery and isolate a suitable fascicle of the median nerve at the level of the elbow and use it to innervate the free muscle transfer. The principle of this is akin to the ulnar nerve to biceps transfer procedure advocated by Oberlin to obtain elbow flexion in upper trunk brachial plexus palsy [15]. Proximally, the muscle is attached to the lower end of the humerus and distally to the flexor digitorum profundus (FDP) tendons proximal to the carpal tunnel. Ideally, a separate free muscle transfer should be used to restore thumb flexion. We have not been satisfied with the functional outcome when using the same muscle to power the flexors of both the fingers and the thumb. In spite of obtaining good range of movement of the fingers and the thumb, adjusting tension to synchronize the movement of the thumb and the fingers for pinch is difficult. Because a separate free muscle transfer for thumb flexion may be impractical or impossible, we prefer using a free functional muscle transfer to restore finger flexion coupled with selective arthrodesis of thumb joints in a functional position.

Zones B and C

In our series, 70 % of forearm replant patients have good intrinsic recovery. This is attributed to the shortening of the bones during the primary procedure that allows for a proper and tension-free nerve repair and a shorter distance for the axons to travel to their final destination. In lower third forearm- and wrist-level replants (zone B), direct tendon repair is possible resulting in substantially better functional results. Tenolysis may be required at this level secondarily.

In transmetacarpal-level amputations, after the repair of the flexor tendons, it can be sometimes impossible to repair the extensor tendons. While many patients will be functionally competent without extensors [16], we prefer to reconstruct the extensor tendons when possible. In such instances, extensor reconstruction is carried out secondarily. Tendon grafts are frequently required, and fascia lata is a good source for tendon grafts. Tension in the grafts during extensor reconstruction must be adjusted in such a way that flexion is not compromised. The authors maintain the interphalangeal joints in flexion, with both the metacarpophalangeal joints and the wrist in neutral position while suturing in the tendon grafts. In this way, the flexion of the fingers will not be compromised. In crush amputations, the skin on the dorsum of the hand may not be adequate and a flap for soft tissue coverage may be needed prior to tendon reconstruction.

In contrast to extensor tendons, we prefer to always perform primary repair of the flexor tendons. Other authors have performed two-stage flexor reconstructions by placing tendon rods in the flexor sheaths in proximal finger replants during the primary procedure [17]. As mentioned in prior chapters, we prefer skeletal shortening to allow primary repair of the flexor units.

Bridging Gaps in Nerves

A critical determinant of functional outcome is the quality of nerve recovery. If nerves are not repaired primarily, early secondary repair is advocated [13]. The proximal end of the nerve is identified by Tinel's sign, and distal identification is made easy if there has been documentation of its position in the original operation notes. If primary repair is not feasible during the original replantation, then the nerve ends should ideally be dissected and brought to a superficial level and anchored to the surrounding soft tissues. Their position is photographed, and the skin corresponding to that level is marked by tattooing or scarring the skin with a small X (Fig. 14.5a–j). During secondary reconstruction, incisions are made along the marked areas, the nerve ends are identified and prepared, and nerve grafts are tunneled under intact skin. This reduces the length of the access incisions needed and makes the procedure safer. Nerve grafts can pass along nonanatomical pathways. Many nerves, like the ulnar nerve and common digital nerves, pass closely along the vessels, and isolating the nerve ends and positioning them at a superficial and easily accessible level at the primary procedure make the secondary procedure easier.

In proximal replants, an attempt is made to repair all the nerves if possible. The radial nerve is the nerve that is most frequently missed. At the arm level, secondary reconstruction of median and ulnar nerves yields good results, particularly for recovery of the long flexors. Muscle recovery obviously depends on the ischemia time during the primary procedure, with more viable muscle fibers available for recovery with shorter ischemia time [18, 19]. Whenever possible, both the median and ulnar nerves are reconstructed. If only one nerve is available proximally or if the available graft material is insufficient to graft both nerves, then the nerve grafts are shared to reconstruct both the ulnar and the median nerve. Four to five nerve grafts can be attached to the proximal end with two or three grafts shared distally between the median and ulnar nerve. We find that reconstruction of both the median and ulnar nerves provides a better outcome than isolated reconstruction of either nerve. While the median nerve is most important, providing sensation to a critical area of the hand and sometimes thenar muscle recovery, ulnar nerve repair often leads to recovery of the thumb adductors and significantly adds to the functional capability of the hand [1, 20].

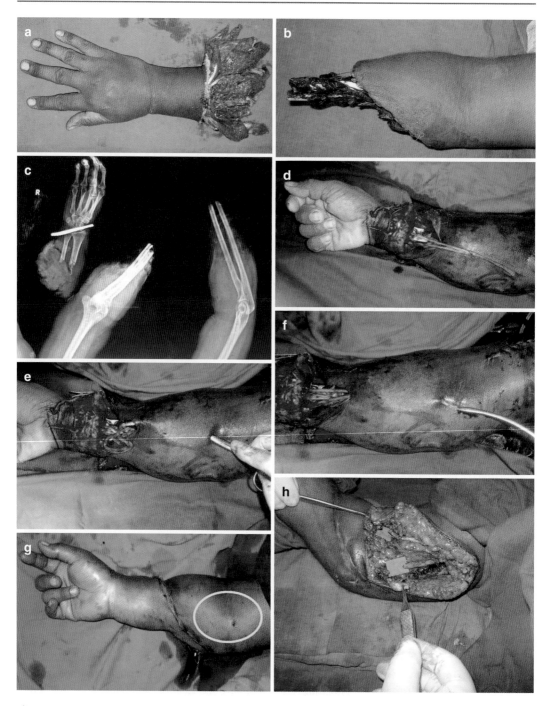

Fig. 14.5 (**a**, **b**) Avulsion amputation of the forearm. (**c**) Radiograph showing the skeletal level of injury. (**d**) Replant done, and there is a long segment of median and ulnar nerves available distally. (**e**, **f**) A tendon tunneler passed in the subcutaneous plane to get the nerves in a direct pathway. (**g**) The site of the distal end of nerves marked with a small x scar on the skin. (**h**) During secondary repair, it is easy to identify the distal end. Mobilization of the proximal end allowed primary repair of the median nerve and a short segment graft for the ulnar nerve. (**i**, **j**) Patient able to hold a cup of coffee and have enough power grip, a 2PD of 10 mm, and achieved Chen grade 2 outcome

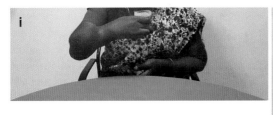

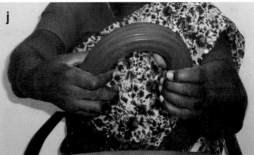

Fig. 14.5 (continued)

Group 2 Procedures: Procedures to Promote Healing or Enhance Function of Structures Repaired During the Original Procedure

Procedures to Promote Bone Healing

Primary bone union is a significant determinant of outcome, and ideally, there should be very few occasions when secondary procedures for bone healing are needed. Nonetheless, the incidence of bone nonunion has been reported as high as 10 % in digital replantation [21]. Bone shortening, which is an integral part of replantation in our experience, helps to reduce the incidence of nonunion [20]. Sabapathy et al. in their report of 20 successful major replantations found that the average bone shortening in the forearm and arm was 7.4 cm (range 5–10 cm), and that in three cases bone shortening was achieved by proximal row carpectomy. With such significant shortening, they did not have a single case of nonunion. If bone grafting is required, the timing will depend upon the need for reconstruction of other structures. If nerves or tendons also need secondary reconstruction, then bone grafting is done between 8 and 12 weeks after the primary procedure. If all other structures have been well repaired, rehabilitation of the tendons is the priority and the bone grafting is done between 3 and 6 months after the original procedure [22].

Tendon Surgery

Tendon surgery is the most common late secondary procedure performed after replantation, followed by surgeries for joint mobility and skeletal reconstruction [23, 24]. Tenolysis is indicated when the passive range is more than the active range, and no further progress occurs in spite of good therapy over a period of 6 weeks [25]. Ross et al. found that tendon function and motion after digital replantation can be improved with early mobilization protocols and two tendon repairs, although many surgeons disagree and prefer to suture only the FDP during the original procedure. Zone 1 and 5 flexor tendon repairs had better total active motion than injuries in Zones 2, 3, or 4 [26]. Lengthy incisions may be needed to expose the entirety of the flexor tendons, and, therefore, this procedure is done after the wound is soft and supple. Though it may be safe to do it by 4 months, usually it is done much later. Jupiter et al. found that the average time at which flexor tenolysis occurred was 10 months after replantation (range 5–19 months), which is consistent with other published studies [25, 27, 28]. Since tenolysis should be followed by early postoperative mobilization, it should be performed only after all the procedures requiring immobilization are completed and the overlying soft tissue is supple. The risk of tendon rupture, which is dependent on the quality of the original repair and the progress of tendon healing, can be significant and must be carefully taken into consideration [28, 29].

The previous surgery scars dictate access incisions. Zigzag incisions incorporating part of the original surgical scars are usually planned. This allows good exposure and facilitates the release of adhesions. Tenolysis of flexors in the digits is best performed under local anesthesia. The completeness of the procedure can be checked by having the patient actively flex the finger. When the procedure is done under general anesthesia or regional nerve block, the "traction flexor check" recommended by Whitaker et al. is practiced [30].

Through a proximal wrist incision, the tenolysed tendon is exposed and traction is applied to verify the range of movement. If there is restriction, the pressure used at the time of pull can break up minor adhesions. At proximal levels, a handheld Doppler is used to map the course of the vessels so that the incision could be planned safely (Fig. 14.6a–g). At exploration, major nerves in the region are first isolated and protected. Tenolysis is done and the completeness of the procedure is checked by obtaining full flexion on passive pull

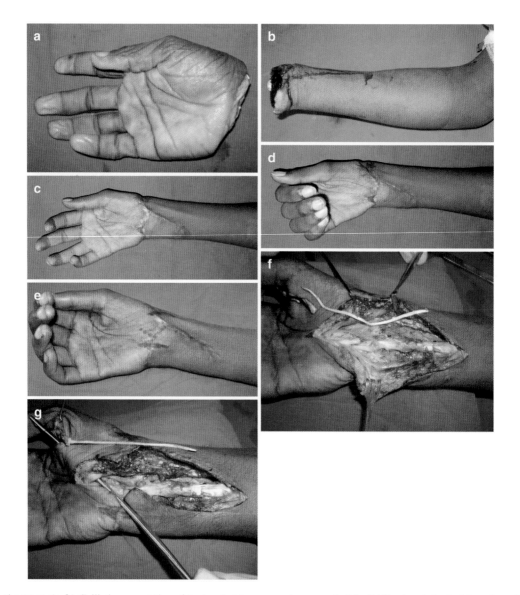

Fig. 14.6 (**a**, **b**) Guillotine amputation of the hand at the wrist level. (**c**, **d**) At 6 months, good finger function achieved, but no thumb flexion. (**e**) Preparatory to exploration with a handheld Doppler, the lines of the repaired vessels are marked (*solid lines*) and the incision planned (*dotted line*). (**f**, **g**) FPL was found ruptured, and it was reconstructed with a tendon graft. Being aware of the line of the repaired vessels makes secondary reconstruction safe

of the tendon from a site proximal to the replantation level. If there has been significant edema in the immediate postoperative period at the time of replantation, fibrosis and adhesions will be present all along the tendon, and extensive exposure may be needed. Pulley reconstruction or tendon reconstruction using tendon grafts may be needed [31]. Obviously, tendon surgery needs to be followed by regular and supervised physiotherapy [32].

Flexor tenolysis after replantation is often coupled with extensor tenolysis. This is contrasted with isolated flexor tendon injury, which typically only requires isolated flexor tenolysis. Even if the extensors were not repaired, adhesions around the distal end can limit the motion of the flexors and the adherent ends must be released to gain flexion. This usually occurs in transmetacarpal replants, where we feel that the incidence of extensor tenolysis is very similar to that of flexor tenolysis [33]. Flexor tenolysis may also need to be combined with joint procedures such as a capsulotomy of the metacarpophalangeal and interphalangeal joints.

Jupiter et al. reported their results after tenolysis in 37 replanted fingers and four thumbs. They noted an increase of total active motion from 72° to 130° ($p<0.001$). Their results were not as encouraging when the procedure was done for the thumb. Poor results were also noted in crush/avulsion amputations, hands with more than two digits amputated, and those requiring proximal interphalangeal joint capsulotomy [28]. Yu et al. reported an increase in total active motion from 119 to 159°. Only one of their 21 patients had deterioration of total active motion after tenolysis [6]. To date, no authors have reported loss of the replant after tenolysis.

Group 3 Procedures: Procedures Not Part of the Normal Steps of Replantation but Which Are Done Secondarily to Enhance Function and Cosmesis

After the secondary procedures which are directly linked to the primary repair are completed, there comes a phase in the rehabilitation of the replant patient where the focus shifts to enhancing function or cosmesis through alteration of the existing anatomy. These procedures are done later and usually involve the soft tissues and the skeleton.

Skin and Soft Tissue Procedures

These include skin grafts, Z-plasties, local flaps, and fat grafting to correct contractures, widen the web spaces, and correct contour deformities [34, 35].

Tendon Procedures

Tendon transfers, which are extensively used for the improvement of function in complex injuries, are less common in replantation as both the flexor and extensor compartments are injured and there is a paucity of uninjured donor tendons. One occasion where it may be used is for the reconstruction of the extensors after transmetacarpal replants. A wrist flexor can be extended with fascia lata tendon grafts and used to power the extensors. We have found that this gives better results than using individual interposition tendon grafts to the proximal extensor cut ends, due to the shortening and fibrosis of the extensor muscle fibers. Since muscle excursion is linked to the muscle fiber length, a contracted muscle loses its excursion potential. When we use an uninjured muscle as the motor, the potential for range of movement is much higher.

Another specific indication for secondary tendon transfer is the correction of a claw deformity after a transmetacarpal replant. At this amputation level, the lumbricals and interossei may be lost either during the initial injury or subsequent debridement. In such instances, only the long flexors and extensors are functioning. Even though both the PIP and MP joints may obtain a full range of movement, their function is not coordinated, with the interphalangeal joints flexing before the metacarpophalangeal joints. This leads to finger flexion pushing objects out of the palm rather than surrounding them in a grip. A claw correction procedure done for such patients tremendously improves their outcome. The extensor carpi radialis longus is extended by a fascia lata tendon graft. Although normally it is routed through the volar side of the wrist, in this specific patient population, it is passed though a dorsal route to avoid injury to the repaired vessels and nerves. The tendon graft passes volar to the transmetacarpal ligament (Fig. 14.7a–k).

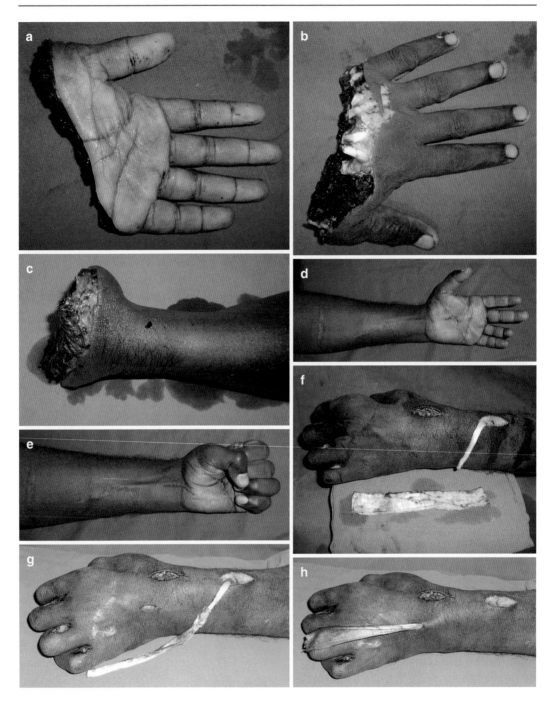

Fig. 14.7 (**a–c**) Transmetacarpal amputation of the hand. (**d, e**) Full range of movement obtained, but there is no pinch activity possible because the interphalangeal joints flex first. (**f**) Extensor carpi radialis longus (ECRL) tendon harvested and a strip of fascia lata taken. (**g**) Fascia lata strip attached to the ECRL tendon. (**h, i**) Tunneled to the level of the wrist and the fascia lata divided into four strips. (**j**) The route of the transfer. (**k**) The patient is now able to oppose each of the fingertips and pick up objects

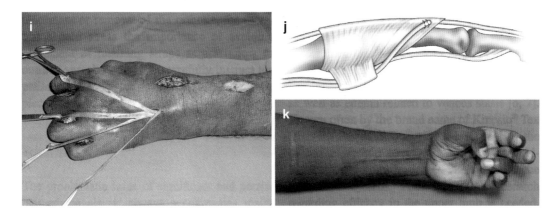

Fig. 14.7 (continued)

Procedures on the Bones and Joints

Selective arthrodesis of the finger joints is done to provide stability and maximize the function of the recovered muscles and is a useful procedure in major replants. In these proximal replants, recovery of the long flexors is more predictable than the recovery of the intrinsics, due to the long distance the axons have to travel to reinnervate the intrinsic muscles [33, 36, 37]. Recovery is even worse in the smaller muscles like lumbricals and interossei compared to the thenar muscles and the adductors of the thumb. In many cases of major replants, patients recover good flexion at the interphalangeal joints but the fingers assume a claw position and only a hook grip is possible, and the fingertips do not meet the thumb pulp. In such instances, we have arthrodesed the proximal interphalangeal joints in about 10° of flexion and the CMC joint of the thumb in an abducted position. The force of the long flexors then acts on the metacarpophalangeal joints, and there is better prehensile activity. The value of the procedure is assessed by casting the proximal interphalangeal joints in the proposed position of immobilization. After a few days, the patient can determine if this procedure would enhance their hand function.

Lengthening of the Replanted Part

Bone shortening is an integral part of replantation. This will vary according to the site of replantation and the type of injury. In guillotine and clean-cut amputations, there is less need for bone shortening, but bone loss or shortening may be significant in the forearm and arm segments in crush and avulsion amputations. As mentioned in prior chapters, we advocate bone shortening as it facilitates skeletal fixation, obviates the need for vein and nerve grafts (which can shorten ischemia time and decrease the incidence of fasciotomy), and allows primary skin closure without tension [38]. Up to 5 cm of shortening in the forearm and arm segments are easily accepted. Chuang et al. described an average of 5 cm and 7 cm of bone shortening in forearm and arm amputations, respectively [13]. We have done shortening of 10 cm in these areas and still obtained satisfactory functional results, but the length discrepancy remains easily visible to even casual observers. In digits, shortening of border digits is more easily acceptable than the central digits. Due to its complexity, distraction lengthening of the replanted part has been mainly used in the thumb and the long bones of the upper limb and in the leg [39].

Kempton et al. performed a metanalysis of distraction osteogenesis in the hand and found that, on average, it takes 116 days to achieve a lengthening of 2.2 cm, with a complication rate of 26.4 %, and 6.4 % of cases needed bone grafting. In addition, distraction after traumatic injuries had an even higher complication rate of 36.8 % compared to congenital cases where the complication rate is 21.8 %. The incidence of complications was 35.8 % in thumb metacarpal distraction compared to 27.1 % in other metacarpals and 24.2 % for phalangeal distraction [40].

Studies have shown that distraction of repaired vessels and nerves is possible without compromise of function [41]. Unal et al. reported a case of lengthening of a thumb distal phalanx replanted on its metacarpal because of loss of the proximal phalanx. There was a shortening of 4 cm in their case, and they performed 2.5 cm of lengthening using a unilateral mini distraction device at 6 months post replantation. The distraction was started on the tenth day after surgery at an interval of 1 mm/day until a length of 25 mm was achieved. The fixator was kept in place for 4 months to allow ossification of the callus, and no bone grafting was required. At the time of removal of the fixator, the first web was deepened and the patient had a good result. Distraction works well in situations where increased length is the only goal. In the thumb, it is useful when there are functioning thenar muscles. In fingers it is much less useful [42, 43]. Vucetic reported a case of forearm elongation after hand replantation in a patient who required 13 cm shortening during replantation because of segmental tissue damage. At 6 months post replantation, they used an Ilizarov apparatus to lengthen the forearm by 7 cm and correct the ulnar deviation and flexion deformity of the wrist, with a satisfactory final cosmetic and functional outcome [44].

In lower extremity replantation, shortening over 3 cm would usually need secondary bone lengthening. Normally, the leg length discrepancy is addressed as a secondary procedure, and the site of distraction is proximal to the site of amputation. Proximal metaphyseal osteotomy and callus lengthening can be done between 2 and 3 months after replantation, although it has been described after this initial period [45, 46].

There is only one report of immediate lengthening at the site of bone contact. In a replantation of the proximal third amputation of the leg, Mirzoyan et al. performed primary massive shortening of 13 cm and Ilizarov frame application. Distraction was started on the 20th day at the site of osseous approximation, with a subsequent corticotomy. Full length of bone was achieved 332 days after replantation. On the tenth postoperative day, a free flap was necessary for skin necrosis and infection. This case proved that distraction can occur at the sites of the neural and vascular repairs [41].

Conclusion

The goal of replantation is to provide the patient with a better functional limb than what could be achieved with closure of the amputated stump and the usage of the best available prosthesis. Primary repair of all the structures to achieve primary healing followed by a good rehabilitation protocol continues to be the gold standard. Accumulated experience over the last five decades has proven that secondary procedures done at the appropriate time are useful to improve the functional grading. Secondary procedures are no doubt challenging because they have to be done without injuring the critical structures, and many replanted extremities depend on the repaired vessels for a long period of time. Awareness of the potential benefits of secondary procedures at times will help in extending the indications for replantations particularly in crush and avulsion amputations. Deciding the ideal timing of secondary reconstruction, limiting the access incisions and taking care to avoid injury to the critical structures followed by supervised physiotherapy are the key to achieving success.

References

1. Sabapathy SR, et al. Replantation surgery. J Hand Surg Am. 2011;36(6):1104–10.
2. Matsuzaki H, Kouda H, Maniwa K. Secondary surgeries after digital replantations: a case series. Hand Surg. 2012;17(3):351–7.
3. Fufa D, et al. Digit replantation: experience of two U.S. academic level-I trauma centers. J Bone Joint Surg Am. 2013;95(23):2127–34.
4. Yaffe B, et al. Major upper extremity replantations. J Hand Microsurg. 2009;1(2):63–7.

5. Carlsen BT, Prigge P, Peterson J. Upper extremity limb loss: functional restoration from prosthesis and targeted reinnervation to transplantation. J Hand Ther. 2014;27(2):106–13.

6. Yu JC, et al. Secondary procedures following digital replantation and revascularisation. Br J Plast Surg. 2003;56(2):125–8.

7. Sabapathy SR, Bhardwaj P. Secondary procedures in replantation. Semin Plast Surg. 2013;27(4):198–204.

8. Griffin PA, Tan E, Katsaros J. Late arterial thrombosis in a replanted thumb: a case report. J Reconstr Microsurg. 1989;5(1):75–7.

9. Zhou M, et al. Vacuum assisted closure therapy for treatment of complex wounds in replanted extremities. Microsurgery. 2013. doi:10.1002/micr.22178. Epub ahead of print.

10. Buncke HJ, Jackson RL, Buncke GM, Chan SWL. Surgical and rehabilitative aspects of replantation and revascularization of the hand. In: Scheider LH, Hunter JM, Mackin EJ, Callahan AD, editors. Rehabilitation of the hand: surgery and therapy. 4th ed. St. Louis: Mosby; 1995.

11. Haas F, et al. Immediate functional transfer of the latissimus dorsi myocutaneous island flap for reestablishment of elbow flexion in upper arm replantation: two clinical cases. J Trauma. 2004;57(6):1347–50.

12. Chaudhry S, Hopyan S. Bipolar latissimus transfer for restoration of elbow flexion. J Orthop. 2013;10(3):133–8.

13. Chuang DC, et al. Traction avulsion amputation of the major upper limb: a proposed new classification, guidelines for acute management, and strategies for secondary reconstruction. Plast Reconstr Surg. 2001;108(6):1624–38.

14. Sabapathy SR, Elliot D. Complex injuries to the flexor mechanism in the hand and the forearm. In: Cheema E, editor. Complex injuries of the hand. 1st ed. London: JP Medical Publishers, 2014;115–16.

15. Oberlin C, Béal D, Leechavengvongs S, Salon A, Dauge MC, Sarcy JJ. Nerve transfer to biceps muscle using a part of ulnar nerve for C56 avulsion of the brachial plexus: anatomical study and report of four cases. J Hand Surg Am. 1994;19:232–7.

16. Quaba AA, Elliot D, Sommerlad BC. Long term hand function without long finger extensors: a clinical study. J Hand Surg Br. 1988;13(1):66–71.

17. Scott FA, Howar JW, Boswick Jr JA. Recovery of function following replantation and revascularization of amputated hand parts. J Trauma. 1981;21(3):204–14.

18. Dec W. A meta-analysis of success rates for digit replantation. Tech Hand Up Extrem Surg. 2006;10(3):124–9.

19. Lin CH, et al. Hand and finger replantation after protracted ischemia (more than 24 hours). Ann Plast Surg. 2010;64(3):286–90.

20. Morrison WA, McCombe D. Digital replantation. Hand Clin. 2007;23(1):1–12.

21. Pomerance J, et al. Replantation and revascularization of the digits in a community microsurgical practice. J Reconstr Microsurg. 1997;13(3):163–70.

22. Sabapathy SR, et al. Technical considerations and functional outcome of 22 major replantations (the BSSH douglas lamb lecture, 2005). J Hand Surg Eur Vol. 2007;32(5):488–501.

23. Wang H. Secondary surgery after digit replantation: its incidence and sequence. Microsurgery. 2002;22(2):57–61.

24. Wang H, Oswald T, Lineweaver W. Secondary surgery following replantation. The mutilated hand. Philadelphia: Elsevier; 2005.

25. Schneider LH. Tenolysis and capsulectomy after hand fractures. Clin Orthop Relat Res. 1996;327:72–8.

26. Ross DC, et al. Tendon function after replantation: prognostic factors and strategies to enhance total active motion. Ann Plast Surg. 2003;51(2):141–6.

27. Dy CJ, et al. The epidemiology of reoperation after flexor tendon repair. J Hand Surg Am. 2012;37(5):919–24.

28. Jupiter JB, Pess GM, Bour CJ. Results of flexor tendon tenolysis after replantation in the hand. J Hand Surg Am. 1989;14(1):35–44.

29. Eggli S, et al. Tenolysis after combined digital injuries in zone II. Ann Plast Surg. 2005;55(3):266–71.

30. Whitaker JH, Strickland JW, Ellis RK. The role of flexor tenolysis in the palm and digits. J Hand Surg Am. 1977;2(6):462–70.

31. Lehfeldt M, Ray E, Sherman R. MOC-PS(SM) CME article: treatment of flexor tendon laceration. Plast Reconstr Surg. 2008;121(4 Suppl):1–12.

32. Sandvall BK, et al. Flexor tendon repair, rehabilitation, and reconstruction. Plast Reconstr Surg. 2013;132(6):1493–503.

33. Weinzweig N, Sharzer LA, Starker I. Replantation and revascularization at the transmetacarpal level: long-term functional results. J Hand Surg Am. 1996;21(5):877–83.

34. Friedrich JB, Katolik LI, Vedder NB. Soft tissue reconstruction of the hand. J Hand Surg Am. 2009;34(6):1148–55.

35. Muzaffar AR, Chao JJ, Friedrich JB. Posttraumatic thumb reconstruction. Plast Reconstr Surg. 2005;116(5):103e–22.

36. Paavilainen P, et al. Long-term results of transmetacarpal replantation. J Plast Reconstr Aesthet Surg. 2007;60(7):704–9.

37. Hanel DP, Chin SH. Wrist level and proximal-upper extremity replantation. Hand Clin. 2007;23(1):13–21.

38. Gelberman RH, et al. Digital sensibility following replantation. J Hand Surg Am. 1978;3(4):313–9.

39. Matev I. Thumb metacarpal lengthening. Tech Hand Up Extrem Surg. 2003;7(4):157–63.

40. Kempton SJ, McCarthy JE, Afifi AM. A systematic review of distraction osteogenesis in hand surgery: what are the benefits, complication rates, and duration of treatment? Plast Reconstr Surg. 2014;133(5):1120–30.

41. Mirzoyan AE. Reimplantation and lengthening with use of the Ilizarov apparatus after a traumatic amputation of the leg. A case report. J Bone Joint Surg Am. 1996;78(3):437–8.

42. Unal MB, Cansu E, Parmaksizoglu F. Lengthening of a thumb distal phalanx replanted to its metacarpus because of loss of the proximal phalanx: case report. J Hand Surg Am. 2011;36(4):661–4.

43. Matev IB. Thumb reconstruction after amputation at the interphalangeal joint by gradual lengthening of the proximal phalanx. A case report. Hand. 1979;11(3):302–5.

44. Vucetic CS. Forearm elongation after hand replantation. A case report. J Bone Joint Surg Am. 2005;87(1):181–6.

45. Nisanci M, et al. Replantation of a crush amputation of distal tibia followed by lengthening with Ilizarov circular external fixator: two-year follow-up. Microsurgery. 2002;22(7):295–9.

46. Betz AM, et al. Primary shortening with secondary limb lengthening in severe injuries of the lower leg: a six year experience. Microsurgery. 1993;14(7): 446–53.

Rehabilitation Following Replantation in the Upper Extremity

15

Sarah A. Ezerins, Carol J. Harm, Steve J. Kempton, and A. Neil Salyapongse

Introduction

The goal of rehabilitation following upper extremity replantation is to optimize functional outcomes for the patient while protecting the repaired structures during the healing process. Several factors need to be taken into account when implementing postoperative therapy for any level of injury after replantation. Paramount is an established postoperative rehabilitation team consisting of the patient, hand surgeon and surgical team, hand therapist, and others (i.e., family, friends, caregivers, etc.). Effective communication among team members ensures continuity of care in order to maximize the patient's recovery and outcomes. Rehabilitation psychology may also be recommended for consultation as replantation injuries may have a significant, life-altering impact on the patient.

The therapist's skill is an important consideration as a substantial knowledge base of anatomy, physiology, and experience is required in order to set realistic expectations for functional outcomes and to make the necessary clinical judgments regarding the response to treatment and the appropriate progression of the treatment program. An integral part of this skillset includes the conscious "use of self" or the ability of the therapist to become "an effective tool in the evaluation and intervention process" [1]. One mantra in hand surgery is that only half of the outcome from any reconstruction is due to the surgery; the remainder comes through the efforts of the patient and therapist. As noted in prior chapters, the process of returning to functional status following replantation requires great time and effort even after the replant survives. An effective relationship between the therapist and patient will make all postoperative interventions more likely to succeed.

Patient participation and compliance is of key importance. The patient must understand the necessity for therapy including attending all appointments, compliance with using prescribed protective orthotics, following through with the home exercise programs, and adherence to precautions as instructed by the surgeon

S.A. Ezerins, OTR, MS
Occupational Therapy Department,
University of Wisconsin Hospital and Clinics,
Hand and Upper Extremity Clinic, Madison, WI, USA
e-mail: sezerins@uwhealth.org

C.J. Harm, BS, OT, OTR, CHT
Department of Occupational Therapy, University of Wisconsin Hospital and Clinics, Hand and Upper Extremity Clinic, Madison, WI, USA
e-mail: charm@uwhealth.org

S.J. Kempton, MD
Division of Plastic Surgery, University of Wisconsin Hospital and Clinics, Madison, WI, USA
e-mail: skempton@uwhealth.org

A.N. Salyapongse, MD (✉)
Division of Plastic Surgery,
University of Wisconsin Hospital and Clinics,
Madison, WI, USA
e-mail: a.salyapongse@uwmf.wisc.edu

and therapist. Rehabilitation psychology may be particularly helpful if the patient is experiencing any stress factors affecting participation in the treatment program. These factors may include pain, changes in body image, family stress, availability of transportation to therapy, and financial concerns.

Due to the complexity of any replant, the hand therapist must utilize clinical reasoning and problem-solving skills in order to balance protection of healing structures with orthotics and implementation of early mobilization. It is the use of early controlled motion which prevents adhesion of the tendons and the potential for joint contracture. The following factors [2] should be taken into consideration:

• Nature of the injury
• Flexor and extensor tendon involvement, including quality and tension on repair
• Fracture(s), including type and stability of fixation
• Joint mobility
• Nerve involvement, including quality and tension on repair, muscular innervations, and sensory status
• Vascular involvement, including quality, tension, and location of arterial and vein repairs
• Level of soft tissue involvement (muscle, ligament, wounds, scar formation, grafts, flaps, etc.)

Should there be any particular concerns about the quality of repairs or tension/stability across structures, the surgeon and therapist should discuss this in detail prior to beginning the rehabilitation regimen. Review of the various repaired structures may be helpful to the therapy team to improve familiarity when undertaking the treatment of the replantation patient. Being able to visualize the location of repairs unique to the patient will facilitate monitoring of progress and identification of complications as rehabilitation progresses.

Throughout the course of rehabilitation, the therapist and surgeon will continue to monitor perfusion, wound healing, and sensory recovery of the replanted part; however, the area of most direct intervention by the therapist will be the musculotendinous system. Vascular and neural repairs need to be protected, wounds must be attended to, but ultimately, therapy cannot increase vascular patency or accelerate nerve regrowth. Motion, on the other hand, remains the domain of the hand therapist.

Tendon Rehabilitation

Historically, rehabilitation began with a period of immobilization followed by passive motion programs. This approach led to significant problems with limited motion due to scarring. To combat the problem of scar adhesion, surgeons and physicians began to experiment with "early active" motion programs. Today, we refer to these protocols as "early controlled motion" allowing for graded stresses to the healing tissues utilizing both active and passive glides of the tendons through forming scar tissue.

Although timelines for progression of exercises and use of orthoses can provide general guidelines, the patient's individual tissue response should be considered in any therapy program. Groth [3] established a clinically useful model for determining an individualized regime of exercises known as the "Pyramid of Progressive Force Exercises" (Fig. 15.1).

The Pyramid of Progressive Force provides a systematic method to determine progression of therapeutic exercises designed to provide the appropriate level of force to the healing flexor tendon to achieve tendon glide with the minimal amount of force needed to affect the desired excursion. When adhesions preventing tendon glide occur during rehabilitation, this presents clinically as a plateau or decrease in range of motion. Exercises in the pyramid represent a series of specific rehabilitation levels arranged according to the amount of load being placed on the healing tendon in order to affect excursion of the tendon through the wound site.

This approach differs from traditional, time-regimented protocols in that the tendon excursion or "glide" dictates the advancement of the exercises based on patient's response to the exercises. Initial exercises begin with those that provide the lowest level of force to the tendon

Fig. 15.1 The Pyramid of Progressive Forces. Rehabilitation exercises generally begin at the base, where stress on tendons will be least. Stress increases as the exercises move up the pyramid, with resistive, isolated joint motion at the pinnacle (Used with permission from Groth [3])

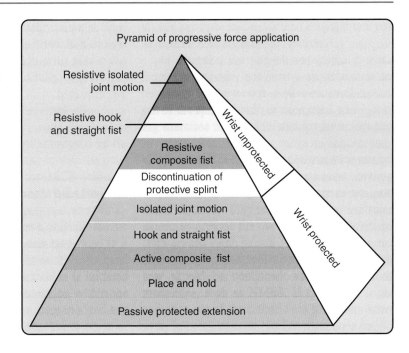

repair and progress only as needed to gain the desired tendon excursion. Protected passive motion of the digit promotes distal excursion of the tendon, whereas passive wrist extension promotes proximal tendon excursion. These glides provide the lowest level of force to achieve tendon excursion while remaining within the tensile strength of the repair. If the patient demonstrates improving range of motion to this level of load application, they should remain at the existing level of exercise force. If the patient's tendon excursion is not responsive to the load application at that level, the exercises should be progressed upward to the next level on the pyramid.

Wound Care

Following replantation, the most common types of wounds that may be encountered by the treatment team include closed incisions, open wounds, abrasions, and skin grafts. It is important to know how each of these is managed to ensure that proper dressing care is provided during hand therapy sessions.

Incisions and Abrasions

Closed incisions will be sutured and have bulky postoperative dressings, which may be taken down as soon as postoperative day one as reepithelialization of the wound typically occurs in the first 24 h. Dressings should be changed daily or as needed. Incisions and abrasions may be cleaned with soap and water, though submersion of the hand should be avoided.

Skin Grafts

Skin grafts are used to cover soft tissue defects once the concern for gross contamination is eliminated. Skin grafts may either be full thickness (epidermis and dermis) or partial thickness (epidermis and part of the dermis) and may be meshed in order to increase surface area, prevent fluid collection, and aid in graft contouring (Fig. 15.2a, b). Skin grafts heal by way of diffusion (imbibition) from the underlying wound bed and from alignment of existing vessels (inosculation) and ingrowth of new blood vessels (angiogenesis). The critical time for this to occur is in the first 5 days where a pressure dressing is kept in place (bolster or vacuum-assisted dressing). Occasionally, when the graft rests directly on top of venous outflow from the replanted digit, no compressive dressing will be applied. In this setting, great care must be taken during dressing changes at therapeutic visits so as not to disturb the skin graft.

Factors that result in early graft failure include seroma, hematoma, and graft shear. Shearing forces are the most important for the therapist to consider, and caution should be particularly observed when designing and securing a custom orthosis. Ideally, any orthotic used within the first 1–2 weeks following skin graft placement should either avoid contact with the graft or, alternatively, have a wide distribution of pressure over the entire area.

Assessment of initial graft take should be made 5–10 days following the graft. Skin graft take is always assessed in follow-up with the hand surgeon, and dressings should be left in place during initial therapy sessions. If a graft has not successfully taken within this time frame, it is unlikely to ever take. Indicators of skin graft take

include a graft that is adherent to the underlying wound bed with no necrosis and color matching of the skin surrounding the original donor site. In the event of graft loss, local wound care should be instituted with nonadherent dressings and antibiotic ointment to prevent desiccation of the deep tissue, allowing for granulation and secondary healing.

Neural and Vascular Monitoring

Sensation should be assessed as soon as feasible, and patient education regarding sensory precautions should be initiated early in the process. Clearly, more proximal levels of replantation will require longer periods of time to demonstrate any sensory return to the fingertip. Sensory testing should include Semmes-Weinstein monofilament testing to determine quality of sensation. Other tests, such as moving and static two-point discrimination, may be used; however, the discrimination of return of sensation is likely to be less accurate than monofilament testing (Fig. 15.3).

Management of the vascular status of the replant largely consists of monitoring, avoidance of stressors that might increase sympathetic tone, and avoidance of compression. The patient should be instructed to avoid temperature extremes as well as to monitor circulation by observing the color and capillary refill of the replanted part. When instructing the patient in

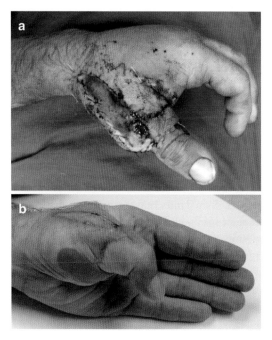

Fig. 15.2 (a) The appearance of a full-thickness skin graft over a replanted thumb as observed during the first dressing change at postoperative day 3. (b) The same graft and thumb at 3 months postoperatively

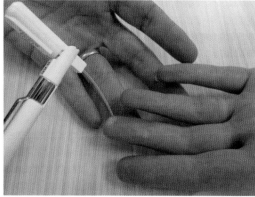

Fig. 15.3 Semmes-Weinstein filament (SWF) testing. Pressure is applied with the tip of the filament until the filament bends into a "C" shape. The finest filament that can be sensed in this fashion defines sensibility by SWF criteria

placement or removal of the orthotic, the therapist should stress the importance of avoiding placement of retaining straps across inflow or outflow vessels and should carefully instruct the patient in the appropriate level of tension to be placed on the retaining straps.

Edema

The problematic issue of significant and persistent edema almost always accompanies major trauma. Because persistent edema increases tissue resistance and limits the progression of both active and passive range of motion postoperatively, effective edema management strategies are paramount to all rehabilitation protocols. Edema management techniques include elevation, icing, active ROM, and light compression [4]. Interventions such as icing and compression in the setting of replantation may be contraindicated due to poor sensation and fresh vascular reconstructions. Thus, elevation is the treatment of choice at the initial posttrauma and postsurgical phase.

Depending on patient tolerance and the level of the replant, manual lymph drainage (MLD) may provide an early technique to decompress the hand and fingers. In order to perform MLD, light surface massage should be performed starting proximally at the shoulder near the site where the lymphatics drain into the subclavian system. The massage should move distally along the arm and forearm to just proximal to the level of replantation. Efficacy of this procedure in decreasing hand/wrist edema in the setting of external fixation of distal radius fractures has been shown [5].

Kinesthetic taping is another modality that has shown promise in treating posttraumatic edema as well as edema related to venous stasis [6, 7]. Known often by the brand name of Kinesio® Tex (Kinesio Precut, Albuquerque, NM) taping, the procedure appears to improve edema by providing increased mobilization of fluids through the lymphatic system. Although more research regarding efficacy in the upper limb is needed, we have had good success in reducing edema with this method in a wide range of hand and wrist injuries complicated by swelling. One advantage appears to be that taping does not restrict circulation in any way when correctly applied. Sensitivity to adhesives is a contraindication to using Kinesio tape.

Scar Management

Scar management may begin as soon as the wound has sufficiently healed. The therapist may apply light compression wraps and begin retrograde massage if vascularity allows. Adjunctive therapy to manage scar restrictions may include the use of ultrasound, a modality frequently employed in multiple scar conditions. Silicone gel sheeting (Fig. 15.4a, b) or elastomer putty products (Fig. 15.5) may be helpful with scar maturation by maintaining hydration of the new collagen tissue. These topical treatments are primarily useful for improving the clinical appearance of the

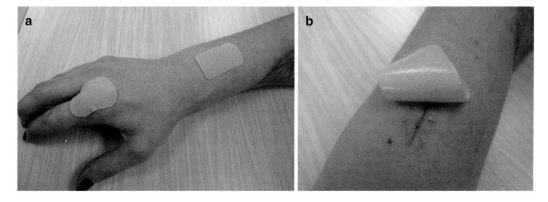

Fig. 15.4 Silicone gel sheeting may be useful in managing cutaneous scar healing. Appropriately sized segments may be cut from larger, over-the-counter sheets (**a**) or self-adherent patches (**b**) may be used

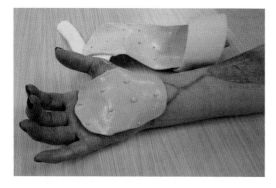

Fig. 15.5 Elastomer putty allows scar compression and maintains cutaneous moisture. Advantages include the ease of molding the putty into virtually any configuration and the ability to place the elastomer mold into a compression garment

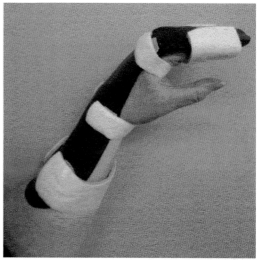

Fig. 15.6 Dorsal block splinting (orthosis). A standard for protection of flexor tendon repairs, the orthotic should be fabricated with finger position determined in consultation with the surgical team so that excessive stress is not placed on either extensor or flexor tendon repairs

scar rather than addressing any contribution of the scar to the function of the underlying structures [8]. Scar support, through linear, longitudinal taping or compression garments, shows some promise in preventing scar hypertrophy [9]. Compression garments for scars should only be implemented only after vascular perfusion has been firmly established.

Rehabilitation by Level of Replantation

Digital Replantation

Initial Protected Active and Passive Motion (Days 3–21)

Rehabilitation following digital replantation (flexor zones 1 and 2) should begin as early as possible after postoperative day 3. Early motion of the involved digit prior to this time is not recommended due to postoperative pain and inflammation [10–12]. This short delay does not affect outcomes, as the risk of adhesion formation in the very early postoperative period is low, since collagen formation does not typically begin until day 3.

Prior to initiating therapy, the bulky surgical dressings should be removed to allow for the fitting of a custom orthosis. An assessment of the wound can be done at this time with any concerns

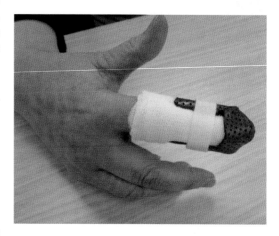

Fig. 15.7 Distal replants may occasionally be protected solely by a finger-based orthotic

being relayed to the surgical team. A dorsal blocking orthosis is then fabricated, placing the wrist in neutral, the metacarpophalangeal (MCP) joints in approximately 60–70° of flexion, and the interphalangeal (IP) joints in full extension (Fig. 15.6). These positions may be modified depending on any repairs requiring primary arthrodesis of finger joints. If the injury is to the fingertip only, a finger-based splint may be fabricated (Fig. 15.7).

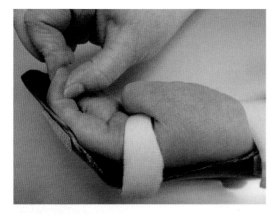

Fig. 15.8 PROM distal glide exercises for the DIPJ. Passive flexion of the DIPJ is performed using the unaffected hand to feel light resistance, then extended to the limit of the splint

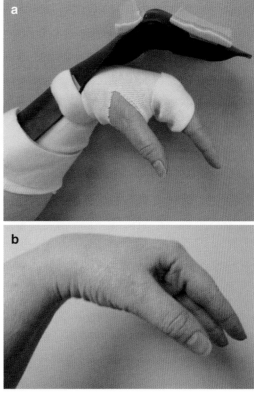

Fig. 15.10 Passive tenodesis exercises for tendon glide begin in the orthotic (**a**) and gradually progress to similar maneuvers outside of protection. (**b**) Wrist flexion, either actively or by gravity, results in passive extension of the fingers

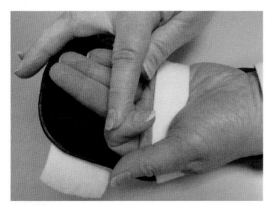

Fig. 15.9 PROM distal glide exercises for the PIPJ. Passive flexion of the PIPJ is performed using the unaffected hand to feel light resistance, then extended to the limit of the splint

Early motion of the replanted digit may begin 3–5 days after surgery. Therapist-directed passive range of motion is helpful in order to "warm up" the tissues and decrease overall tissue resistance due to edema and immobility [12]. The patient is instructed to passively flex and extend the DIP joint and the PIP joints in turn for several repetitions within the dorsal blocking orthosis (Figs. 15.8 and 15.9). These passive ROM exercises also serve to promote distal glide of the tendons.

Tenodesis exercises promote proximal glide of the flexor tendons. These exercises are performed in a limited range of motion and begin with gravity-assisted passive wrist flexion, resulting in finger extension (Fig. 15.10a, b) followed by active wrist extension, which produces finger flexion (Fig. 15.11a, b). The dorsal block orthosis should be used initially for these maneuvers; however, the patient can gradually progress to limited PROM out of the orthosis.

The initiation of active ROM requires discussion with the surgical team. When approved, early active motion may be performed by flexing the digits to midrange using a submaximal effort [11] to no more than approximately 45° at each of the three finger joints (MCP, PIP, and DIP). Full active flexion is not advised as it could increase tension at the repair and risk rupture. Full active extension is allowed within the constraints of the orthotic. Exercises should be performed four times a day. Additionally, active

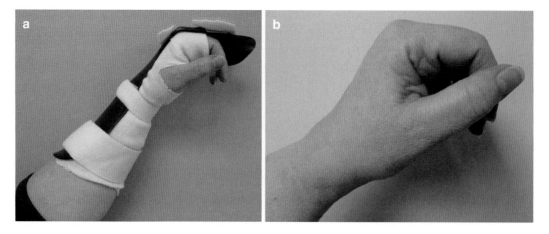

Fig. 15.11 Active wrist extension results in passive finger flexion. Exercises begin in the orthotic (**a**) and continue after orthotic removal (**b**)

range of motion of uninvolved structures, including the elbow and shoulder, should be encouraged to maintain mobility for function.

When the patient is 2.5 weeks out from surgery, the thermoplastic dorsal blocking orthosis may be modified to extend the wrist to 20–30°. Therapeutic exercises continue to emphasize both active and passive finger flexion. Passive ROM for distal glide of the tendon should continue prior to active motion exercises. Active flexion up to two-thirds of full range is encouraged with continuation of submaximal effort so that it is resistance free. Active flexion into the final one-third of full range of motion results in resistance which is 5–10 times that of the previous two-thirds and consequently carries a greater risk of tendon rupture [10,11]. If any resistance to active flexion is encountered, gentle passive motion into the end ROM may be implemented. Awareness of resistance in both the flexors and extensors should be continuously monitored; when new resistance is encountered at a point that provided smooth glide at prior sessions, formation of adhesions may be suspected. Resistance at the end points of motion, especially full flexion, may represent tightness or shortening of the extensor repair. While adhesions may prompt a move up the pyramid of exercises in order to prevent progression, attempting to force past a shortened tendon will likely only lead to gap or rupture.

Though function of the flexor tendons has traditionally overshadowed the role of the extensor tendons, extensor function should not be neglected. As in the case of isolated extensor repairs, early active motion may be beneficial. The necessity of protecting the flexor tendon repair precludes the use of relative motion splinting; however, protected active extension *in concert* with the uninjured digits may allow incorporation of some of the benefits of relative motion splinting without compromising the flexor repair. Ultimately, some degree of extensor tendon PROM will be achievable through the implementation of the flexor protocol.

Progressive Tendon Excursion Phase (Weeks 3–6)

At the 3-week postoperative time point, the patient may be instructed to begin working toward full active finger flexion with the wrist positioned in neutral to slight extension. Gentle blocking exercises and differential tendon gliding exercises may be introduced if deficits in range of motion remain. In the presence of flexor tightness, a volar extension orthosis (either static or static progressive) with low-load prolonged stretch [13] may be fabricated for the patient to wear for extended periods during the day or at night. At 5 weeks, active and passive range of motion of the wrist beyond neutral position (flexion and extension) should be encouraged.

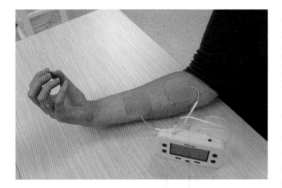

Fig. 15.12 Neuromuscular electrical stimulation can assist with strengthening and retraining as the patient progresses to a point where the tendons can be safely stressed

Light compression wraps and retrograde massage should be continued for the management of edema [2]. Neuromuscular electrical stimulation (NMES) (Fig. 15.12) may be implemented to promote pull through of the tendons and assist with strengthening of previously denervated muscles as nerve innervation returns. Motor points of the innervated muscles are utilized to facilitate the needed action potential for muscle contraction to occur. The additional training required for use of NMES can typically be obtained through the vendor.

At 6 weeks, the use of the protective orthosis can be discontinued and light activities of daily living (ADL) are allowed. The patient is advised to continue splint use for protection during heavier activities or when in potentially vulnerable situations. The patient may begin using their involved extremity to perform light functional activities at home such as eating finger foods or using the hand as a light assist for dressing. Forceful gripping, lifting, or pinching activities are not allowed until greater tensile strength is obtained in the tendon.

If not previously assessed, a sensory evaluation including a Semmes-Weinstein monofilament test should be conducted at this time to determine the patient's baseline and/or to continue to monitor nerve regeneration. Loss of sensation is a risk factor for other injuries, and if not previously done, sensory precautions need to be emphasized with the patient as they begin to reintegrate use of their extremity into daily living

activities. Compensatory strategies to reduce risk include avoiding temperature extremes as well as prolonged positioning, which could result in pressure ulceration. Visual compensation is often recommended in order to perform tasks safely.

Graded Strengthening (Weeks 8–12)

At 8 weeks, light resistive exercises may be implemented. Exercise resistance may progress as the patient tolerates, understanding that tendon is typically not considered to have regained full tensile strength until at least 12 weeks post repair [14]. Graded functional activities may continue with the precaution to continue to avoid full composite extension with resistance such as in weight-bearing activities.

At 12 weeks, work simulation may be implemented to promote functional use as the patient transitions back to their normal work demands [2]. A dynamic or static progressive orthosis may be used if necessary to help resolve any remaining deficits in passive range of motion. Sensory reeducation should continue every 4–6 weeks to determine the patient's nerve recovery.

Thumb Replantation

The thumb contributes approximately 40 % of the overall function of the hand [2]. For this reason, the thumb constitutes one of the most commonly replanted digits. While many of the principles described for rehabilitation of the digits will apply to the thumb, there are a few differences that warrant discussion.

Initial Protected Active and Passive Motion (Days 3–21)

The protocol for thumb replant is very similar to digital replantation, focusing on early controlled motion for joints that are not pinned. This is particularly important in that the thumb tolerates loss of motion at the interphalangeal joint (IPJ) better than the remaining digits. Given this, it will not be uncommon to encounter a patient whose thumb replant has been stabilized with a K-wire traversing the IPJ. A custom dorsal blocking thumb orthosis should be fabricated on postoperative days 3–5, ideally positioning the wrist in neutral and the thumb in abduction midway between radial and palmar abduction. The MP and IP joints of the thumb should be positioned in approximately 15° of flexion if possible to avoid tension on the replanted structures. Similar to digital replants, when both flexor and extensor tendons are involved, treatment should be biased in favor of the flexor tendons while maintaining awareness of the extensor involvement.

Rehabilitation efforts should approximately be 3–5 days following surgery. Passive range of motion should be performed for several repetitions to decrease overall resistance whenever possible. If distal motion is not possible due to pinning of the IP or MP joints, wrist tenodesis exercises should be initiated. Full active flexion should be avoided; however, the patient can be instructed to flex the thumb to midrange of motion by "flickering" using light effort or no more than 50 % effort [11]. Full active extension is encouraged up into the constraint of the splint. Patients are instructed to perform all exercises four times a day. Active range of motion of uninvolved structures, including the uninvolved digits, forearm, elbow, and shoulder, is encouraged to maintain function.

Progressive Tendon Excursion Phase (Weeks 3–6)

At the 2.5-week postoperative time point, both active and passive thumb flexion are emphasized. The patient should be reminded to continue to perform passive warm-up exercises prior to active motion. Resistance-free active flexion up to two-thirds of full range is the goal at this stage, with subsequent passive motion to achieve full flexion. Thumb extension should not be neglected, and the patient's ability to achieve full active extension should be monitored throughout this stage of rehabilitation.

At 4–5 weeks, composite flexion of thumb motion at the CMC, MCP, and IP joints is initiated. If necessary, neuromuscular electrical stimulation (NMES) may be used to facilitate excursion of the flexor pollicis longus. Full AROM and PROM of the wrist beyond the neu-

tral position should be achieved at this time. The patient may begin gentle blocking exercises of the thumb at 5 weeks and may remove the orthosis to perform light functional activities as tolerated. No forceful grasping or pinching is permitted.

The patient may be allowed to discontinue the thumb orthosis at 6 weeks; however, continued use of the splint is strongly recommended for protection during heavy activities and when in vulnerable situations. Use of a web space orthosis may be also considered to reduce any residual adduction contracture if needed. The patient should be instructed to wear this splint only at night to avoid limiting functional use during the day. Dynamic splinting should be implemented if there is residual joint stiffness that limits functional use.

Graded Strengthening (Weeks 6–12)

Between 6 and 12 weeks, the primary focus of therapy is to maximize the patient's functional use of the replanted thumb. From 6 to 8 weeks, the patient is encouraged to begin using the thumb for light prehensile activities of a functional nature. This may include eating finger foods, picking up light items, using a spoon or fork, and writing (which may require a built-up grip). By 8 weeks, a light resistive strengthening program may be implemented such as with light therapy putty or a hand exerciser. Once again, it is important that the patient be instructed in sensory reeducation and desensitization techniques as needed.

At 12 weeks, a work-conditioning program may be considered in preparation for return to work. Along with conditioning and strengthening, it is important to incorporate prehensile and dexterity activities to maximize the patient's hand function and to problem solve through activities that are difficult to perform.

Hand Replantation at the Transmetacarpal Level

According to Jones et al. [2], excellent functional outcomes can be achieved following transmetacarpal amputation. Bony fixation takes precedence at this level of injury. Longitudinal K-wire fixation is commonly used in children, whereas rigid internal fixation with plates and screws is more likely seen in adults.

Initial Protected Active and Passive Motion (Days 3–21)

Postoperative day 3–5, the patient should be fitted with a dorsal protective orthotic with the wrist positioned in neutral with the MCP joints at approximately 60° and IP joints in full extension. Depending on the level of injury and what structures were involved, the degrees of MCP flexion desired in the protective orthosis may vary, so it is important to clarify preference with the hand surgery team. Gentle passive motion is initiated for both finger flexion and extension within the constraints of the splint, taking care to avoid any tissue resistance during motion. Active range of motion of uninvolved joints, such as the elbow and shoulder, should be implemented at this time. Limited motion secondary to tissue edema is likely with more proximal amputation, and management with elevation should be reinforced with the patient.

Progressive Tendon Excursion Phase (Weeks 3–6)

By 3 weeks, gentle active motion exercises of the fingers and thumb should be encouraged within the constraints of the dorsal blocking orthotic. Gentle wrist tenodesis exercises may begin outside of the splint. Due to the level of injury, there may be significant denervation of the intrinsic muscles; therefore, gentle tendon excursion exercises should include intrinsic plus and intrinsic minus without forcing motion. The patient should continue wearing the orthosis between exercises and at night. Patients should be encouraged to perform exercises often, approximately 10-min sessions every 1–2 h. Edema management may progress to retrograde massage if necessary.

By 4–5 weeks, blocking exercises within the constraints of the splint may be introduced for the PIP joints if limitations in active range of motion are present. Active exercises may also begin with wrist flexion and extension, for which the dorsal blocking orthotic may be removed. The orthotic

should continue to be worn in between exercise sessions and at night for protection.

At 6 weeks, the patient may begin to wean from the orthotic, continuing to wear it when necessary for protection. Active range of motion out of the splint should be continued, and blocking exercises may be initiated for the MCPs and IP joints. Gentle passive range of motion may also begin at this time, provided that such manipulation will not place undue stress across healing fractures. If the patient exhibits signs of extrinsic flexor tightness, they may be fitted with a volar extension orthotic for use at night or as tolerated with graded light stretch [13]. Therapy for the management of residual edema and or restrictive scar should be continued, adding the use of modalities, such as NMES, if applicable. Light activities out of the orthotic are permitted; however, full resistance to the flexor tendons should be avoided until 12 weeks postoperatively due to limited tensile strength.

Graded Strengthening (Weeks 8–12)

At weeks 8–10, gentle resistive strengthening may commence. Work simulation activities may begin in preparation for potential return to work. Despite return of function through extrinsic musculature, the small muscles of the hand may remain denervated. The team should continue to monitor for intrinsic minus contractures and, when noted, should fabricate orthoses to substitute for lack of intrinsic function (dorsal blocking for the metacarpophalangeal joint) and to avoid deformity (first web space splint). Sensory reeducation should continue and should be reassessed at least every 4 weeks.

The need for secondary procedures is common at the transmetacarpal level due to the number of structures involved. For this reason, the hand therapist should pay close attention to slow or failed range of motion progression and communicate this information to the surgical team. Simultaneous rehabilitation of flexion and extension of the fingers is difficult to achieve, and it is important to maximize both throughout the therapy progression in order to reduce the likelihood of a secondary procedure such as a tenolysis.

Hand Replantation at the Wrist Level

Amputation at the wrist level is often the result of a guillotine type of injury. Beyond what has been discussed thus far in this chapter, the greatest challenge of rehabilitating the wrist-level replant patient is the certain loss of innervation to the intrinsic muscles and an increased time frame for motor and sensory nerve recovery.

Initial Protected Active and Passive Motion (Days 3–21)

Therapy again may begin 3–5 days postsurgical repair. As discussed previously, bony fixation dictates the progression of rehabilitation efforts. Consistent with previous amputation levels, a protective dorsal blocking orthosis is fabricated with the wrist in neutral, MPs in 60–70° of flexion and full extension of the IP joints allowed. If the distal radial ulnar joint (DRUJ) is involved, limiting forearm pronation and supination may be warranted. This can be achieved through fabrication of a Munster-style splint with a dorsal block extension as dictated by the need for positioning of the fingers. Constrictive straps should be avoided in order to facilitate the protection of early vascular anastomoses along with control of edema. Wide straps to distribute pressure evenly or other light wide wraps to hold the orthotic in place can reduce risk of constricting blood flow.

When cleared by the surgical team, early controlled motion may begin with gentle passive range of motion and "flickering" of the digits. Tenodesis exercises can commence once the surgical team is satisfied with bony fixation and status of bone healing.

Progressive Tendon Excursion Phase (Weeks 3–6)

At 3–6 weeks, there can be gradual reduction in use of the protective orthotic, which is typically discontinued by week 6. Gentle stretching and static progressive splinting may be considered to improve any limits to ROM. Once the dorsal blocking orthosis is discontinued, a functional positioning orthotic will likely be necessary due to loss of intrinsic function. The functional orthosis should be fabricated in approximately 60° of MP flexion to prevent contractures, which would otherwise occur due to the loss of lumbrical function. Consideration should be given to adding a thumb post, positioning the thumb in functional opposition if needed. Additionally, static progressive splinting may be desirable to reduce any residual contractures. While the therapeutic relationship requires a certain degree of optimism and encouragement, the team should also educate the patient regarding the slow and often incomplete return of intrinsic muscle function.

Active range of motion exercises and muscle reeducation exercises for any returning muscle groups should be performed at this time. Any resistive manual muscle testing should be performed carefully as full force to the tendons should be avoided until maximal return of tensile strength has been achieved at approximately 12 weeks.

Graded Strengthening (Weeks 8–12 and Beyond)

At 8–10 weeks, light resistive strengthening may begin. Due to the proximal level of amputation, patients may require ongoing therapy to monitor reinnervation of the intrinsic muscles. Additional strengthening exercises may be needed upon return of motor innervation to these muscle groups.

Arm Replantation

Amputation at the forearm level or above can be very complex due to the mechanism of injury, affecting a number of structures at varying levels of injury. The extensive damage to the residual limb requires thorough debridement to avoid infection.

Initial Protected Active and Passive Motion (Days 3–21)

Early in the postoperative course (Day 3–7), a custom dorsal elbow/wrist protective orthotic should be fabricated with positioning dependent on the level of injury and the structures involved. Typically, the elbow will be positioned in 70° of flexion with the forearm and wrist positioned in neutral. In the likely event of nerve repair, the orthotic should extend to include the metacarpophalangeal joints and thumb as described for replants at the level of the hand. Active range of motion of all uninvolved joints may be initiated. Edema management should also begin, and the patient should be instructed to elevate the involved arm above the heart.

At week 1–2, passive range of motion to the fingers, thumb, and wrist may be initiated. It is important for the therapist to begin instruction in one-handed compensatory techniques to assist in activities of daily living, as this may be a long-term necessity. Education for various adaptive equipment needs is also recommended.

During weeks 2–4, gentle active and passive range of motion for the elbow and shoulder should be initiated. If the patient has undergone a distal humeral-level replant, elbow range of motion will be based on the stability of fixation and the quality of repair of the biceps and triceps tendons. Gentle passive motion is initiated first and progresses to active motion as the patient tolerates. For replantation proximal to an intact elbow joint, transition to a locking, hinged orthosis may facilitate home exercises within the "safe" range by the patient. Continued edema management with gentle compression wrapping of the hand and fingers may also be implemented as needed.

Progressive Range of Motion (Weeks 4–8)

By 4 weeks following replantation, active range of motion may begin for the entire involved upper extremity. The patient should be instructed to continue to use the protective orthotic between exercises and at night to prevent deformity in the joints. Due to the substantial number of muscles denervated by more proximal amputation, liberal use of an assortment of orthoses should be considered. One common example would be a forearm-based, dorsal orthotic that includes extensions to protect against intrinsic minus posture. Levels of injury that spare proximal forearm muscles may demonstrate earlier function. In this setting, neuromuscular electric stimulation (NMES) may assist in retraining, but it is important to remem-

ber that the muscles distal to the nerve repair will be denervated. When proximal amputations result in significant denervation, the initial focus should be on passive range of motion rather than active motion at this stage of rehabilitation.

The subsequent few weeks should include active-assist as well as passive range of motion for the elbow, forearm, wrist, and hand. The protective orthotic may be discontinued around this time, but it is strongly recommended that the patient continues to use it when in vulnerable situations. Loss of passive range of motion or positional deformities can be addressed either through static progressive splinting or dynamic splinting. Resting orthoses to maintain functional positioning and prevent further deformity should continue until more distal muscle function returns. Throughout the process, return of motor innervation should be monitored and active exercises added to facilitate recovering muscles in preparation for return to functional activities.

Graded Strengthening (Weeks 8–12 and Beyond)

At 8 weeks, gentle resistive strengthening may begin for any returning musculature with a muscle grade of fair or higher. Prior to implementing resistive strengthening, the therapist must ascertain that passive range of motion is present throughout the planned strengthening arc of motion. Forceful motion against the fixed end point of a joint contracture may place undue stress on musculotendinous repairs, some of which may consist of fascial repairs proximal to musculotendinous junctions. Motor recovery will typically take 4–6 months or longer following replantation surgery. If not implemented earlier, modalities such as NMES may be helpful in assisting motor recovery.

At 12 weeks and beyond, it is not uncommon to continue dynamic splinting due to intrinsic paralysis. A functional orthosis with MPs blocked in flexion is ideal to prevent deformity due to lumbrical weakness. Incorporating a thumb opponens component may also be beneficial to aid functional use while awaiting nerve recovery (Fig. 15.13).

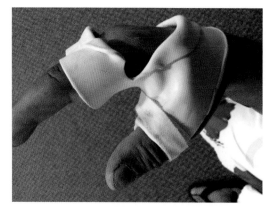

Fig. 15.13 When intrinsic weakness occurs, an orthosis blocking MPJ extension may assist in preventing a claw deformity. Thumb opposition via the same splint can place the digits in a position that allows better function from the extrinsic musculature

Secondary Procedures

As upper extremity replantation survival rates improve, the expectations for functional recovery have increased. Secondary elective operations are often required as an adjunct to hand therapy to optimize recovery and meet the demands of the motivated patient. For this reason, the treatment team should not look at another operation as a hindrance to rehabilitation efforts.

The time frames provided for secondary procedures and any continued immobilization following these procedures may vary depending on the level of injury and the stage of recovery in which it was performed. Communication between the therapist and surgeon must occur prior to beginning rehabilitation and should include detailed discussion regarding the procedures performed, the quality of the tissues (especially the status of prior tendon repairs and the flexor pulley system), and the expectations for motion based on the intraoperative findings.

The hand therapist plays a critical role in determining the ideal timing of secondary surgery. Ideally, secondary procedures should be avoided until nerve, joint, and tendon functions are stable and the overlying skin envelope is supple. However, when functional improvement levels off, a secondary operation may be considered to gain

function. The therapist's communication of therapy progress with the surgery team is of utmost importance. The following sections detail aspects of therapy that may need to be modified following the more common secondary operations.

Tendon

Tenolysis is the most common operation performed after upper extremity replantation. For flexor tenolysis, early active range of motion is essential in the postoperative period and should start on postoperative day one under hand therapist supervision. This consists of active and passive ROM exercises and differential gliding exercises for 10 min each hour. Over the first month following tenolysis, a resting extension orthosis may be used between exercise sessions and at night in order to decrease the risk of the extrinsic muscle tension resting the fingers in a flexed posture. In addition, if the process of tenolysis requires reconstruction of the pulley system (typically the A2), a thermoplastic ring orthosis should be used to help protect the new pulley during exercise. If passive extension of the fingers is easy but active flexion is limited, dynamic splinting may be initiated to increase passive flexion. At 4 weeks, the patient may begin to wean from the orthosis/dynamic splint as long as active range of motion is achieved in flexion and extension. By 6 weeks, strengthening exercises should be initiated and may include light resistive putty or a foam ball.

Extensor tenolysis in zones 1 through 5 is managed similarly to the release of flexor tendons. Active and passive range of motion should be initiated on the first postoperative day. Reverse blocking should be done with passive extension of the MP joints and active extension of the IP joints. An extension orthosis may be worn at night and between exercises. Neuromuscular electrical stimulation (NMES) may be added on postoperative days 3–5. At 4 weeks, hand strengthening may be introduced slowly, and use of the extension orthosis should be gradually reduced. Independence from the orthosis and/or dynamic splint and return to normal activities by 6 weeks should be the goal. When the tenolysis occurs more proximally through zones 6 through 8, exercises are modified in that NMES can be started on day 1 and dynamic or static progressive flexion splinting should be used to achieve passive full available MP and IP joint flexion.

Secondary tendon repair and tendon grafting should follow the same early active motion protocol as primary tendon repair as previously described in the chapter.

Contractures

Following dorsal and volar MP and PIP capsulotomy/capsulectomy, the dressing should be removed on postoperative day one, and initiation of unrestricted active and passive range of motion exercises is initiated for 10 min every hour. Exercises should focus on composite flexion and extension involving the IP, MP, and wrist joints. Intrinsic stretching and abduction and adduction should also be performed. A custom safe position orthotic should be fashioned for dorsal release and an extension splint fitted for volar release to be worn during rest and at night. If the patient demonstrates good passive range of motion of the digits but strength appears to limit excursion, dynamic splinting may be initiated. Dynamic flexion and extension splinting should be worn four to six times per day for 45 min for dorsal and volar release, respectively. At 4 weeks, weaning from the splint may begin along with strengthening exercises as long as passive range of motion is preserved. Discontinuation of the splint and return to normal activity is expected by 6–8 weeks post release.

It is not uncommon for the need to release a skin contracture with or without capsulotomy/capsulectomy. Following skin contracture release, early passive and active range of motion protocol will be important. If a skin graft is in place, it is ideal to wait 7–10 days prior to initiation of therapy.

Bone and Nerve

Therapy following bone grafting and revision for nonunion depends on the rigidity of the fixation. If stable fixation is achieved, then therapy should be similar to therapy following internal fixation after a fracture. Following 4–6 weeks of immobilization, the splint/cast is removed and active range of motion initiated. Passive range of motion exercises should be done at this time in the joints directly distal and proximal to the area of fixation. Splinting is typically in the intrinsic plus position with MP joints blocked into flexion. At 5–6 weeks, passive range of motion can be initiated in joints proximal and distal to fixation as long as there is evidence of clinical healing. Strengthening exercises may start at 7–8 weeks.

Nerve grafts and nerve transfer procedures are set under no tension and should not interfere with therapy.

Conclusion

Rehabilitation of a replant is a complex process in which a multitude of factors may affect the outcome. Even in the most ideal of situations, unforeseen factors may arise affecting the outcome. The level of injury and the greater number of structures involved will have a direct impact on the length of rehabilitation and the final functional outcome of the replanted extremity. The skill of the surgeon and the therapist with active participation of the patient working together is essential to minimize potential problems to achieve the best possible outcome for the injury.

References

1. Mosey AC. Psychosocial components of occupational therapy. 1st ed. Philadelphia: Lippincott Williams & Wilkins; 1986. p. 199.
2. Jones NM, Chang J, Kashani P. The surgical and rehabilitative aspects of replantation and revascularization of the hand. In: Skirven T, Osterman AL, Fedorczyk J, Amadio P, editors. Rehabilitation of the hand and upper extremity. 6th ed. Philadelphia: Elsevier Mosby; 2011. p. 1262–71.
3. Groth GN. Pyramid of progressive force exercises to the injured flexor tendon. J Hand Ther. 2004;17(1): 31–42.
4. Sorenson MK. The edematous hand. Phys Ther. 1989;69(12):1059–64.

5. Härén K, Backman C, Wiberg M. Effect of manual lymph drainage as described by Vodder on oedema of the hand after fracture of the distal radius: a prospective clinical study. Scand J Plast Reconstr Surg Hand Surg. 2000;34(4):367–72.

6. Bialoszewski D, Wozniak W, Zarek S. Clinical efficacy of kinesiology taping in reducing edema of the lower limbs in patients treated with the Ilizarov method–preliminary report. Ortop Traumatol Rehabil. 2009;11(1):46–54.

7. Aguilar-Ferrándiz ME, Castro-Sánchez AM, Matarán-Peñarrocha GA, Guisado-Barrilao R, García-Ríos MC, Moreno-Lorenzo C. A randomized controlled trial of a mixed Kinesio taping-compression technique on venous symptoms, pain, peripheral venous flow, clinical severity and overall health status in postmenopausal women with chronic venous insufficiency. Clin Rehabil. 2014;28(1):69–81.

8. O'Brien L, Jones DJ. Silicone gel sheeting for preventing and treating hypertrophic and keloid scars. Cochrane Database Syst Rev. 2013;9:CD003826.

9. Widgerow AD, Chait LA. Scar management practice and science: a comprehensive approach to controlling scar tissue and avoiding hypertrophic scarring. Adv Skin Wound Care. 2011;24(12):555–61.

10. Tang JB. Indications, methods, postoperative motion and outcome evaluation of primary flexor tendon repairs in zone 2. J Hand Surg Br Eur Vol. 2007;32E(2):118–29.

11. Lalonde D. How the wide awake approach is changing hand surgery and hand therapy: inaugural AAHS sponsored lecture at the ASHT meeting, San Diego, 2012. J Hand Ther. 2013;26(2):175–8.

12. Lalonde DH, Martin AL. Wide-awake flexor tendon repair and early tendon mobilization in zones 1 and 2. Hand Clin. 2013;29(2):207.

13. Flowers KR, LaStayo PC. Effect of total end range time on improving passive range of motion. J Hand Ther. 2012;25(1):48–55.

14. Cooper C. Fundamentals of hand therapy: clinical reasoning and treatment guideline for common diagnoses of the upper extremity. St. Louis: Mosby; 2006.

Index

A

Acellular dermal matrix, 62
Advanced trauma life support (ATLS)
  child and adolescent replantation, 140, 141
  digit replantation, 52
  forearm/arm replantation, 84, 86
Amputations, finger
  avulsion, 50, 51
  bone fixation techniques, 58
  classification, 50
  demographics, 49
  guillotine, 50
  heparin, 64
  multidigit, 51
  zigzag Bruner incisions, 55
Anticoagulation, 64, 96
Arm replantation. *See also* Forearm/arm
  graded strengthening, 203, 204
  initial protected active and passive motion, 202–203
  progressive tendon excursion phase, 203
Arterial insufficiency, 83, 112, 113, 165
Arterial repair, 57–58, 93–94
Arterial shunting, 92
Artificial nerve conduits
  allografts, 35
  biodegradable conduits, 33
  bridging, segments, 34
  collagen, 34
  cytokines and growth factors, 34
  FDA-approved devices, 34
  morbidities, 33
  silicone and PTFE, 33
Avulsion/crush injury, 69
Axonotmesis, 27

B

Bair Hugger™, 63
Bilateral forearm amputation, patient, 77–78
Bone fixation
  digits replantation, 55–56
  forearm/arm, 92–93
  radiocarpal joint, 73–78
Bridging gaps surgery
  in nerves, 181–183

skin and soft tissue
  replanted hand, abdomen, 177–178
  transmetacarpal amputation, 175, 176
  web contracture, 179
tendons
  arm, 179
  forearm-level replantations, 180
  zones B and C, 180–181

C

Child and adolescent replantation
  amputated part, sterile gauze, 140
  anatomic and physiologic differences, 138–140
  antibiotic prophylaxis, 141
  ATLS, 140
  avulsion-type amputation, 137, 138
  crushing and avulsion amputations, 141
  mechanism and etiology, 137–138
  microsurgical anastomosis, 141
  multiple digit crush amputation, 137, 139
  PALS, 140
  postoperative management, 142
  psychosocial adaptation, 141
  revascularization procedures, 142
  sympathetic nervous system, 142
  traumatic amputations, 137
Chuang classification
  avulsion amputations, 90
  grading replantation functional outcomes, 97
Complications
  cold intolerance, 169
  radiocarpal joint, 79

D

Darrach-type resection, 93
Dextran
  branched polysaccharide, 96
  head and neck microvascular
    reconstruction, 107
  hypovolemia, 107
  Leuconostoc mesenteroides streptococcus, 107
  pulmonary edema, 125
  usage, 107–108

A.N. Salyapongse et al. (eds.), *Extremity Replantation: A Comprehensive Clinical Guide,*
DOI 10.1007/978-1-4899-7516-4, © Springer Science+Business Media New York 2015

Digits/digital replantation
    active and passive motion, 196–198
    amputation injuries, 49
    avulsion amputations, 50
    classifications, 50
    graded strengthening, 199
    intraoperative technique
        amputated part preparation, 53–55
        arterial repair, 57–58
        bone fixation, 55–56
        nerve repair, 60–62
        principles, 53
        proximal stump preparation, 55
        skin closure and dressings, 62–63
        tendon repair, 56–57
        venous repair, 58–60
    microsurgical anastomosis, 49
    microvascular anastomosis, 50
    patient selection
        injury-related factors, 50–51
        patient-related factors, 51–52
    postoperative care, 63–64
    prehospital care, 52
    preoperative evaluation, 52–53
    progressive tendon excursion phase, 198–199
    socioeconomic and psychological impact, 49
    vessel anastomosis, 49
Disseminated intravascular coagulation (DIC), 95–96
Distal radio ulnar joint, 77–78
Doppler probes, 96, 111
Dorsal tendon repairs, 78

E
End-to-side nerve repair, 32
Epineural repair, 29, 30
Epineural sleeve repair, 30, 31
Esmarch tissue protector, 57
Euro-Collins (EC) solutions, 88
Extremity replantation
    anatomy, 9–11
    arm, crocodile belly, 6, 7
    bilateral leg amputation, 6
    bone fixation, 3
    face and scalp avulsion, 5
    fracture fixation
        cancellous bone graft, 15
        diaphysis, 14
        hypertrophic nonunions, 15
        intraosseous wire techniques, 12, 13
        Kirschner wires (K-wires), 13
        open reduction and internal fixation, 14
        osteosynthesis, 12
        screw fixation, 14
    healing, 11–12
    micro-instrument development, 4
    microvascular techniques, 4
    primary adhesion, 3
    Saints Cosmas and Damian, 2
    secondary tendon reconstruction, 20
    tendon anatomy, 15–16

    tendon healing, 16
    tendon repair
        epitendinous suture techniques, 17, 19
        extensor shortening, 20
        extracellular matrix protein
            expression, 19
        gap formation, repaired tendon, 17
        grasping and locking, 17, 19
        suture anchoring, 17
        vascular and neural, 16
    vascular repair, 3

F
Fascicular repair, 31–32
Flagyl®, 85
Flexor tendon repair, 58, 74
Flexor tenolysis, 75
Foley catheter, 85, 95
Forearm/arm
    amputations, 83
    complications, 97–98
    crossover limb replantation, 99
    distal injuries owing, 83
    evaluation, 84–85
    expectations, 96–97
    fasciotomies, 84
    near amputations, 83
    patient selection
        amputated parts, preservation, 88–89
        amputation level, 90–91
        description, 85–86
        ischemia time, 88
        mechanism/extent of injury, 89–90
        patient condition, 86–88
        replantation vs. prosthesis, 86
    physiology, 84
    postoperative care, 95–96
    secondary procedures, 98
    sharp mechanism, 83–84
    soft tissue contamination, organic
        and inorganic material, 84
    surgical treatment
        arterial repair, 93–94
        arterial shunting, 92
        bone fixation/shortening, 92–93
        digital- and hand-level replantations, 92
        early revascularization, 91–92
        geographic restrictions, 92
        meticulous debridement, 91
        muscle adjacent, 91
        musculotendinous repair, 94–95
        myonecrosis, 91
        nerve repair, 95
        skin coverage, 95
        upper limb replantations, 91
        UW solution, 91
        venous repair, 94
    temporary arterial bypass shunting, 84
    temporary ectopic replantation, 98–99
    upper extremity amputation, 84

H

Hand replantation
    bony fixation, 200–201
    graded strengthening, 201
    initial protected active and passive motion, 201
    progressive tendon excursion phase, 201
    wrist level, 202
HDR. *See* Heterotopic digital replantation (HDR)
Heparin-induced thrombocytopenia (HIT), 106, 108
Heterotopic digital replantation (HDR)
    flexor digitorum superficialis, 133, 134
    metacarpal hand, 134
    mid-hand gap, 134, 135
    multiple radial/ulnar digit amputations, 134
    mutilating hand injuries, 133
    ODR, 133
    precision grip, 134
    spare parts surgery, 134, 135
    thenar muscles, 133, 134
Hirudin, 108, 113, 165–166
HIT. *See* Heparin-induced thrombocytopenia (HIT)

I

Intraosseous 90-90 cerclage, 57

K

Kessler core sutures, 58

L

Leech guidance, engorged finger, 61
Lidocaine, 108
Limb replantation, 99
Lister technique, 56, 57
LMWH. *See* Low-molecular-weight heparin (LMWH)
Lower limb replantation
    arterial catheter perfusion, 146
    bone shortening, 157
    crushing injury, 148
    definitive wound coverage, 148
    extremity amputations, 145
    heel, calcaneal and sole amputations, 147
    heterotopic/"crossover" replantation, 152–153
    injury-related factors, 147
    knee joint preservation, 147
    leg avulsion, 153
    pediatric injuries, 147
    perioperative considerations, 155–156
    plantar sensation, 145
    proactive treatment strategy, 157
    prosthetic fitting, 153, 154
    risk-benefit ratio, 146
    salvage, 153–155
    sharp injury, 146
    skeletal lengthening
        distraction osteogenesis, 149
        ring fixator, 149, 150
        tubular external fixator, 149
    soft-tissue coverage and bone lengthening, 147
    soft-tissue management, secondary
        debridement, 146
    soft-tissue necrosis, 156
    temporary ectopic
        contralateral femoral artery
            and saphenous vein, 150, 151
        contralateral posterior tibial
            vessels, 150, 152
        monorail fixator, 150, 152
        skin-edge necrosis, 150, 153
    transtibial, 153, 154
    vascular and neural repairs, 157
    X-ray, healed tibia and calcaneus, 153, 155
Low-molecular-weight heparin (LMWH),
        64, 96, 106–107

M

Management, complications
    bleeding, 164–165
    bone, 162–163
    cold intolerance, 169
    extensor and flexor tendons, 163
    nonunion and malunion treatment, bone, 166–169
    preparation and prevention, 161–162
    primary nerve repair, 164
    reconstructive managements, 166
    stiffness, finger, 166, 169
    tenolysis, 166
    vascular, 163–164
Meticulous debridement, 91
Musculoskeletal repair. *See* Extremity replantation
Musculotendinous repair, 94–95
Myonecrosis, 91

N

Nerve conduits
    autografts, 32
    biological repair, 33
    tensionless repair, 32
Nerve repair, 60–62, 95
Nerve repair and neural recovery
    aberrant regeneration, 26
    amputation, 25
    assessment and reporting process, 35
    axonotmesis, 27
    axons and fascicles, 26
    classifications and descriptions, injury, 26, 27
    epineural *vs.* fascicular, 25
    intrinsic and extrinsic factors, 35
    nerve conduits (*see* Nerve conduits)
    neuropraxia, 26–27
    neurotmesis, 27
    peripheral nerve trauma, 25
    peripheral repairs, 36
    topography, 36
    types, 29–32
    Wallerian degeneration and axonal
        regeneration, 27–29

Neural and vascular monitoring, 194–195
Neuropraxia, 26–27
Neurotmesis, 27
Non-vital tissue, 71–73

O
Orthotopic digital replantation (ODR), 133, 136
Osteosynthesis
    abduction and adduction, 42–43
    interosseous wiring, 42
    Kirschner wires, 42

P
Papaverine, 58, 108
Partial thromboplastin time (PTT), 79, 106, 107
Pediatric advanced life support (PALS), 140, 141
Pedicled latissimus flap, 87
PIP. *See* Proximal interphalangeal (PIP)
Pistachio conveyor belt, 69
Postoperative care, forearm/arm, 95–96
PRC. *See* Proximal row carpectomy (PRC)
Prosthesis *vs.* replantation, 86
Proximal interphalangeal (PIP), 2, 118, 185, 197, 201, 205
Proximal row carpectomy (PRC)
    arthrodesis, 67
    transcarpal replantations, 79
    wrist salvage, 73–74
Proximal row carpectomy and fixation, 75–76
Proximal stump, 55
PTT. *See* Partial thromboplastin time (PTT)

R
Radiocarpal joint
    avulsion/crush injury, 69
    bony fixation, 73–78
    care and challenges, 67
    clinical examination, 68
    complications, 79
    dorsal tendon repairs, 78
    flexor tendon repair, 74
    laboratory values, 69
    non-vital tissue, 71–73
    operative sequence, 69–70
    part and amputation stump, 68
    part preparation, 70–71
    postoperative care and monitoring, 79
    PRC, 79–80
    social and psychological effects, 67
    traction, crush and degloving injuries, 69
    transcarpal and radiocarpal amputations, 67
    transmetacarpal amputations, 67
    upper extremity replantation, 67
    veins, 78–79
    vessels and nerves, 74, 76
    wrist level amputations, 68
    x-ray images, 68
Radio carpal ligaments, 75–76

Rehabilitation
    arm replantation, 202–204
    digital replantation, 196–199
    edema, 195
    hand replantation (*see* Hand replantation)
    load application, 193
    patient participation and compliance, 191
    problem-solving skills, 192
    proximal tendon excursion, 193
    scar management, 195–196
    secondary procedures
        bone and nerve, 205
        contractures, 205
        tenolysis, 204–205
    thumb replantation, 199–200
    transportation to therapy and financial concerns, 192
Reperfusion injury, 98
Replantation, child and adolescent.
        See Child and adolescent replantation

S
Salvage
    arterial insufficiency, 113
    crush/avulsion injuries, 112
    intravenous bolus, 113
    microvascular anastomosis, 112
    vascular thrombosis, 112
    venous insufficiency, 113–114
Secondary procedures, replantation
    avulsion amputation, left forearm, 171–173
    bone healing, 183
    bones and joints, 187–188
    bridging gaps surgery, tissues, 175–183
    classification, 174
    documentation, 174
    functional restoration, 171
    skin and soft tissue procedures, 185–187
    tendon surgery, 183–185
    tenolysis and contracture release, 171
    timing, 174–175
    types, 174
    upper limb prosthesis technology, 174
Second-toe transfer
    distal index finger, 124
    right index and middle finger, 124
    and third-toe transfer, 125
Semmes-Weinstein filament (SWF) testing, 194
Skin closure and dressings, 62–63
Skin coverage, 95
Sunderland classification, nerve injury.
        See Nerve repair and neural recovery

T
Temporary ectopic replantation, lower limb
    contralateral posterior tibial vessels, 150, 152
    femoral artery and saphenous vein, 150, 151
    monorail fixator, 150, 152
    skin-edge necrosis, 150, 153
Tendon repair, 56–57

Tensionless nerve repair
  nerve tube, 62
  vein conduit, 61
Thumb replantation
  avulsion injury, 39, 40
  bone repair, 43
  digital nerves, 40
  functional impairment, 39
  graded strengthening, 200
  initial protected active and passive motion, 199–200
  mechanism of injury, 39
  microvascular repair, 43–45
  osteosynthesis, 41–43
  postoperative management
    arterial thrombosis, 45
    interphalangeal joint, 47
    Kirschner wires, 46
    proximal joints, 47
  preoperative management, 40–41
  progressive tendon excursion phase, 200
  tissue coverage, 45
Toe-to-hand transplantation
  complication, 127
  crushing/avulsion injuries, 119–120
  donor site morbidity and potential loss, 118
  donor site rehabilitation, 126
  drawback, 117
  finger and thumb amputations, 117
  foot cosmesis, 118
  heterotopic replantation, 119
  implications, 118
  index and middle fingers, 118
  methods, 117
  microanastomoses, 118
  microsurgical toe transfer, 118
  motor rehabilitation, 126
  outcomes
    measurement, hand function, 127
    thumb replantation and great-toe transplantation, 126–127
  PIP, 118
  postoperative care
    Chang Gung Memorial Hospital, 125
    dextran and heparin, 125
    donor foot, 126
    Doppler ultrasound and laser Doppler, 125–126
    dressing, 125
    toe flap monitoring, 125
  primary and secondary transfer, 119
  second-toe transfer, 124
  sensory rehabilitation, 126
  single-/multiple-digit amputations, 117–118
  surgical technique
    donor site closure, 122
    nerve repair, 122
    recipient site preparation, 121
    skeletal fixation, 121
    skin closure, 122
    tendon repair, 121–122
    toe harvest, 120–121
    vascular anastomosis and wound closure, 122

  tissue preservation, 120
  trimmed great-toe transfer, 122–123
Transhumeral amputation, 87
Traumatic amputations, 76
Trimmed great-toe transfer
  degloving injuries, 122
  proximal phalanx/metacarpal bone, 122
  thumb amputation, proximal phalanx, 122, 123
T shunt, 68

U
University of Wisconsin (UW) solution, 88, 91
Upper extremity replantation, 67
Upper limb replantations, 91

V
Vascular patency
  back table preparation, 103–104
  description, 103
  intra- and postoperative pharmacology
    acetylsalicylic acid (aspirin), 107
    anticoagulant drugs, 105
    catecholamines, 105
    clinical data and outcomes, 105
    dextran, 107–108
    fibrinolytic agents, 108
    heparin, 105–106
    hirudin, 108
    lidocaine, 108
    LMWH, 106–107
    papaverine, 108
  ischemia time, 114–115
  meta-analysis, 114
  microsurgical techniques, 103
  microvascular patency, 114, 115
  monitoring
    clinical evaluation, 110
    fluorometry and fluorescence imaging, 112
    handheld Doppler ultrasonography, 111
    implantable Doppler devices, 111
    nursing staff, plastic and reconstructive surgery, 112
    perfusion/vascular thrombosis, 110
    pulse oximeter, 112
    surface temperature, 110–111
    tissue oximetry, 111
  postoperative care
    brachial plexus blockade, 109
    brachial plexus catheters and indwelling catheters, 110
    cold intolerance, 109
    smoking, 109
    thumb replantation, 109
    vasoconstriction, 109
    vasopressors, 109
  salvage (*see* Salvage)
  vein grafting, 104, 105
  venous flaps, 105

Veins, 78–79
Venous repair, 58–60, 94
Vessels, 74, 76
Volar and dorsal approach, 72
Volar veins, 56

W
Wallerian degeneration and axonal regeneration
    distal and proximal stumps, 27
    extracellular matrix proteins, 29

    intracellular calcium, 27
    motor end plates, 29
    peripheral nerve transection, 29
Wound care
    incisions and abrasions, 193
    skin grafts, 193–194
Wound coverage, lower limb
    bone shortening, 148
    circumferential skin necrosis, 148